W9-CBD-594

Prevention's
THE SUGAR SOLUTION®
COOKBOOK

RODALE
LIVE YOUR WHOLE LIFE™

Every day our brands
connect with and inspire
millions of people to live
a life of the mind, body,
spirit — a whole life.

Prevention's

THE SUGAR SOLUTION®
C O O K B O O K

More Than 200 Delicious Recipes to Balance Your Blood Sugar NATURALLY

By the Editors of Prevention® magazine
with Ann Fittante, MS, RD

RODALE

About *Prevention* Health Books

The editors of *Prevention* Health Books are dedicated to providing you with authoritative, trustworthy, and innovative advice for a healthy, active lifestyle. In all of our books, our goal is to keep you thoroughly informed about the latest breakthroughs in natural healing, medical research, alternative health, herbs, nutrition, fitness, and weight loss. We cut through the confusion of today's conflicting health reports to deliver clear, concise, and definitive health information that you can trust. And we explain in practical terms what each new breakthrough means to you, so you can take immediate, practical steps to improve your health and well-being.

Every recommendation in *Prevention* Health Books is based upon reliable sources, including interviews with qualified health authorities. In addition, we retain top-level health practitioners who serve on our board of advisors. *Prevention* Health Books are thoroughly fact-checked for accuracy, and we make every effort to verify recommendations, dosages, and cautions.

The advice in this book will help keep you well informed about your personal choices in health care— to help you lead a happier, healthier, and longer life.

Notice

This book is intended as a reference volume only, not as a medical manual. The information given here is designed to help you make informed decisions about your health. It is not intended as a substitute for any treatment that may have been prescribed by your doctor. If you suspect that you have a medical problem, we urge you to seek competent medical help.

Mention of specific companies, organizations, or authorities in this book does not imply endorsement by the publisher, nor does mention of specific companies, organizations, or authorities imply that they endorse this book.

Internet addresses and telephone numbers given in this book were accurate at the time it went to press.

Rodale books may be purchased for business or professional use or for special sales. For information, please write to: Special Markets Department, Rodale Inc., 733 Third Avenue, New York, NY 10017

Printed in the United States of America
Rodale Inc. makes every effort to use acid-free ⊗, recycled paper ♻.

Photography by Mitch Mandel
Food styling by Diane Vezza
Book design by Christina Gaugler

ISBN-13 978–1–59486–519–0
ISBN-10 1–59486–519–1

Distributed to the book trade by Holtzbrinck Publishers

2   4   6   8   10   9   7   5   3   1   hardcover

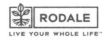

We inspire and enable people to improve their lives and the world around them

For more of our products visit **rodalestore.com** or call 800-848-4735

CONTENTS

THE SOLUTION
TO YOUR WEIGHT WOES

Heavenly slices of French toast, stuffed with a creamy banana filling and dusted with confectioners' sugar. Savory mini pizzas oozing with cheese. Soul-satisfying french fries. Macaroni and cheese. It sounds like a menu made in heaven. But in reality, these dishes—and many more—are part of a way of eating that can satisfy your tummy and slim your waistline. Without hunger. Without deprivation. And without food cravings that wake you out of a sound sleep at 2 a.m.

It's The Sugar Solution weight-loss program. This cookbook, the companion to the successful *The Sugar Solution*, has more than 200 delicious recipes to help you bring the principles of this satisfying way of eating into your daily life. Think you might not have time to cook a separate meal for yourself every day? All the recipes are family friendly, and many are ready in less than 15 minutes, while many others can be prepared in 20 minutes or less.

And everyone in your family stands to benefit. The Sugar Solution is a safe and effective way of eating that can improve your body's ability to convert blood sugar—your body's primary source of energy—into fuel, rather than store it as fat. Ultimately, because the program prevents the dramatic surges and ebbs in blood sugar (also called glucose) that lead to food cravings, you're likely to find that you're satisfied with less food, and that your yen for sugary, fatty foods fades away.

In this book, you'll find all the information you need for experiencing the benefits of The Sugar Solution program for yourself.

- Get the latest news on the connection between blood sugar, insulin, and body weight.
- Learn why certain foods tend to blunt appetite and cravings—and why others keep you continuously ravenous.
- Try the 21-Day Lifestyle Makeover—a month's worth of tempting menus that will help melt away those extra pounds.
- Be inspired to balance your blood sugar with activities and stress-management techniques that are fun and simple.

Best of all, The Sugar Solution will help you enjoy the foods you love while the pounds melt away. Page through the recipes in this cookbook and you'll find plenty of well-loved favorites—pasta, potatoes, bread, rice, and even cookies. That's right, you'll be enjoying carbohydrates. It's not necessary to banish carbs from your diet, if you choose the right ones in the right amounts. You'll find specific advice on finding the right carbs on page 2.

Ready to get started? Give *The Sugar Solution Cookbook* a try and chances are, you'll be rewarded with a slimmer, healthier body—for good.

CHAPTER 1

THE SUGAR SOLUTION STRATEGY: A BEHIND-THE-SCENES GUIDE TO SUCCESSFUL WEIGHT LOSS

If you're like many people, you've tried low-fat diets, high-protein diets, and the get-thin-quick diets found in popular magazines. But have they helped you lose weight and keep it off? In fact, if you're like most people who eventually quit them in frustration, you may have gained even *more* weight after following one of these diets.

Sound familiar? Don't beat yourself up. The problem may be in your blood—specifically, your blood sugar. Fortunately, so is the solution.

Let's begin with a rundown of what happens in the bloodstream when you eat. It's the first step toward understanding exactly how The Sugar Solution can help you lose weight.

It's in the Blood: The Science behind The Sugar Solution

Everyone has glucose in their blood. Glucose is the fuel that powers every cell in the body. When you eat, your body breaks down the food into glucose so it can enter the bloodstream. That process then triggers the pancreas to produce the hormone insulin. Think of insulin as a key that unlocks the cells, allowing glucose to enter. Once in the cells, glucose is either used for fuel or stored in the liver or muscles for future use.

How much insulin is needed to unlock cells depends on what we eat. Some foods take longer than others to break down into glucose. Those that break down slowly provide a lower amount of glucose for your body to absorb over a longer period of time; the pancreas responds by releasing insulin more slowly, too. Even better, when blood sugar rises gradually, it declines just as slowly over time. This gentle rise and fall actually discourages food cravings. However, when foods break down and enter the bloodstream quickly, the pancreas must quickly crank out a lot of insulin to ferry glucose from the blood into the cells. And once insulin has pushed glucose from the blood, glucose drops so low that it triggers cravings, overeating, and weight gain.

Essentially, the faster glucose enters the blood, the faster insulin rises—and the faster blood sugar plummets once that insulin begins to work. This pattern of rapid spikes and dips in your blood sugar level is a problem, both for your overall health and your weight.

Over time, the overeating that results can lead to excess body fat, which can cause cells to ignore insulin's signal to take glucose from the blood. In this condition (insulin resistance), glucose is locked out of the cells and converted to fat, which takes up even more real estate on the hips, waist, and behind.

Many advocates of low-carbohydrate weight-loss plans blame "carbohydrates" as the cause of our country's obesity epidemic. But in reality, no one gains weight by eating too many apples or too much oatmeal.

It's more accurate to say that different types of carbohydrates have different effects on blood sugar and the release of insulin. And those carbohydrates that cause the most dips and spikes in your blood sugar levels can leave you with terrible hunger pangs. Moreover, it's the excess calories consumed due to hunger-inducing fluctuations in blood sugar that cause weight gain.

Quick Carbs, Slow Carbs: How the Right Foods Can Help You Lose Weight

To better understand which foods are broken down into glucose more quickly than others, let's talk about carbohydrates. There are two basic categories of carbohydrates: unrefined and refined. Although they're both converted to glucose and raise blood sugar, they aren't converted at the same rate. How fast they're absorbed—and how much—is what impacts your weight.

Unrefined carbohydrates—found in plant foods like legumes, starchy vegetables, and whole grains—are rich in fiber and take longer to digest, which ultimately helps slow the body's absorption of the carbohydrates that these foods contain. Hence, these *slow carbs*, which delay the conversion of carbohydrates into glucose.

Refined carbohydrates—the kind in white bread, pasta, crackers, and baked goods—are a different story. Lacking the fiber that was removed when the grains were milled, these foods speed through the intestines and flood the bloodstream with glucose, causing insulin levels to zoom upward. Eat too many of these *quick carbs* and your body gets more glucose than it needs. That excess is turned into fat.

Even worse is that spike in insulin followed by a drop in blood sugar, which causes false "hunger" that is too often satisfied with even more quick carbs. It's a vicious cycle: You reach for quick carbs because you're hungry; your blood sugar and insulin skyrocket; then your blood sugar plunges leaving you blindsided by cravings, so you reach for more quick carbs because you're hungry—and your weight goes up, up, and away.

5 REASONS TO EAT THE SUGAR SOLUTION WAY

The healthy benefits of switching over to The Sugar Solution formula can be almost as dramatic as they are quick. Follow it faithfully, and here's what you can expect:

- Weight loss of $1/2$ pound to 2 pounds a week
- Fewer cravings for the sugary, fatty foods that cause weight gain
- More energy that lasts throughout the day
- Increased level of emotional well-being, self-confidence, and self-esteem
- Reduced risk of heart disease, diabetes, and cancer; researchers estimate that losing just 5 to 10 percent of body weight can reduce the risk of heart disease by lowering your blood pressure and cholesterol levels

It doesn't have to be this way. The Sugar Solution way of eating will wean you off the junk carbs at the root of your bottomless hunger. You'll learn how and what to eat to manage your blood sugar so you feel satisfied, not stuffed.

Lose Weight, Eat Great

The Sugar Solution way of eating is so satisfying that you'll never experience feelings of deprivation that can come with diets that restrict carbohydrates or fats. That's because this program is built around an irrefutable fact: Lasting weight loss isn't about eliminating *all* carbohydrates or avoiding every gram of fat that you find. It's about making smart choices.

On this program, you limit quick carbs and consume moderate amounts of slow carbs, lean proteins, and healthy fats. You'll also practice portion control and eat smaller, more frequent meals. All of these strategies help the insulin "key" efficiently go about its business of unlocking cells, leaving little surplus glucose hanging around to be stored as fat. As a bonus, normalizing glucose and insulin levels tend to boost energy. You'll have more incentive to work out regularly and be less inclined to reach for sweets at midafternoon.

Ann Fittante, MS, RD, a certified diabetes educator, has designed a second 21-Day Lifestyle Makeover exclusively for this cookbook, which uses many of the 200 recipes in these pages. Best of all, you don't have to endure 2 weeks of no-carb living to start dropping weight—it often happens within the first week.

As in the first book, *Prevention's The Sugar Solution*, the recipes and meal plans in this cookbook are based on the glycemic index (GI), which ranks foods based on how swiftly and how much they raise blood sugar. The meal plans are also relatively low in calories (1,400–1,600 calories per day) and contain a balance of carbohydrates, protein, and fat, which will help slow absorption of carbohydrates.

Foods with a low GI—typically healthy, slow carbs—are converted to glucose more slowly than those with a medium or high GI (typically quick carbs). Eating lower on the GI scale benefits insulin and blood sugar levels, which in turn discourages fat storage. And because fiber-rich, low-GI foods stay in your system longer, they keep you full and

Sweet Success
BETH SHAW

Thirty-eight-year-old yoga instructor Beth Shaw was skinny as a rail until she turned 16. "I had a sedentary after-school job, and a good part of my income went to burgers, Chinese food, and pizza," says the resident of Hermosa Beach, California. In a matter of months, Beth had gained 25 pounds.

With diet and exercise, the 5-foot-11 woman shed those pounds—and more—and stayed slender for a few years. "In college, I weighed 135 pounds. I was borderline anorexic," she says. Eventually, however, the scale headed north once again.

Beth was at her highest weight—185 pounds—in 1989, when she moved from her native New York City to Los Angeles. Alone in an unfamiliar place, toiling at a stressful job, food was her consolation. "I sat from 6:45 a.m. to 5 p.m. but was constantly tired and stressed," she says. "I felt fat, helpless, and depressed. My weight—and my life—were out of control."

Determined to ease her stress, Beth began to practice yoga. Something clicked. "It put me in touch with my body, reduced my stress, and improved my mood." She began to study yoga and in 1993 began to teach it. Shortly thereafter, she created YogaFit, a hybrid style of yoga that emphasizes fitness.

But though her business was a smashing success, Beth was still battling her extra pounds. Her weight seesawed until 1995 when she met a personal trainer at one of her yoga retreats. On his advice, the 175-pound Beth began an eating plan that emphasized low-glycemic carbohydrates.

Breakfast was two eggs with oatmeal or a protein drink. At midmorning, she nibbled on a low-carb snack bar. Lunch was sushi or a green salad with tuna or chicken. In the midafternoon, Beth snacked on a piece of fruit with a handful of nuts or a protein drink. For dinner, she enjoyed fish, chicken, or steak; a salad; and a small sweet potato. Beth also lifted weights and did cardio along with her yoga.

"My weight began to drop instantly," she says. A year later, she was 20 pounds lighter.

Beth now weighs between 150 and 153 pounds and wears a size 6–8. She lifts weights twice a week, walks with her dogs, and practices some form of yoga 5 days a week. Last fall, she ran a half-marathon. "I feel calm and in control," she says.

discourage the overeating that leads to weight gain. The recipes in this cookbook are prepared with lower-GI ingredients such as beans, grains, and whole-grain flours and pastas. If you follow the 21 days of menu plans, you'll never feel deprived with six tasty, filling meals and snacks a day. Here are just some of the mouthwatering recipes you'll enjoy.

- All-American Pot Roast (page 242)
- Apricot-Ginger Buttermilk Scones (page 83)
- Blueberry-Ginger Crumb Pie (page 348)
- Carrot Cake Pancakes with Maple–Cream Cheese Spread (page 76)
- Curried Sweet Potato Salad (page 165)
- Oven-"Fried" Chicken (page 262)
- Shaved Barbecue Beef Sandwiches with Spicy Slaw (page 147)
- Shepherd's Pie (page 243)

SLEEP MORE, LOSE MORE

If you sleep less than 8 hours a night, getting more Zs may help you lose weight. Sleep deprivation disrupts your body's normal ability to process and control various weight-related hormones, including glucose and cortisol. This imbalance encourages cells to store excess fat, lowers your body's fat-burning ability, and may make it tougher to control cravings.

But just 9 hours of sleep for 3 consecutive nights can reverse this, making weight loss easier. Here's a trio of sleepy-time tips.

Take a brisk, after-dinner walk. Regular exercise—30 minutes most days of the week—reduces stress and raises body temperature, which primes you for slumber.

Each evening, prep for sleep. Take a bath, listen to relaxing music, and make sure your bedroom is dark, cool, and quiet.

Nap to nip cravings. If you've endured a sleepless night, take a 10-minute nap the next day. It will improve both your mood and your ability to stick to your diet.

OUR DIET'S SAFETY FEATURES

Ever struggled through a low-carb diet and shed your hair along with the pounds? Or felt like death warmed over on one of those 800-calorie-a-day fad diets? Unlike these kinds of nutritionally unbalanced, overly stringent weight-loss plans, The Sugar Solution program was designed with your health in mind, as well as your satisfaction. Here's why:

- **It's not a fad.** The Sugar Solution plan is based on the current recommendations in medical and nutritional literature. It doesn't exclude major food groups (hint: carbohydrates) or advocate pricey supplements.

- **It's nutritionally sound.** On this plan, you get the nutrients you need for energy and good health—not the case with many low-carb or low-calorie diets. Each meal is packed with vitamins, minerals, fiber, and health-promoting plant compounds from a balanced mix of complex carbohydrates, lean proteins, and good fats.

- **It contains enough calories.** You'll consume between 1,400 and 1,600 calories a day. This range is low enough to promote safe weight loss but not low enough to slow your metabolism or cause you to feel ill or exhausted.

- **It won't lead to hair loss.** Some women on low-carb plans complain of losing their hair along with their excess pounds, perhaps because these diets skimp on nutrients. With this program, your hair stays on your head.

- **It won't cause gallstones.** Very low calorie diets of 800 calories or less are associated with gallstones. These solid chunks of material form in the gallbladder—the pear-shaped organ that produces bile, which aids in digestion—and can get stuck in the gallbladder duct, causing pain and infection. (It's thought that rapid weight loss reduces the gallbladder's ability to contract and send bile into the intestine.) On The Sugar Solution plan, weight loss is slow, which reduces the risk of gallstones.

- **It's safe for people with diabetes.** Low-carb diets can cause ketosis, in which the body burns fat for fuel instead of carbohydrates. Ketosis is dangerous for some people with diabetes. On this plan, you never go into ketosis, because at least half your diet is carbohydrates. (However, people with diabetes who follow *any* weight-loss plan should step up their blood-glucose monitoring and contact their doctor if they experience low blood sugar.)

Putting the Plan into Action: The Sugar Solution's Triple Threat

Unless you're a master juggler who spins plates for a living or a ballet dancer who can stand *en pointe* for hours at a time, you know that it's hard to balance anything on one leg for long. That same fact applies when you're trying to lose weight—expecting lasting results from food changes alone is more than likely to leave you stumbling from time to time. That's why The Sugar Solution is designed to function like a stool supported by three legs: an eating plan that helps normalize blood sugar and insulin levels, regular physical activity, and stress management. All have beneficial effects on insulin and weight and, when used together, can improve your odds of achieving lasting weight loss.

Cardiovascular exercise, such as brisk walking, and resistance training, or lifting weights, both burn calories, help reduce body fat, and increase muscle mass, all of which

A SUPERCHARGED METABOLISM: JUST ADD WATER

Want to supercharge your calorie-burning potential? Drink up, says Ann Fittante, MS, RD. It seems that fluids—especially plain water—really can support weight-loss efforts. Researchers in Germany measured the resting metabolism of 14 men and women before and after they drank just over 16 ounces of water. Within 10 minutes, their metabolisms began to rise, and after 40 minutes, their average calorie-burning rate was 30 percent higher. And it stayed elevated for more than an hour.

Researchers don't understand why, but they calculate that drinking eight cups (64 ounces) of water a day—the generally recommended amount—can burn off almost 35,000 calories a year, or about 10 pounds.

But you don't need to drown in the stuff. A recent National Academy of Sciences report found that most women need 11 cups (88 ounces) of fluid a day, but it doesn't all have to be water. A cup of tea counts, as does juice or the occasional diet cola. (Limit or eliminate sugary sodas and juices, though. Studies show that liquid calories don't register on your hunger radar and can sneak up on your waistline.) It's safe to drink a total of 8 to 12 cups a day. And drink it cool—part of the increased calorie burn occurs as the body warms the liquid to body temperature.

help cells become more sensitive to insulin. Lifting weights also helps build muscle, which burns more calories per pound than fat. In our 21-Day Lifestyle Makeover, look for the "Get Yourself Moving" box, which contains an easy way to put more movement into your day. Add one or more of these simple steps to your life, and you could burn 100 or more extra calories a day. That adds up to more than 10 pounds a year.

Stress also affects the way the body uses blood sugar and insulin. Under chronic stress, the body releases higher-than-normal amounts of a stress hormone known as cortisol. These increased cortisol levels not only signal the brain that it needs food but also tell the body to store as much fat as possible—and to hold on to it. One study led by a researcher at Pennsylvania State University found that women who secreted higher levels of cortisol in reaction to a stressful event were more likely to snack on high-fat foods than those who produced less cortisol in reaction to the same event. Because the short-circuiting of stress can pay off in a slimmer waistline, each day of our 21-day plan features one simple, yet effective, way to short-circuit stress.

To feel fitter and healthier than ever before, pair the tasty menus and recipes in these pages with regular, moderate-intensity physical activity—such as a brisk 30-minute walk daily—and stress-control tactics. Follow the tips and strategies in the 21-Day Lifestyle Makeover that starts on page 44, and you'll hit the ground running.

CHAPTER 2

THE SUGAR SOLUTION PLAN: 4 SIMPLE PRINCIPLES (AND 16 EASY TIPS) FOR SUCCESS

Now that you understand the science behind The Sugar Solution program, it's time to put the plan into practice. Follow the 21-Day Lifestyle Makeover, and you're off to a great start. Have more weight to lose after 21 days? Repeat the program, or simply live and cook by the simple principles below. The weight will continue to melt away, along with your food cravings and fatigue, if you follow the basic advice that lies at the heart of The Sugar Solution program.

Principle 1: Upgrade Your Carbs

Craving a juicy McIntosh apple or a warm and crunchy slice of whole grain toast? Enjoy. On The Sugar Solution program, you don't eliminate carbohydrates, you upgrade them— that is, trade in the quick carbs that encourage weight gain for the slow carbs that dampen your appetite and discourage excess body fat. Live by this principle, watch your portion sizes, and you'll find it's easier not only to lose weight but to keep it off. You'll also eat hearty with none of the deprivation of most low-carb menu plans, and your body will get the vitamins, minerals, and other substances essential to good health.

As you'll see, we've upgraded the carbohydrates in our recipes with mouthwatering results. Our Carrot Cake Pancakes (page 76) and Mexican Wedding Cookies (page 329) are made with whole grain pastry flour. The Spicy Corn and Sweet Potato Chowder (page 117) lends an old-fashioned favorite—traditionally made with white potatoes—a new and tasty twist. Love chocolate cake? Turn to page 345 to see how we've made a good thing even better with low-fat, low-glycemic ingredients.

Upgrading your carbs is simpler than you think. Here are four easy ways to do it. As you'll see, sometimes the glycemic index (GI) of a particular food matters less than its content of vitamins, minerals, and health-protective plant chemicals.

- Upgrade from white to sweet potatoes. Of course, you can eat a small spud every now and again. But there are good reasons to make the moist, orange-fleshed spud a regular indulgence. Not only is the GI of a sweet potato much lower than that of a regular potato (54 versus 85), but sweet potatoes are packed with beta-carotene, vitamins C and E, and fiber. Try a small, baked sweet potato, sprinkled with cinnamon and artificial sweetener. Or bake up some sweet potato fries. Preheat the oven to 450°F. Coat a baking sheet with cooking spray. Slice 2 medium sweet potatoes or yams (peels on, for extra fiber) into $\frac{1}{2}$"-thick wedges. Combine the potatoes, 1 tablespoon of olive oil, $\frac{1}{4}$ teaspoon of salt, and $\frac{1}{8}$ teaspoon of pepper in a bowl and toss well. Arrange the potatoes in a single layer on the baking sheet. Bake for 30 to 45 minutes, turning halfway through. Serve immediately.

- Upgrade from white to whole grain pastas. Their GI is nearly identical (41 for white spaghetti, 37 for whole wheat). However, the latter contains more fiber and healthy plant nutrients than the former. They pack more flavor, too—many people come to love the chewy, nutty-tasting whole wheat pastas. If you don't, Eden Foods offers a hybrid pasta that combines 60 percent whole grain flour with refined flour. You'll find it in natural food stores or in some large supermarkets, or visit www.edenfoods.com. And check the stores for other whole grain pastas made with brown rice, corn, spelt, and buckwheat.

• Upgrade from white to whole grain bread. Again, both varieties of bread are similar on the GI scale, because when fiber is finely ground, as it often is in whole wheat flour, it doesn't present enough of a digestive challenge to lower the GI of foods made with it. However, whole wheat bread is a healthier choice because of its extra fiber and other nutrients. Best bets include Pepperidge Farm 100% Stone Ground Whole Wheat Bread, Wonder Stone Ground 100% Whole Wheat Bread, and Thomas' Sahara 100% Whole Wheat Pita Bread. Tried 'em and don't like 'em—or can't get used to 'em? When you make a sandwich, do some sleight of hand: Put a slice of your favorite bread on top, and use whole grain bread on the bottom. Or use whole grain bread to make your own bread crumbs.

Discover one new whole grain a month. From amaranth to wild rice, there's a dazzling array of whole grains from around the world to bring to your table. For example, cooked quinoa (pronounced KEEN-wa) is excellent in casseroles, soups, stews, and stir-fries (and cooks in about 15 minutes). You can even cook it in fruit juice and enjoy it as a breakfast cereal, or use it cold in salads. And bulgur is delicious as a side dish that doesn't require stove-top cooking. Your local natural food store will have 'em all. To field-test these great grains, try our delicious Curried Couscous Salad (page 177), Quinoa with Raisins, Apricots, and Pecans (page 226), and Mediterranean Couscous (page 231).

Principle 2: Eat Less, More Often

Mom probably told you to eat three square meals a day, but that may be bad advice when you're trying to lose weight. Research has found that women who eat large meals may burn 60 fewer calories per day than those who eat smaller amounts of food every few hours. And while 60 calories a day may not sound like much, it's the equivalent of 6 pounds a year.

On The Sugar Solution program, you eat small amounts more frequently—every 3 hours or so. These mini-meals can keep your blood sugar on an even keel, which dampens food cravings and prevents the spikes in insulin that promote fat storage. And there's plenty of compelling evidence that this eat-less-more-often strategy works. Researchers at the

University of Massachusetts in Worcester found that people who eat four or more times daily—generally three meals and one or two snacks—are less likely to be obese than those who eat fewer meals.

Eating every few hours may seem an unlikely way to save calories, if you usually skip meals or starve yourself to lose weight—until you consider that these methods actually slow your metabolism. It's true. When you starve yourself, the body senses that food is scarce and conserves its reserves, slowing its metabolism to hold on to what it has until the next big meal comes along.

TEAM YOUR WILLPOWER WITH SKILLPOWER

When it comes to weight loss, you need more than willpower. You need skillpower—the ability to solve problems and strategize when things get tough and your resolution to be good evaporates. Willpower is like a car's engine: It gets you revved up to go. But skillpower is the steering wheel that helps you navigate obstacles. These tips can help you hone this expertise.

Set smaller, more doable goals. In the beginning, willpower is strong and intoxicating. You think you'll do everything perfectly—no more sweets, an hour-long workout a day, skimpy portions—and by summer, you'll look like a *Sports Illustrated* swimsuit model. Skillpower says forget the bikini and focus on fitting into last year's shorts. Rewarding yourself for achieving small goals like this keeps skillpower sharp and motivation high.

Plan ahead to avoid danger zones. Hanging out with friends at a coffeehouse while your mouth waters over the chocolate croissants requires iron willpower. The smarter skillpower way: Get your coffee to go and chat while you take a brisk, croissant-free walk together.

Catch yourself quickly. If you raid the office vending machine at 4 p.m., you're likely to hit the cookies when you arrive home from the office. Use skillpower to get back on track and eat a healthy dinner. A Brown University study of 142 people reports that if you get back on the diet-and-exercise track immediately after a binge, your weight loss efforts won't suffer.

For success on The Sugar Solution plan, follow these mini-meal do's and don'ts.

Avoid portion distortion. The idea is to feed your body enough to keep your hunger at bay and your metabolism revving. If you overfuel, you defeat the whole purpose of eating small. To make sure your mini-meals are truly mini, use a salad plate as a dinner plate and a coffee cup as a bowl. As you'll see, the meals in the 21-Day Lifestyle Makeover are rarely more than 600 calories, and snacks top out at 150 calories.

Follow the formula. Each mini-meal should contain a balance of nutrients, including slow carbs, protein, and healthy fat. Don't worry about looking up nutrition guidelines to calculate the exact ratios—just make sure that all three nutrients are included in what you select. For example, a healthy mini might be half a turkey sandwich (no cheese) on whole grain bread with ½ teaspoon of light mayo and a piece of fruit; or a mini-pita with 1 tablespoon of hummus and 5 baby carrots.

Start your day with a mini-meal. Studies show that breakfast eaters tend to lose more weight when dieting than do breakfast skippers. But that's not a green light to order the Farmer's Breakfast Special at the diner every morning. Instead, apply the mini-meal formula here, too. You might scramble two egg whites with spinach and wrap it in a small whole grain tortilla, or enjoy ½ cup of oatmeal with half an orange and a cheese stick.

Choose maxi-nutrient minis. Don't be tempted by the small packages that lurk in the snack aisle or inside vending machines. A tiny bag of chips or half a candy bar might look mini, but you'll be cheating yourself out of nutrients—and put yourself right back on that blood sugar roller coaster. Ditto for the new snack products that tout only 100 calories per serving. It's not always calories that count: You'll need to weigh your selections by the amount of quick carbs they contain as well.

Principle 3: Eat One Bowl of High-Fiber Cereal a Day

Cereal lovers, rejoice! Not only does The Sugar Solution allow this breakfast favorite on the menu, it encourages you to enjoy it. That's because eating just 1 serving a day can provide as much as 15 grams of fiber—half, or more than half, of the 25 to 30 grams experts recommend.

Of course, adding more fiber to your diet is a healthy choice. But it's also a smart move if you're looking to drop some weight. In a 2003 study, researchers at the Harvard School of Public Health linked diets high in whole grains to lowered weight gain.

Over a 12-year period, the researchers followed the eating habits of more than 74,000 women to study the association between whole grain intake and weight gain over time. What they found: The more whole grains the women consumed, the less they tended to weigh. Moreover, women who ate the most fiber had a 49 percent lower risk of weight gain than women who consumed the lowest amount of fiber. It may be that whole grains promote weight loss because they give that tummy-satisfying feeling of fullness (researchers call it satiety) or because they influence the body's use of insulin.

If you plan to follow our makeover, feel free to swap any of the suggested snacks for your bowl-a-day. You can also opt to have cereal for breakfast as many times a week as you wish. And try these tips.

Spoon up the right portion. Successful weight loss begins with correct portion sizes. Eat 1 serving of cereal for breakfast, ½ serving for a snack (with ½ cup of fat-free or soymilk). Use a measuring cup for a week until you're certain you know what 1 serving really looks like.

THE SUGAR SOLUTION CEREAL SAFARI

Finding a whole grain cereal got easier in 2004, when General Mills announced that it would make all its cereals with whole grains. Opt for a brand that contains at least 7 grams of fiber. The cereals that follow are low in calories and sugar and are good sources of appetite-blunting slow carbs.

- All-Bran with Extra Fiber (1 cup) 100 calories, 15 grams fiber
- Fiber One (½ cup) 118 calories, 14 grams fiber
- Kashi Seven Whole Grains & Sesame (¾ cup) 90 calories, 8 grams fiber
- General Mills Multi-Bran Chex (1 cup) 200 calories, 8 grams fiber

Sweet Success
CARSON REDWINE

Carson Redwine, a welfare worker in Muncie, Indiana, started to gain weight after his 30th birthday. "I was less active than I used to be and didn't change my eating habits," says Carson, now 53. As he continued to gain, he tried to cut back on doughnuts, bread, chips, and cookies. Unfortunately, he failed. By 2000, Carson carried almost 300 pounds on his 6-foot-1 frame.

"I knew I had a problem," he says. "I woke up at night short of breath. Taking my daily walk with my wife, Anna, was becoming more difficult. When I bent over to tie my shoelaces, it was hard to breathe. My weight made me self-conscious, and I was upset with myself for allowing myself to get so heavy." He vowed to lose weight for good.

In March 2003, he turned his eating habits around, abandoning the quick carbs that contributed to his weight gain and low energy levels. "At first, I was miserable," says Carson. But it wasn't long before he started to feel better, physically and mentally.

Carson started his day with slow carbs: a cup of oatmeal topped with a handful of walnuts or pecans or slices of fresh fruit. Sometimes, he enjoyed two organic eggs prepared with olive oil and his own homemade, fiber-full whole wheat toast. Lunch was a piece of fruit, a slice of cheese, a slice of his bread spread with peanut butter, and a glass of milk, or a bowl of his homemade bean or chicken-vegetable soup. For dinner, he enjoyed broiled or baked fish or chicken, a baked sweet potato, salad, and a green vegetable. Between meals, Carson snacked on nuts and fruit and drank plenty of water and green tea.

Over a 20-month period, Carson lost almost 50 pounds, and he now weighs 247 pounds. He'd like to get down to 170 pounds—his weight when he got married at age 19—and is "actively pursuing that goal."

Carson has continued his daily walks, which have become much easier. "Anna and I walk 2 to 3 miles a day," he says. "We also do Leslie Sansone's Walk Away the Pounds. Her workouts are excellent for people of all ages."

Carson says that his life has changed for the better. "I no longer doze off when I sit down," he says. "I sleep better. I'm more active. And I'm in control, not the potato chips and soft drinks. Now I think about what I eat."

Make your cereal berry sweet. Give your cereal an extra blast of flavor as well as fiber, with berries. Just ½ cup of fresh raspberries contains 4 grams of fiber; ½ cup of frozen blueberries has 2 grams of fiber. (Feel free to use a sugar substitute as well.)

Splash on the soy. Both regular and vanilla low-fat soymilk are a delicious twist on regular skim milk and a good option if you're lactose intolerant or allergic to cow's milk. Look for calcium-fortified brands with calcium and vitamin D at about the same levels as dairy milk: 300 milligrams of calcium, 100 IU of vitamin D per 8 ounces. A few to try: Silk Vanilla, 8th Continent Vanilla, or WestSoy Plus Vanilla.

Sprinkle on the flax. Mixing 1 tablespoon of high-fiber, ground flaxseed into your cereal can help curb your appetite and eliminate calories. Flaxseed is also a rich source of alpha-linoleic acid (ALA), an important omega-3 fat that protects against high cholesterol, diabetes, and high blood pressure. You'll find flaxseed at health food stores or natural food supermarkets. Refrigerate promptly since the delicate oil in flaxseed can go rancid easily.

Principle 4: Don't Skimp on Good Fats

If you've tried the popular high-protein diets, you're probably sick of the sight of bacon, steak, and pork rinds. That's good, because much of the fat on these plans is derived from the unhealthy saturated fats found in butter, fatty red meats, and full-fat dairy products. Many quick carbs—cookies, cakes, and crackers—tend to contain trans fats, which are just as unhealthy as saturated fats, if not more so. Trans fats—created when hydrogen gas reacts with oil—raise bad LDL cholesterol, like saturated fats do, but also crush heart-protective HDL cholesterol. Further, these "frankenfats" have been linked to cancer and diabetes.

However, a diet stripped of fat isn't healthy, either. Your body needs fat to function properly. Dietary fat also stabilizes blood sugar levels, which helps you feel full and satisfied for hours.

On The Sugar Solution program, you'll consume from 25 to 30 percent of your total daily calories from fat, most of that derived from healthy fats such as olive oil, natural peanut butter and other nut butters, and avocados. Cold-water fish such as salmon, walnuts, almonds, flaxseed, and canola oil contain heart-healthy omega-3 fatty acids.

As you'll see in the recipes, we swap butter for olive oil, forgo full-fat cheese and sour cream for the reduced-fat kind, and use the leanest cuts of beef and pork. So go ahead, dig into the Grilled Peppered Steak with Multigrain Texas Toast (page 240). You'll consume just 5 grams of fat per serving.

If you're following the 21-day program, we've calculated your fat budget for you. Once you're on your own, however, there are simple ways to make sure you choose good fats over bad. Trade your grilled steak or burger for grilled salmon once a week, and ditch the bacon bits on your salads and top them with nuts or seeds for a flavorful crunch.

Keep the following tips in mind and you'll be sure to get the good fats you need.

Eat a good-fat appetizer to crush cravings. Marshall Goldberg, MD, an endocrinologist at Thomas Jefferson University Medical College in Philadelphia, found that spreading 2 teaspoons of olive oil on half a slice of bread eaten 15 to 20 minutes before a meal helps his patients control their cravings. Olive oil is known to stimulate the release of cholecystokinin (CCK), a gut hormone that signals the brain to stop eating. It may be that olive oil also slows stomach contractions, which creates a sense of fullness. (Of course, make your bread whole grain.)

Feast on fatty fish twice a week. Salmon is an easy way to get your omega-3s, called eicosapentaenoic acid (EPA) and docosahexaenoic acid (DHA). A serving of salmon the size of a deck of cards (about 3 ounces) will bring you almost 2 grams of EPA and DHA. Or have a tuna salad sandwich. Buy canned white albacore tuna in water (light tuna has less omega-3s). Use low-fat mayo or mayo made from canola oil.

Go nuts. Sprinkle 2 tablespoons of toasted, chopped nuts a day on your whole grain cereal, low-fat yogurt, salads, or stir-fries. And feel free to indulge in 1 serving (2 tablespoons) of all-natural peanut butter, which doesn't contain trans fats or added sugar.

Switch to trans free margarines. A few to try: Land O' Lakes Light Country Morning Blend, I Can't Believe It's Not Butter with Yogurt!, Promise Ultra Spread, and Spectrum Naturals Spread (sold in natural food stores).

Sweet Success
MARY KONIZ ARNOLD

Mary Koniz Arnold, 43, gained weight after getting married and having kids. "My food choices changed. I went from choosing skinless chicken to bratwurst, brown rice to biscuits," she says. Her stressful job at a nonprofit agency included food at every special event and meeting.

Mary felt fit and stayed active—"I walked or jogged every day, swam at the Y, rode my bike, and danced." But by 2000, the 5-foot-1 Mary weighed 217 pounds. Around that time, she bought a pair of size 20 pants and felt compelled to buy a girdle for her 20-year high-school reunion.

The weight began to come off when Mary made modest changes in her diet and started teaching gymnastics part-time. "I took my daughter to her class one day, and they were short-staffed," she says. "I had done gymnastics as a child, and I could still do the moves, so I offered to help."

Her first year teaching gymnastics, she lost 10 pounds. Changing jobs in 2002—Mary is now a writer/photographer at a community college in Poughkeepsie, New York—helped her lose another 10. "I walked more and had less access to food," she says.

Mary kept off those 20 pounds and even completed a half-marathon in 2003. In the spring of 2004, before training for a full marathon, she developed a knee problem. An orthopedist recommended physical therapy—and weight loss. "Exercise wasn't enough anymore. I had to change my diet drastically," she says. She was at 197 pounds.

She joined a weight-loss program offering support meetings and guidance in food choices. A typical breakfast: oatmeal with fruit, ½ cup of fat-free milk, and ⅓ cup of fat-free cottage cheese. Lunch was brown rice and beans with salsa and fat-free cheese, or lean meat and a salad. Dinner: 2 ounces of lean meat, 1 cup of whole grain pasta or brown rice, salad, and cooked vegetables. Snacks included fruit, fat-free cheese, raw veggies, and whole grain cereal with fruit and skim milk.

In 8 months, she lost another 60 pounds and now weighs 137 pounds. "Yesterday I bought a pair of pants—size 2!" she says.

She's running again, and dropping 80 pounds has allowed her to surpass her childhood gymnastics skills. "I always loved the balance beam, but now I do the uneven bars, too—pullovers, back hip circles, mill circles, and jumping to the high bar," she says. "I'm still working on my back handspring."

CHAPTER 3

STOCKING THE SUGAR SOLUTION KITCHEN

The Sugar Solution lifestyle doesn't just transform your body, it transforms your kitchen. Since you'll be spending less time at the drive-through window and more time preparing your own healthy, tasty meals, there's a good chance that your pantry, refrigerator, and freezer need a drastic overhaul. Fortunately, our Kitchen Makeover—which takes just minutes—will make losing extra pounds and adopting healthier eating habits much easier.

The biggest benefit? Having the right foods on hand prevents slips and binges that can slow your weight loss or derail your efforts altogether. When you don't keep quick carbs and bad fats in your house, they can't undermine your good intentions. Similarly, if you stock your kitchen with slow carbs and good fats, you won't break into your husband's chips or your children's lunchbox snacks because there's nothing else to eat.

What's more, cooking and eating at home takes much less time than you think. You might spend 5 minutes planning your weekly menu, 30 minutes a week at the supermarket, and 20 minutes a day in the kitchen preparing dinner (less for breakfast and lunch). When you think about it, preparing healthy meals takes about as much time as sitting in your car at the drive-through or waiting in line at the local takeout place.

This chapter is a guide to stocking your kitchen with Sugar Solution–friendly foods.

When you shop smart, you put the makings for fresh, healthy meals right where you need them: in your pantry, refrigerator, and freezer. Follow our easy three-step Kitchen Makeover and you'll be able to whip up meals that please your tastebuds (and your waistline) in less time than it takes the pizza guy to ring your doorbell.

Step 1: Put Your Kitchen on a Diet

In this step, you ferret out the quick carbs and bad fats lurking in your pantry, refrigerator, and freezer. Toss the following waist-thickening foods, or box up unopened items and donate them to charity.

- Boxed dinner mixes or high-fat, high-calorie frozen dinners
- Bread, bagels, or English muffins that are not whole grain
- Frozen convenience foods, such as french fries and fish sticks
- Full-fat ice cream
- Full-sugar jellies and jams
- High-fat lunchmeats (salami, bologna, pepperoni)
- High-fat meats
- High-fat processed meats, such as bacon, sausage, and hot dogs
- Most canned soups, stews, and pasta meals
- Most salad dressings (unless they're free of trans fats)
- Packaged cookies, baked goods, and other sweets
- Pasta and noodles made from white flour
- Processed cheese in cans
- Salty snack foods
- Stick margarine (unless it's free of trans fats)
- Sugar-coated cereals, or those that are not whole grain
- Sugar-sweetened yogurt
- Sugary soft drinks and juices

Step 2: Restock with Healthy Foods

When you've completed Step 1, you should be left with mostly slow carbs and good fats. These foods include:

- All-natural peanut butter or other nut butter
- Eggs
- Fresh or frozen fish, such as tuna, sardines, or salmon, or canned tuna and salmon in water
- Fresh or frozen fruits and vegetables
- Frozen juice bars with no sugar added
- Lean meats and poultry (chicken, turkey breast, or very lean ground beef)
- Low-fat bottled marinara sauce
- Low-fat dairy or soy products
- Nuts prepared without salt or fat (raw almonds, walnuts, no-salt peanuts)
- Olive, flax, and canola oils
- Whole grain breads, cereals, and pastas

Step 3: Go Forth and Shop!

You say your cupboards (and fridge and freezer) are bare? It's time to restock them with healthy fare. Below you'll find lists of foods to fill them with, by category, along with some tasty cooking tips. No need to buy every item listed: Let your personal tastes guide your selections. But do be adventurous and buy items you've never tried before.

FRUITS AND VEGETABLES

Buy these:

- Canned or frozen legumes
- Canned vegetables (optional; buy low-sodium, or drain and rinse before use)

- Edamame (Japanese whole soybeans)
- Fresh fruit (apples, bananas, blueberries, exotic fruits, grapefruit, grapes, melon, oranges, strawberries)
- Fresh herbs (basil, cilantro, parsley, rosemary, tarragon, and thyme)
- Fresh vegetables (broccoli, cabbage, carrots, celery, collard greens, cucumber, green/red/yellow peppers, kale, mushrooms, onions, squash, tomatoes, zucchini)
- Frozen berries
- Frozen vegetables prepared without fat or fatty sauces
- Packaged greens (including spinach) for salads
- Scallions (green onions)
- Sweet potatoes
- Winter squash

Tasty tips:

- Because frozen veggies are frozen at the peak of ripeness, they're often more nutritious than the fresh stuff that's been languishing in the produce bins. Go for Asian stir-fry or other mixes that include one or more of the following: broccoli, carrots, cauliflower, and Brussels sprouts.
- Tuck veggies in every sandwich—and not just a token lettuce leaf. Pick up prewashed bagged greens with big flavor power, such as baby spinach, arugula, and mesclun mix. Or try precut coleslaw mix (shredded cabbage and carrots).
- Kale, mustard and turnip greens, and Swiss chard are delicious, chock-full of healthy phytochemicals, and easy to prepare. Just wash, cut off the tough bottom stems, and sauté until limp in olive oil seasoned with garlic, ginger, or other spices.
- Fresh herbs and scallions add zip and flavor to many foods. Snip and top on salads.
- Crushed, peeled tomatoes or plain diced tomatoes in juice can be used in a wide variety of dishes. No-added-salt tomato sauce can be used on pizza or mixed with a commercial pasta sauce to lower its sodium content.

- Like veggies, fruits are flash-frozen at their ripest. Your best-tasting and most nutritious bets: berries (loaded with antioxidants) and mangoes (with beta-carotene). Toss ½ cup each of blueberries and raspberries into a smoothie, or add to pancakes and breads.

- Edamame is available at most natural food stores either fresh or frozen. Cook in the pod and serve as an appetizer.

- Cut sweet potatoes lengthwise into eight wedges per potato. Place in a bowl and toss with a little olive oil and paprika. Spread on a baking sheet that has been coated with nonstick spray and bake in a 450°F oven, turning once, for 30 to 45 minutes, until golden brown.

- Stir unsweetened applesauce or a little curry powder into cooked, solid-pack frozen squash and serve as a side dish.

WHOLE GRAIN BREADS, CEREALS, AND PASTAS

Buy these:

- Barley
- Brown rice
- Bulgur
- High-fiber/low-sugar hot and cold cereal
- Oatmeal (whole oats) or steel-cut oats
- Whole grain bread and English muffins
- Whole wheat couscous
- Whole wheat or corn tortillas
- Whole wheat or whole grain pasta

Tasty tips:

- Heat small whole wheat or corn tortillas briefly in a skillet, then roll with a combination of diced cooked chicken, cooked pinto beans or black beans, diced scallion, roasted red pepper, and a bit of cheese. Heat until the cheese melts.

- To make a crispy snack, brush 1 whole wheat tortilla with a teaspoon of olive oil, and sprinkle with your favorite seasonings (chili powder, garlic, salt, pepper). Cut into 12 wedges. Arrange on a lightly oiled baking sheet. Bake at 350°F for 5 to 10 minutes, until crisp. Cool on paper towels and enjoy. Makes 1 serving.

- Couscous is a form of pasta usually made from refined wheat flour. Use the whole wheat kind (available in natural food supermarkets), and you'll score 7 grams of craving-busting fiber per serving, compared with just 2 grams in regular couscous.
- Toasting barley gives it a light, nutty flavor. Place the barley in a nonstick skillet over medium heat. Cook, stirring or shaking constantly, for 5 minutes, or until grain is golden.
- Bake brown rice! Combine rice and liquid (chicken, beef, or vegetable broth) in a casserole dish. Cover and bake at 375°F for 25 minutes, or until the liquid is absorbed.

LOW-FAT DAIRY PRODUCTS

Buy these:

- Fat-free milk or soymilk
- Fat-free or low-fat cottage cheese
- Fat-free or low-fat yogurt (plain or flavored)
- Reduced-fat cheese (as well as lower fat cheeses like goat cheese and part-skim mozzarella)
- Small amount of highly flavored cheese, such as Parmesan, Blue cheese, or Cheddar (used as a condiment)

Tasty tips:

- Reduced-fat cheese has come a long way—the quality and taste are better than ever. Try low-fat cheese on whole grain crackers and sandwiches, or shred some over your veggies at dinner.
- A number of cheeses, such as aged sharp Cheddar, feta, and grated Parmesan or Romano, add a lot of flavor in small amounts. Use as you would a condiment—approximately 1 tablespoon to flavor eggs, pasta, or salads.
- Use fat-free or low-fat plain yogurt as a lower-fat, higher-calcium stand-in for sour cream or mayonnaise.
- Don't use a lot of yogurt? Buy an 8-ounce container and replace as needed.

Sweet Success

FRAN EHRET

On Valentine's Day 2002, Fran, then 60, received a sugary surprise. But it wasn't a heart-shaped box of chocolates. It was a diabetes diagnosis from his doctor.

The retired postmaster from Hellertown, Pennsylvania, was told that his blood sugar was a staggering 190 mg/dl. (Diabetes is diagnosed at 126 mg/dl.) Moreover, at 5 feet 8 inches and 200 pounds, Fran was obese. If he didn't lose weight, his doctor said, he'd have to take insulin.

"That scared me," says Fran, now 62. His brother, a diabetic, had passed away at 62. His father, also a diabetic, had died of a heart attack at 63.

"I was a time bomb waiting to happen," says Fran. "I used to not care about what I ate or when I ate it." His biggest weakness was eating at night. His cravings typically started right after dinner, when he snacked on potato chips, sausage, or bologna and cheese, and ended only when he nodded off in front of the TV.

"I wasn't ready to die," Fran says. Determined to take charge of his health, he overhauled his eating habits.

Instead of the quick carbs he usually ate for breakfast—doughnuts and sugar-laden coffee, or a cheesesteak omelet, home fries, and white toast slathered with butter—he had a bowl of whole grain cereal with 1 percent milk and a cup of tea. Lunch was tuna salad (made with low-fat salad dressing) on whole wheat bread rather than a sandwich piled high with lunchmeat. For dinner, Fran switched from red meat, mashed potatoes, and white bread to fish, chicken, or whole wheat pasta and two vegetables prepared without fat.

As Fran trimmed his diet, he ramped up his activity levels. He began to walk an hour a day, either outdoors or on his treadmill, which he moved from the basement into the sunroom so that he could use it while watching TV.

In just a few months, Fran shed 30 pounds. Napping during the day or nodding off in front of the TV was a thing of the past. "My energy levels were through the roof," he says. Three years later, Fran has kept off every last pound, continues to stick to his healthy diet and daily walks, and still has energy to burn. "And the last time my doctor checked my blood sugar, it was normal," says Fran. "No insulin for me."

LEGUMES

Buy these:

- All varieties of beans—garbanzo, pinto, white, navy, black
- Lentils

Tasty tips:

- Some supermarkets carry legumes, such as black beans or pinto beans, in the frozen foods section. If you find them, snap them up. Frozen legumes are lower in sodium and have a firmer texture than canned beans. Also, you can add small amounts of frozen beans to your dishes without wondering what to do with the rest of the can.

---

5 SMART WAYS TO DO SOY

Slash waist-thickening (and artery-clogging) saturated fat with these great-tasting soy versions of meat and cheese favorites. Daily saturated fat limits: women, 12 g; men, 15 g.*

Instead of . . .	. . . Try Soy	Saturated Fat Savings Per Serving
Armour Homestyle Italian Meatballs	Veggitinos Wholesome Vegetable Meatballs	9 g
Weaver Chicken Nuggets	Morningstar Farms Chik Nuggets	3 g
Stouffer's Five Cheese Lasagna	Amy's Tofu Vegetable Lasagna	5 g
Red Baron Four Cheese Pizza	Amy's Organic Crust & Tomatoes Pizza	4 g
Weaver Hot Wings	2 Morningstar Farms Buffalo Wings	2 g

Based on 1,500 calories per day for women; 2,000 calories per day for men.

- To save money, boil dried legumes or use a pressure cooker and freeze the extra portions.
- If you prefer canned beans, rinse and drain before using to reduce sodium.
- Mix white beans with drained tuna, chopped red onion, cooked macaroni, and vinegar and olive oil.
- Add white beans, quick-frozen spinach, and rounds of cooked Italian turkey sausage to reduced-sodium chicken broth for a quick and hearty soup.

MEAT, POULTRY, AND FISH

Buy these:

- Boneless, skinless chicken breasts
- Canned salmon and tuna
- Extra-lean ground beef or ground turkey
- Fish and seafood (frozen or fresh)
- Lean boneless pork chops
- Soy or veggie burgers

Tasty tips:

- Cut raw or leftover chicken breast into chunks. Sauté in 1 to 2 teaspoons of taco or fajita seasoning or jarred curry paste. Add sliced raw onions and peppers and continue to sauté until the veggies are soft. Serve on salad greens and top with salsa and a dollop of fat-free sour cream (optional). You can use leftover pork chops or extra-lean ground beef or turkey, too.
- Here's another great way to use a leftover chicken breast or pork chop. All you need is a package of whole wheat wonton wrappers (available in natural food stores). Preheat the oven to 350°F. Shred chicken (there should be enough for 2 wrappers). Place lengthwise in wrappers, roll, and seal. Coat an ovenproof baking dish with olive or canola oil spray. Bake for 15 to 20 minutes, until the wrappers are crisp. Enjoy plain or with salsa, reduced-sodium soy sauce, or chutney. Makes 1 serving.
- To avoid exposure to mercury and PCB contaminents common to oily fish, choose light tuna packed in water (instead of albacore) and wild salmon (versus farmed).

- For salmon patties, mix drained, flaked salmon with chopped onion and a beaten egg white. Add enough fresh whole wheat bread crumbs to make a moist, but not runny, mixture. Form into patties and sauté in a nonstick skillet with a little olive oil until brown on both sides and heated through.
- Have a bit of leftover salmon? Cut it in chunks and toss with hot whole grain pasta, a tablespoon of olive oil, and fresh garlic. Even better if you have a handful of grape or cherry tomatoes toss them in, too.

NUTS

Buy these:

- 1 to 2 varieties of your favorite nuts; choose from the following: almonds, Brazil nuts, hazelnuts, peanuts, walnuts

Tasty tips:

- Try a wide variety of nuts—you'll diversify your health benefits. For example, walnuts contain heart-healthy omega-3s. And most varieties of nuts—including walnuts, almonds, peanuts, and hazelnuts—contain beta sitosterol and campesterol, two chemicals that can lower harmful blood cholesterol levels.
- To reduce your sodium intake, choose unsalted nuts.
- For the best flavor, toast almonds or walnuts lightly in a heavy skillet.
- Add 1 tablespoon of nuts to cooked vegetables, tossed salads, or grains.
- Nuts pack plenty of calories—about 180 calories an ounce—so keep portion sizes small (one handful equals 1 serving or 1 ounce).

CONDIMENTS, HERBS, AND SPICES

Buy these:

You already may have many of these items, but check your spice rack to see if you need to restock—or try something new.

- Basic seasonings: bay leaves, cinnamon, cumin (whole seeds), Italian seasoning, nutmeg, oregano, paprika, parsley (dried and fresh), rosemary, thyme
- Capers
- Chili sauce
- Cooking wine
- Dijon mustard
- Flax oil (store in the refrigerator)
- Horseradish
- Hot-pepper sauce
- Low-sodium soy sauce
- Natural sweeteners: honey, apple butter
- Olive and canola oils
- Salsa
- Sun-dried tomatoes
- Tahini
- Vinegars: balsamic, red wine, rice wine
- Worcestershire sauce

Sweet Success

JASON HENDERSON

Before he graduated from college with a major in wildlife management, Jason Henderson, 31, was at his perfect weight. At 5 feet 11 inches, he weighed between 180 and 185 pounds. After college, however, the Virginia resident realized his true calling and enrolled at the prestigious Culinary Institute of America in Hyde Park, New York. "I developed a taste for high-fat, high-sugar foods," says Jason. "And while the life of a chef can be tough, there isn't much exercise involved."

After graduating from culinary school in 1998, Jason found work as a chef in Germany. "The fats and carbs were plentiful, and the beer flowed freely," he says. By 2001, when he returned to the United States, he was 15 to 20 pounds heavier. Two and a half years later, when he started working for the army as an executive chef and analyst, he weighed in at 215 pounds.

On New Year's Day 2004, he stepped on the scale: He weighed 230 pounds. "It blew my mind," he says. He lost 20 pounds in 20 days on a low-carbohydrate diet. But then his weight loss stalled, and over the next year, he gained back 6 pounds.

In 2005, stuck at 216 pounds, Jason decided to try again. But this time, he traded in the no-carb approach for the slow-carb approach.

He ate six times a day to keep his blood sugar on an even keel, and he selected foods packed with fiber and slow carbs. Breakfast was oatmeal mixed with protein powder and applesauce. Lunch was a salad with lean meat, chicken, or fish. Dinner might be a peanut butter sandwich on whole grain bread, a portion of whole wheat pasta, or a serving of lean meat and vegetables. Between meals, Jason snacked on low-carbohydrate bars and smoothies made with fresh berries and low-fat milk or yogurt. He also started to exercise, lifting weights and pedaling an elliptical trainer two or three times a week.

Three months later, Jason was 26 pounds lighter. "Now I maintain at around 190 pounds, plus or minus a pound or two," he says. He still hits the gym and the cardio machines two to three times a week.

And he's maintained his weight in spite of being a chef. "Even working around food every day, I'm able to find foods that fit my way of eating," says Jason. "Some days, I find myself looking at my watch and saying, 'It's time to eat again?' My plan now is eating to live rather than living to eat."

CHAPTER 4

FREQUENTLY ASKED QUESTIONS

While individual results will vary among people who adopt any eating program, the same questions seem to come up for a lot of people. Ann Fittante, MS, RD, a certified diabetes educator, offers the answers that can help.

1. I'm 41 and have 40 pounds to lose. I follow the program exactly, but the weight is coming off very slowly. What's going on?

Lots of factors affect how quickly a woman in general—and you in particular—loses weight, including gender and age. Somewhere in her 30s, a woman's metabolism slows about 5 percent every decade. That means if a moderately active 35-year-old woman ate a set number of calories a day to maintain a weight of 140 pounds, she might gain weight eating the same number of calories at age 45. For many midlife women, the gain is so gradual they don't notice it until they step into their jeans and struggle with the zipper.

Though you're losing more slowly than you'd like, don't give up. Gradual weight loss is actually healthier, and most women who lose more slowly are more likely to keep that weight lost for good.

The menu plans contain between 1,400 and 1,600 calories a day, an amount that helps most women lose weight. But to speed things up, consider increasing your daily physical activity by 100 to 200 calories a day. We're not talking much activity here. For example, if you're 155 pounds, you'll burn over 200 calories in 30 minutes of swimming.

If walking is your thing, you'll burn about 250 calories just walking the dog for an hour. (If you weigh more than 155 pounds, you'll burn more calories; less than 155 pounds, you'll burn fewer.)

You can also eliminate 200 to 300 calories each day. For example, you might eat smaller portions at dinner and eliminate one snack. But I recommend moving more. As I've said elsewhere, don't starve yourself. Consuming less than 1,200 calories a day will slow your metabolism even more.

2. I love my muffin in the morning. Any suggestions on how to make muffins acceptable on this program?

You bet! You're right to look for an alternative to store-bought muffins. Most are made with white flour and unhealthy trans fats. And if they're as big as softballs, which most of them are, they contain huge amounts of fat and calories.

For a muffin that won't wreak havoc on your insulin and blood sugar levels, try the Peanut Butter and Banana Streusel Muffins on page 81. Or if you'd rather, modify your favorite muffin recipe. Simply substitute half the flour with 100 percent whole wheat flour, reduce the sugar from 1 cup to ¾ cup, and use heart-healthy canola oil. You can also add nuts and/or ¼ cup of ground flaxseed.

3. On this program, I'm never hungry, and the menu plans are delicious. But the week before my period, I crave sweets, especially chocolate. Every month, I indulge and gain back a pound or two. What can I do to fight off these cravings and stick to the program?

It's fine to indulge in a small square of cake or a scoop of real, creamy ice cream now and then, especially when you're premenstrual. To master your monthly cravings for sweets without derailing your weight loss, calculate the caloric value of the treat you crave, and adjust your menu accordingly. For example, ½ cup of ice cream runs about 150 calories.

To accommodate those additional calories, eliminate one or two of your snacks during the day and/or have smaller portions at mealtime.

Here are a few other sweet treats that'll cost you 150 calories or less. Remember, these are "break glass in case of emergency" treats; they're not for everyday consumption.

- 2 Famous Amos Chocolate Chip Cookies (75 calories)
- 2 tablespoons of chocolate chips (140 calories)
- 4 chocolate kisses (105 calories)
- 2 ounces of angel food cake topped with fresh berries (73 calories)

Better yet, make your own healthier sweet treats. My personal favorite: the Oatmeal-Date Bars on page 334.

4. Is it true that consuming artificially sweetened drinks can lead to weight gain? Are they okay to drink on The Sugar Solution program?

Some studies have speculated that artificial sweeteners might stimulate hunger, while others suggested that sucrose (table sugar) might promote weight loss. To find out, Danish researchers asked 41 overweight people to supplement their diets with either sucrose or artificially sweetened drinks. Ten weeks later, the sucrose group gained an average of 3 pounds, while the fake-sweetener group lost nearly 2 pounds. Turns out the sucrose group added more than 400 calories each day to their normal intake. Calories you drink don't help satisfy your appetite. Because you never compensate for the extra calories by eating less, you end up gaining weight.

I think it's fine to consume artificially sweetened drinks in moderation. In my view, however, water is the way to go. Try one of the new, zero-calorie flavored waters, or mix an ounce of your favorite juice into a tall glass of ice water or club soda.

As far as artificially sweetened foods are concerned, check labels carefully. Many sugar-free foods, including cookies and ice cream, have calorie amounts similar to those of the regular brands and are high in unhealthy saturated and/or hydrogenated fats.

5. My husband and I would like to go on the diet together—we both have about 30 pounds to lose. Does the diet work for men, and does it meet their nutritional and caloric needs?

Yes, the program meets nutritional requirements for both men and women. And how wonderful that you've partnered up! There's no doubt that you'll both lose weight (although he might lose a bit more quickly than you will—men usually do, because of their increased muscle mass).

While the meal plans are between 1,400 and 1,600 calories, most men can lose weight on up to 1,800 calories a day. That's because men's bodies tend to be bigger and pack more calorie-burning muscle than women's. So if your husband feels very hungry, he can either eat larger portions at mealtime or eat larger portions of the snacks listed for that day.

6. I absolutely cannot live without bread, pasta, and potatoes. Is there any way I can enjoy them on the diet?

Yes! The Sugar Solution way of eating isn't about eating less but eating smart—and whole grain breads and pastas give your body the slow carbs it needs. Whole grains make your body work harder during digestion, which slows the rise in blood sugar. When blood sugar levels rise and fall gradually, you feel fuller longer and tend not to eat as often.

What's more, whole grain breads and pastas contain more fiber, iron, thiamin, and niacin than the processed kinds, cost only pennies more, and are now widely available in most large supermarkets. Opt for whole grain products that are 140 calories or less per serving and contain 3 or more grams of fiber per serving.

Potatoes are a good source of B-vitamins and potassium and also contain vitamin C and magnesium. Just eat them in sensible portions (one small baked potato, for example) with low-fat toppings like salsa, cottage cheese, or low-fat sour cream. Eat the skin, too—it's a good source of fiber. Better yet, upgrade your carbs and enjoy a sweet potato instead of a white potato.

7. What can I use instead of butter for cooking, on bread, and on vegetables?

I'm glad you recognize that although butter is a zero-carbohydrate food, it's still a saturated fat, which can raise cholesterol levels. I recommend it as a treat rather than as an everyday part of your diet. To reduce its saturated fat content, blend it with canola oil. Use one part canola oil to one part butter (for example, ¼ cup of canola oil blended with ¼ cup of butter). Also, feel free to use one of those butter-flavor sprays that mimic the taste of butter without the fat or calories.

I'm a big fan of olive or canola oil on—and in—just about any food, in place of butter or margarine. Olive oil, in particular, adds flavor without the heart-damaging saturated fats. I love to sauté my veggies in olive oil and garlic and dip my whole grain bread in olive oil. When I bake, I use canola oil.

8. I have a family history of obesity and diabetes, and my 15-year-old daughter is about 25 pounds overweight. Is it safe for her to go on the program? I want to help her protect her future health.

The Sugar Solution isn't designed to meet the nutritional needs of teenagers (or children or pregnant women, either). Their calorie needs are quite high: between 1,800 and 3,000 calories per day for teenage girls, and even more for teenage boys. It's generally healthier for teens not to restrict calories but to reduce the number of empty calories they consume in the form of soda, sweets, chips, and fast foods. Although I can't recommend that your teen follow the program itself, the meal and snack ideas—and the recipes, of course—are healthful choices for the entire family.

9. Can I still eat fruit? I enjoy it, but I've read that it can slow weight loss because it increases insulin and blood sugar levels.

I don't know where these rumors get started. Fruit does not slow weight loss. Consuming too many calories and/or not exercising regularly does. Nor does fruit increase insulin or blood sugar levels to unhealthy levels. An average-size piece of fruit contains between 15 and 30 grams of carbohydrate. To manage blood sugars, I generally recommend that people with diabetes or insulin resistance consume between 30 and 60 grams of carbohydrate for meals and between 15 and 30 grams of carbohydrate for snacks.

Bottom line: Enjoy from 1 to 3 servings of fruit a day. A medium-size piece contains 100 calories or less and loads of fiber and important vitamins.

10. Like many women, I overeat when I'm stressed. The problem is, I'm stressed out every day! I try to be good, but food calms me. How can I put the brakes on my stress eating?

In prehistoric times, anxious eating may have been a smart survival strategy. Your agitated ancestors grabbed berries after the marauding tigers slunk away; you head for the candy machine after the boss roars. Research has found that stress prompts rats to release hormone signals for high-calorie eating, and it may be similar in humans.

Have you begun The Sugar Solution program? If not, you're bound to discover what many women and men who follow it have already learned: Eating sensible portions of high-fiber, nutritionally balanced food every few hours—rather than skipping meals and gorging on fatty, sugary junk—helps control physiological hunger. You may just find that although your stress level stays the same, your urge to eat your way through stressful situations is drastically reduced. More good news: Exercise, sleep, and healthy eating may keep the stress/eat cycle from kicking in.

A brisk, 10-minute walk or other stress-busting technique can also help break the stress-gorging habit. The 21-Day Lifestyle Makeover features one stress management tool for each day. Practice one or all of them regularly, and you'll soon assemble an arsenal of techniques that allow you to manage stress in a healthy way.

11. Do I have to exercise on The Sugar Solution program?

Everyone needs regular exercise, and improved fitness can do more for your body than speed up weight loss. It can also reduce insulin resistance and boost energy.

Cardiovascular exercise—cardio, for short—elevates your metabolism before and after exercise. Resistance training increases muscle mass, which in turn increases the body's ability to burn calories both during activity and at rest.

But before you lace up your walking shoes or heft a dumbbell, get your doctor's okay to exercise. Then choose an activity that you enjoy. Start at 30 minutes and work up to 60 minutes of activity, three to six times a week. Begin slowly and increase as your body becomes more fit.

12. I want to try the program, but I don't think I can eat six times a day. I'm not hungry at breakfast, usually work through lunch, and eat one meal a day: dinner. Do I really have to eat all these meals?

At least give it a try, because skipping meals has derailed many a dieter's weight-loss efforts. Not eating at regular intervals leads to low blood sugar, which leads to hunger and cravings, which leads to binging. On the other hand, spacing meals and snacks evenly throughout the day helps maintain better blood sugar control and prevent overeating. And we're not talking about large meals here—half a turkey sandwich and a piece of fruit, a small grilled-chicken salad, a low-fat yogurt, and a couple of whole grain crackers. These mini-meals are easy to stash in your desk or the refrigerator at work, and they're easy to find in convenience stores, too.

If you just can't manage six times a day, try eating at least three times a day for two weeks. Chances are, you'll have more energy during the day and feel less hungry by evening.

13. Do you suggest taking supplements while on the program?

On The Sugar Solution program, you'll eat nutrient-dense fruits, veggies, and whole grains and modest amounts of low-fat dairy products and lean meat, poultry, and fish. Still, taking a multivitamin is nutritional insurance—one that *Prevention* recommends for everyone. In fact, a panel of nutrition experts recently concluded that all adults should take a multi. Assuming that you take a multi and eat a healthy diet like The Sugar Solution, you're pretty well covered.

Along with a multi (which should contain 400 IU of vitamin D), consider taking 500 mg of calcium as a separate supplement up to age 50. Over 50, consider taking 700 mg separately but not more than 500 mg at a time for best absorption.

Although I believe that supplements can help meet nutritional requirements, I suggest that you avoid the multivitamin supplements marketed to people on low-carbohydrate diets or any other supplement that claims to promote weight loss. They don't work, and they're a waste of your hard-earned money.

14. I dislike the taste and texture of whole wheat pasta. Can I mix regular pasta with the whole grain kind? Or can you suggest another type of whole grain noodle with a taste and texture more like regular pasta?

Many people who swore they'd never give up white flour pasta have come to love the distinctive taste of the whole wheat variety. (It's chewier than pasta made with white flour, with a nutlike flavor.) But if you can't quite manage whole wheat pasta by itself, it's fine to mix it with white pasta.

Your local health food store will contain a variety of whole grain pastas, including those made with corn, quinoa, spelt, and brown rice. You may enjoy the taste and texture of these varieties better.

15. Can I use condiments on the program, like ketchup, barbecue sauce, and relish?

Yes, you can use condiments in the meal plans—just don't go overboard. One tablespoon is considered free and will not contribute greatly to calories, fat, or sodium. But I encourage you to experiment with alternatives to conventional condiments, or use lower-calorie condiments. For example, salsa is delicious on burgers or scrambled eggs, and I know of people who top their baked potatoes with spicy brown mustard!

16. I'm a night eater. I follow the program until 8 p.m. By 11, I've eaten hundreds of extra calories, and my waistline shows it. What can I do?

It's important to identify the reasons for late-night eating. Are you hungry? Are you bored? Or is noshing at night simply a habit? Make sure that your night eating isn't a physiological response to hunger. The large majority of people who struggle with night eating are those who skip meals or don't eat balanced meals during the day. This is a major setup for overeating at night. If you stick to The Sugar Solution formula of three meals and three snacks a day, chances are that you want to eat for reasons other than physiological hunger.

I'd advise you to practice mindful eating—that is, pay attention to what, how, and how much you eat, as well as your sense of fullness or hunger. To eat mindfully, you need to do nothing when you eat but eat—that means don't watch TV, read, or work. The following exercise, which takes all of about 3 minutes, can help you understand what mindful eating is all about.

Place a finger food in your palm—a nugget of cereal, a grape, a baby carrot. Then pick it up with your fingers. Focus on its shape and texture. Think about this piece of food—where it came from, how it grew. Put it into your mouth, but don't bite it: Simply let it stay in your mouth. Roll it around. Explore it with your tongue. Finally, chew it slowly, focusing on its flavor.

It also might help you to plan an activity for after 8 p.m. You might practice meditation or relaxation techniques or a hobby like needlepoint, knitting, or drawing. If all else fails, simply draw a bath, or step into the shower. It's tough to eat with wet hands or nails.

17. I know you recommend dressing salads with the flax oil recipe on page 199, but can I use bottled low-calorie salad dressings? Will they slow down my weight loss?

As long as you don't pour or ladle them on, low-fat, low-calorie dressings shouldn't slow your weight loss. Limit yourself to 1 or 2 tablespoons, and choose brands that are lower in sodium and contain heart-healthy fats.

18. I'm not particularly fond of some of the meals in the menu plans. Can I interchange one meal for another, or eat my favorite meals regularly?

Absolutely! Meals can be interchanged. The caloric values of each of the breakfasts are similar, as are the lunches and dinners. This means you can interchange a breakfast meal for a breakfast meal, lunch for lunch, and dinner for dinner. As for eating your favorite lunches and dinners, whether you're eating out or using a family recipe, try to keep the portions similar to the meals in The Sugar Solution program. That's 2 to 4 ounces of protein; 1½ cups of veggies or salad; 1 cup of grain, pasta, potato, or casserole; and no more than 1 tablespoon of fat like oil, salad dressing, or mayonnaise.

19. I love a glass of wine with dinner. Can I drink alcohol on this program?

Yes. Just be aware that alcohol tends to raise cortisol levels, sending fat to your belly, and the extra calories could slow your weight loss if you don't plan for them. One drink (which equals 4 ounces of wine, 12 ounces of beer, or 1 ounce of hard liquor) contains from 80 to 150 calories. Eliminate one or two snacks during the day, or have smaller portions at mealtime. For health reasons, women should have no more than one alcoholic beverage per day (men, no more than two a day).

Another reason to cut back on drinking: One study found that, compared with juice or water, having one alcoholic drink before a meal led to eating 200 extra calories—on top of the added calories in the drink itself. Subjects ate faster, took longer to feel full, and continued eating even after they were no longer hungry.

20. I don't have time to cook all these meals. What should I do?

It's true that preparing meals involves more time and energy than picking up a pizza or hitting the drive-through. But not much more time, especially if you plan. Dedicate 1 to 2 hours a week to meal planning, and set aside an evening or weekend day to preparing more time-intensive meals such as casseroles, muffins or quick breads, soups, and stews. Try to incorporate one new recipe per week. Cook double batches of favorite recipes so you can freeze the unused portion or have leftovers.

Keep in mind that The Sugar Solution is a *lifelong* program that helps you keep off those extra pounds for good. Would you rather save time picking up a bucket of chicken, or look smashing in a smaller pair of jeans?

Sweet Success
HELEN LEVELS

From the time she was a girl, Helen Levels craved cookies, cake, and candy. But these treats were off-limits. "My parents wouldn't let us kids have anything sweet, except fruit," recalls the 52-year-old San Antonio resident.

Then her mother passed away, and 13-year-old Helen moved in with an aunt whose dietary guidelines were less restrictive. Finally, Helen could indulge her sweet tooth—and indulge she did! Thus began a 22-year love affair with sweets.

After she married her husband, Bruce, and started a family, Helen's sweet tooth remained as active as ever. Unfortunately, her body didn't, and the pounds began to pile on. Having honey buns slathered with butter and sugar for breakfast and bowls of ice cream or frozen yogurt for lunch didn't help. At her heaviest, she carried 193 pounds on her 5-foot-2 frame.

When Helen turned 35, her normally boundless energy drained away. "I didn't have the energy to do anything," she says. "After work, I'd go home, collapse on the couch, and sleep." She was always thirsty, drinking three 32-ounce bottles of water a day and running to the bathroom two or three times in a half hour. More ominously, Helen lost 30 pounds.

One day, she took a bite of cheesecake a neighbor had made and became so tired, "I didn't think I'd make it to the couch." The next day, Bruce took her to the emergency room. She told the doctors her symptoms: fatigue, thirst, frequent urination. They tested her blood sugar. The results: diabetes.

"The doctors said, 'You have to start eating better and exercising now,'" Helen recalls. Alarmed, she immediately replaced the quick-carb sweets in her diet with nutritious, slow-carb fare. Breakfast became a small bowl of bran flakes with milk. Lunch was soup, salad, or fruit salad. On her dinner menu: chicken or fish.

At first, her sweet tooth rebelled. "Sometimes I wanted something sweet so badly I thought I would cry," she says. But her determination—and fear—kept her cookie free.

Helen also purchased a treadmill. Each night after work, she walked—just 15 minutes at first, increasing to an hour over the course of several months.

Within a year, Helen's energy was back and her blood sugar readings vastly improved—without medication. "This morning, my blood sugar was 98 mg/dl," she says. Best of all, Helen lost 43 pounds, now weighing in at 150 pounds. "And I don't crave sweets anymore," she says.

What Helen does crave is staying healthy. "Too many people around me—people younger than I am—are getting sick or dying of diabetes," she says. "I don't want to go through that. If it takes giving up sweets to stay in good health, I'm willing to give them up."

CHAPTER 5

THE SUGAR SOLUTION 21-DAY LIFESTYLE MAKEOVER

Ready to lose up to 2 pounds a week on six tasty, satisfying meals and snacks a day? Get ready for The Sugar Solution Lifestyle Makeover. Based on good nutrition, regular physical activity, and stress management, this 21-day program was created by Ann Fittante, MS, RD, a certified diabetes educator, and the creator of The Sugar Solution.

Each day of the makeover contains three components.

* A menu plan. While you lose weight, you'll eat hearty and enjoy many of your favorite treats and comfort foods—cookies, French toast, mac and cheese, burritos, and pasta primavera, to name just a few. You'll find the dishes featured in the plan in the recipe section. (*Note:* Do not use the menu plans if you're pregnant or have been diagnosed with gestational diabetes.)

* A tip on adding more calorie-burning activity into your day (titled "Get Yourself Moving"), to be used in conjunction with regular physical activity. Experts say that simply being more active during the day can help speed weight loss, and the smallest physical efforts can help move those stubborn pounds—and add enjoyment to your life. Ever hold a "walking meeting" at work or start an office pool to see who can take

the most steps during the week? (Consult your doctor before you begin this or any exercise program.)

- A tip on how to shrug off stress and take some "me time" each day ("Take a Tranquility Break"). No matter how frantic your schedule, our 5-minute tactic is a little pocket of peace you can look forward to each day. Believe it or not, those 300 seconds can add up to a calmer, less-stressed you.

The program itself is stress-free. Follow it faithfully, and chances are, it won't take 30 days to see the rewards of your lifestyle makeover: a slimmer, trimmer, calmer you.

So don't wait another day. Your new body—and life—awaits you.

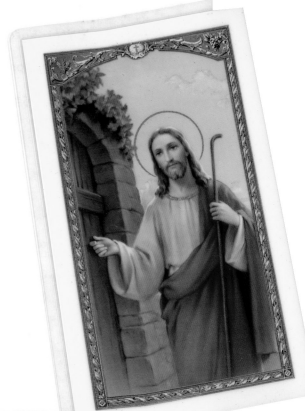

Week 1

RECIPES FOR WEEK 1

Swiss and Turkey Bacon Stratas (page 73)

Super-Easy Barbecue Pulled Pork (page 246)

A Few Less Than a Thousand Islands Dressing (page 192)

Warm Chicken and Cashew Stir-Fry Salad (page 184)

Mediterranean Couscous (page 231)

Grilled Peppered Steak with Multigrain Texas Toast (page 240)

Roasted Ratatouille (page 200)

Skinny Pasta Primavera (page 323)

Apricot-Ginger Buttermilk Scones (page 83)

Dilled Salmon en Papillote (page 298)

Oven-Roasted Brussels Sprouts (page 222)

Sunday

BREAKFAST

Swiss and Turkey Bacon Stratas (page 73)

1 cup sliced kiwifruit and strawberries with a dollop of low-fat vanilla yogurt

LUNCH

Tuna sandwich: Mix ½ cup tuna, 1 tablespoon low-fat mayonnaise, and chopped onion and/or chopped red bell pepper (optional). Spoon onto 1 slice rye bread or toast. Top with spinach leaves or lettuce, 1 slice tomato, and a second slice of rye bread.

1½ cups tossed salad with 1 tablespoon low-fat salad dressing

SNACK

¾ cup applesauce; mix with 1 ounce granola and sprinkle with cinnamon

DINNER

Super-Easy Barbecue Pulled Pork (page 246)

1 medium baked potato with 1 tablespoon low-fat sour cream

1 cup broccoli and carrots sautéed in 1 teaspoon olive oil and garlic

1 cup fortified soymilk (fat-free milk can be substituted)

SNACK

½ cup low-fat vanilla yogurt with ½ cup blueberries

Daily Analysis
Calories: 1,598
Protein: 95 grams
Carbohydrate: 228 grams
Fat: 36 grams
Cholesterol: 238 milligrams
Sodium: 2,229 milligrams
Fiber: 28 grams

Exchanges
Carbs: 15 (7 bread/starch, 4 fruit, 2 milk, 5 vegetable)
Lean Meats: 7
Fats: 3

GET YOURSELF MOVING

Take your partner or kids to the local laser-tag place. Challenge them to a few rounds.

TAKE A TRANQUILITY BREAK

Reconnect before the workweek rush—give your partner or child 15 uninterrupted minutes of your attention before bed. Connection is a potent antidote to the Sunday blues.

Monday

BREAKFAST

¾ cup low-fat vanilla yogurt mixed with
   1 tablespoon almonds

1 slice whole grain bread with 1 teaspoon
   trans free margarine

SNACK

1 orange

LUNCH

1½ cups low-sodium black bean and ham soup

1 small corn muffin (2 ounces)

1 cup raw carrots, cherry tomatoes, and green
   peppers dipped in 2 tablespoons A Few Less
   Than a Thousand Islands Dressing (page
   192) or other low-fat dressing

SNACK

1 cup berries with 2 tablespoons nondairy
   whipped topping or low-fat vanilla yogurt

DINNER

1 serving Warm Chicken and Cashew Stir-Fry
   Salad (page 184)

¾ cup brown rice

SNACK

½ cup cottage cheese mixed with ½ cup
   pineapple

*Note: Save 1 serving of the chicken salad for
tomorrow's lunch.*

Daily Analysis
Calories: 1,557
Protein: 75 grams
Carbohydrate: 221 grams
Fat: 41 grams
Cholesterol: 61 milligrams
Sodium: 1,870 milligrams
Fiber: 46 grams

Exchanges
Carbs: 15 (8 bread/
starch, 4 fruit, 1 milk,
6 vegetable)
Lean Meats: 5
Fats: 4

GET YOURSELF MOVING

Work near a park? Suggest a "mobile meeting" to your colleagues, and walk while you brainstorm. Or
don your sneakers at lunch and do a walking meditation.

TAKE A TRANQUILITY BREAK

Buy a pack of sugarless bubblegum. Blow bubbles at red lights.

Tuesday

BREAKFAST

1 serving high-fiber cereal with 1 cup fat-free
milk

½ cup berries

SNACK

1 cup baby carrots dipped in 2 tablespoons
hummus

LUNCH

1 serving Warm Chicken and Cashew Stir-Fry
Salad

½ cup brown rice

SNACK

1 apple with 2 teaspoons all-natural peanut
butter

DINNER

3 ounces broiled fish topped with 2 tablespoons A Few Less Than a Thousand Islands
Dressing (page 192)

1 serving Mediterranean Couscous (page 231)

1 cup steamed asparagus

SNACK

1 ounce low-fat cheese

1 Asian pear

*Note: Save 1 serving of the couscous for tomorrow's
lunch.*

Daily Analysis
Calories: 1,590
Protein: 99 grams
Carbohydrate: 218 grams
Fat: 40 grams
Cholesterol: 139 milligrams
Sodium: 1,934 milligrams
Fiber: 42 grams

Exchanges
Carbs: 14 (6 bread/
starch, 5 fruit, 1 milk,
7 vegetable)
Lean Meats: 7
Fats: 2

GET YOURSELF MOVING

Today, park 15 minutes away from the office and walk to and from work. If you take public trans-
portation, get off one stop earlier than you normally do.

TAKE A TRANQUILITY BREAK

Make that break for two: Meet your partner or a friend for lunch.

Wednesday

BREAKFAST

1 piece whole grain toast with 1 tablespoon all-natural nut butter

1 cup fortified soymilk or fat-free milk

SNACK

1 serving whole grain crackers

LUNCH

1 serving Mediterranean Couscous

1½ cups mixed green salad with ½ cup kidney or garbanzo beans

2 tablespoons A Few Less Than a Thousand Islands Dressing (page 192) or low-fat salad dressing

SNACK

1 cup fruit salad with 2 tablespoons nondairy whipped topping or low-fat vanilla yogurt

DINNER

Grilled Peppered Steak with Multigrain Texas Toast (page 240)

1 cup steamed Swiss chard or collards

½ cup corn

6 ounces wine or ½ cup low-fat pudding or low-fat ice cream

SNACK

3 cups popcorn sprinkled with 2 tablespoons Parmesan cheese

Daily Analysis
Calories: 1,425
Protein: 72 grams
Carbohydrate: 185 grams
Fat: 41 grams
Cholesterol: 69 milligrams
Sodium: 2,419 milligrams
Fiber: 30 grams

Exchanges
Carbs: 12 (8 bread/starch, 2 fruit, 1 milk, 4 vegetable)
Lean Meats: 6
Fats: 3

GET YOURSELF MOVING

Walk your child to school. If he takes the bus, walk with him to the next stop, then walk back. No child? Walk around the block before work.

TAKE A TRANQUILITY BREAK

Buy a bouquet of daisies at the supermarket. Put them in your traveler's mug, instead of your latte to go.

Thursday

BREAKFAST

Breakfast smoothie: Blend 1 cup fat-free milk or yogurt, 1 banana, 2 tablespoons ground flaxseed, 2 tablespoons protein powder or fat-free dry milk powder, and 2–3 ice cubes.

SNACK

1 ounce mixed nuts (unsalted)

LUNCH

½ turkey sandwich on rye bread (1 ounce turkey, 1 ounce low-fat cheese, ⅛ avocado)

1 cup chicken or vegetable noodle soup

½ cup raw veggies

SNACK

½ small fresh mango (or ½ cup frozen mango, thawed)

DINNER

3 ounces baked chicken

1 serving Roasted Ratatouille (page 200)

1 whole wheat roll with 1 teaspoon trans free margarine

¾ cup low-fat vanilla yogurt sprinkled with cinnamon

SNACK

½ raisin or whole wheat English muffin spread with 2 tablespoons cottage cheese

Note: Bake an extra piece of chicken and save 1 serving of the ratatouille for tomorrow's lunch.

Daily Analysis
Calories: 1,520
Protein: 94 grams
Carbohydrate: 196 grams
Fat: 46 grams
Cholesterol: 142 milligrams
Sodium: 2,655 milligrams
Fiber: 26 grams

Exchanges
Carbs: 13 (7 bread/ starch, 3 fruit, 2 milk, 3 vegetable)
Lean Meats: 6
Fats: 3

GET YOURSELF MOVING

Today, your coffee breaks are walk breaks. If you usually break three times a day for 10 minutes, that's 30 minutes on the move.

TAKE A TRANQUILITY BREAK

At 3 p.m., close your office door and read a chapter of that new bestseller.

Friday

BREAKFAST

1 cup oatmeal with 2 tablespoons walnuts,
1 tablespoon ground flaxseed, and 2 teaspoons maple syrup or brown sugar

SNACK

1 hard-cooked egg, sliced, with ½ tomato

LUNCH

1 serving Roasted Ratatouille

1 serving baked chicken

1 whole wheat roll

1 ounce string cheese

1 Asian pear

SNACK

¾ cup low-fat vanilla yogurt topped with
½ cup peaches; sprinkle with 1 tablespoon
sunflower seeds

DINNER

Skinny Pasta Primavera (page 323); top with
3 ounces grilled shrimp

NO SNACK

Daily Analysis

Calories: 1,575
Protein: 89 grams
Carbohydrate: 200 grams
Fat: 54 grams
Cholesterol: 370 milligrams
Sodium: 1,775 milligrams
Fiber: 36 grams

Exchanges

Carbs: 13 (8 bread/
starch, 3 fruit, 1 milk,
3 vegetable)
Lean Meats: 5
Fats: 5

GET YOURSELF MOVING

Take your dog for a walk tonight. Don't have one? Borrow your neighbor's, or simply walk your "inner dog."

TAKE A TRANQUILITY BREAK

To unwind for the weekend, stop by your church or synagogue for a short prayer, or simply light a candle and gaze at the flame for 10 minutes.

Saturday

BREAKFAST

1 Apricot-Ginger Buttermilk Scone (page 83)

1 cup fat-free milk or low-fat plain yogurt

SNACK

1 banana

LUNCH

Healthy nachos: Top 1½ ounces whole grain tortilla chips with ½ cup beans and 1 ounce shredded low-fat cheese. Bake for 10–15 minutes at 250°F or microwave for 30 seconds until the cheese is melted. Serve with ¼ cup salsa and ¼ cup guacamole.

NO SNACK

DINNER

1 serving Dilled Salmon en Papillote (page 298)

Baked sweet potato with 1 teaspoon trans free margarine

1 serving Oven-Roasted Brussels Sprouts (page 222)

1 cup fat-free milk

SNACK

½ cup ice cream

Note: Save a scone for next week's menu.

Daily Analysis

Calories: 1,464
Protein: 74 grams
Carbohydrate: 198 grams
Fat: 48 grams
Cholesterol: 128 milligrams
Sodium: 2,380 milligrams
Fiber: 32 grams

Exchanges

Carbs: 13 (7 bread/ starch, 2 fruit, 2 milk, 6 vegetable)
Lean Meats: 5
Fats: 4

GET YOURSELF MOVING

Grocery shopping today? Before you take a cart, take a lap around the store.

TAKE A TRANQUILITY BREAK

Declutter a closet, your jewelry box, the kitchen junk drawer. Appreciate that sometimes it's simple to create order out of chaos.

Week 2

RECIPES FOR WEEK 2

Sunday

BREAKFAST

1 Cocoa-Espresso Waffle (page 80) topped with
½ cup sliced strawberries and 1 tablespoon
maple syrup

NO SNACK

LUNCH

1 serving Grilled Ham, Pear, and Gorgonzola
Sandwiches (page 149)

1 ounce potato chips (unsalted, if desired)

SNACK

1 cup raw veggies dipped in 2 tablespoons
Cool Buttermilk Dressing (page 191) or
2 tablespoons low-fat salad dressing

DINNER

3 ounces baked fish

1 serving Roasted Asparagus and Corn
Succotash (page 196)

1 cup brown rice

1 cup fat-free milk

SNACK

Yogurt and fruit parfait: Sprinkle 1 cup low-fat
plain yogurt with ½ teaspoon cinnamon,
½ teaspoon sugar, and 1 tablespoon
chopped walnuts or almonds

Daily Analysis

Calories: 1,597
Protein: 83 grams
Carbohydrate: 215 grams
Fat: 49 grams
Cholesterol: 120 milligrams
Sodium: 2,045 milligrams
Fiber: 27 grams

Exchanges

Carbs: 14 (8 bread/
starch, 1 fruit, 2 milk,
5 vegetable)
Lean Meats: 5
Fats: 5

GET YOURSELF MOVING

Make a list of 5 to 10 things found in nature—a bird's nest, an ant hill, and so on. Then take a 20-minute "scavenger walk" and check them off your list.

TAKE A TRANQUILITY BREAK

Say the Serenity Prayer: "God, grant me the serenity to accept the things I cannot change, courage to change the things I can, and the wisdom to know the difference." Apply it to your life today.

Monday

BREAKFAST

1 serving Strawberry-Mango Smoothie (page 102) with 1 tablespoon ground flaxseed

1 egg, any style, prepared without fat

Note: Save 1 serving of the smoothie for this evening's snack.

SNACK

1 Apricot-Ginger Buttermilk Scone

LUNCH

Greek salad: Toss 2 cups spinach, 2 ounces feta cheese, ½ chopped tomato, ¼ chopped cucumber, ¼ chopped green pepper, and 3 black olives with 1 tablespoon low-fat salad dressing.

1 medium whole grain roll or 2 servings whole grain crackers

SNACK

1 banana sliced in half and spread with 2 teaspoons all-natural peanut butter

DINNER

Speedy Tamale Pie (page 310)

1 cup tossed salad

2 tablespoons Cool Buttermilk Dressing (page 191) or low-fat salad dressing

SNACK

1 serving Strawberry-Mango Smoothie

Note: Save 1 serving of the tamale pie for tomorrow's lunch.

Daily Analysis

Calories: 1,608
Protein: 60 grams
Carbohydrate: 255 grams
Fat: 66 grams
Cholesterol: 347 milligrams
Sodium: 2,331 milligrams
Fiber: 35 grams

Exchanges

Carbs: 17 (8 bread/ starch, 6 fruit, 2 milk, 3 vegetable)
Lean Meats: 4
Fats: 3

GET YOURSELF MOVING

Have a pedometer? Dust it off, clip it on, and aim for 2,500 steps today. If you don't have one, borrow a friend or family member's and use it for 20 minutes.

TAKE A TRANQUILITY BREAK

Nature trumps man-made stress. Whatever the season, do 15 minutes of yard work—rake leaves, pull weeds, pick up sticks and branches, grow an herb garden in tiny pots.

Tuesday

BREAKFAST

½ whole grain bagel spread with 1 tablespoon low-fat cream cheese

1 ounce lox (optional)

SNACK

1 apple

LUNCH

1 serving Speedy Tamale Pie

1 cup celery and carrot sticks

SNACK

1½ cups cubed melon topped with 2 tablespoons whipped topping or low-fat plain yogurt

DINNER

1 serving Savory Turkey Stroganoff (page 268) over 1 cup whole wheat noodles

1 cup sautéed spinach (sauté in 1 teaspoon olive oil and 2 cloves of crushed garlic)

SNACK

1 cup low-fat fruit yogurt

Daily Analysis
Calories: 1,481
Protein: 83 grams
Carbohydrate: 238 grams
Fat: 27 grams
Cholesterol: 99 milligrams
Sodium: 2,447 milligrams
Fiber: 35 grams

Exchanges
Carbs: 16 (8 bread/ starch, 3 fruit, 2 milk, 5 vegetable)
Lean Meats: 5
Fats: 2

GET YOURSELF MOVING

Treat yourself to a "walking lunch"—eat at your desk, then stroll downtown or to the local park.

TAKE A TRANQUILITY BREAK

Who writes letters anymore? You do. Take 5 minutes to write, and 5 minutes to address, stamp, and mail. Cards count.

Wednesday

BREAKFAST

1 serving Fruit and Spice Cut Oatmeal (page 75) with 1 tablespoon ground flaxseed

SNACK

1 ounce roasted unsalted nuts

LUNCH

1 serving Roasted Red Pepper Hummus with Cilantro (page 90, or buy already prepared hummus)

½ large, or 1 small, whole wheat pita bread; stuff with hummus, lettuce, and sliced tomato

1 cup fat-free milk

SNACK

1 ounce whole grain tortilla chips

¼ cup salsa

DINNER

1 serving Rosemary-Scented Swordfish Kebabs (page 297)

1 cup cooked quinoa

½ cup steamed green beans

Tossed salad with 2 tablespoons Cool Buttermilk Dressing (page 191) or low-fat salad dressing

SNACK

1 serving Red Wine–Berry Sorbet (page 359)

Note: Save ½ serving of the hummus for tomorrow's snack and 1 serving of the sorbet for tomorrow's dessert.

Daily Analysis

Calories: 1,537
Protein: 76 grams
Carbohydrate: 201 grams
Fat: 64 grams
Cholesterol: 75 milligrams
Sodium: 2,219 milligrams
Fiber: 28 grams

Exchanges

Carbs: 13 (9 bread/starch, 2 fruit, 1 milk, 3 vegetable
Lean Meats: 5
Fats: 4

GET YOURSELF MOVING

Belong to a book group? Take the meeting outside and walk while you talk. If you don't have a book group, pop an audiobook into your Discman and enjoy. (Don't do this on busy roads.)

TAKE A TRANQUILITY BREAK

Waiting in line can be stressful but not if you compliment a stranger. The smile you receive at the post office, bank, or market will warm you the entire day.

Thursday

BREAKFAST

½ whole wheat English muffin topped with
1 egg, any style, prepared without fat

1 cup low-fat vanilla yogurt

SNACK

½ cup unsweetened applesauce mixed with
½ teaspoon cinnamon

LUNCH

Deli sandwich: 2 ounces lean ham or roast
beef, 2 slices rye or pumpernickel bread,
1 teaspoon mustard, 1 teaspoon mayonnaise,
spinach leaves or lettuce, tomato, and
roasted red pepper

3 cups air-popped popcorn

SNACK

1 cup raw vegetables dipped in ½ serving
Roasted Red Pepper Hummus with Cilantro

DINNER

1 serving All-American Pot Roast (page 242)

Tossed salad with 2 tablespoons Cool
Buttermilk Dressing (page 191) or low-fat
salad dressing

1 serving Red Wine–Berry Sorbet

SNACK

½ serving whole grain cereal with ½ cup fat-
free milk or soymilk and ½ cup raspberries

Daily Analysis
Calories: 1,500
Protein: 86 grams
Carbohydrate: 214 grams
Fat: 52 grams
Cholesterol: 315 milligrams
Sodium: 2,200 milligrams
Fiber: 32 grams

Exchanges
Carbs: 14 (7 bread/
starch, 3 fruit, 2 milk,
6 vegetable)
Lean Meats: 7
Fats: 2

GET YOURSELF MOVING
Grab your kids or friends and go bowling tonight. It's a fun, easy way to move your body.

TAKE A TRANQUILITY BREAK
Surf www.beliefnet.com. Learn something new about your religion or a belief system you know nothing about.

Friday

BREAKFAST

1 cup low-fat plain yogurt

¼ cup granola

1 tablespoon ground flaxseed

¾ cup peaches (fresh or canned in juice)

SNACK

3 cups air-popped popcorn

LUNCH

Burrito: 1 whole wheat tortilla, 1 serving Black Beans and Rice (page 228), 2 ounces ground chicken, and 2 tablespoons salsa

SNACK

1 apple

DINNER

1 serving Linguine with Red Clam Sauce (page 304)

1 cup zucchini and onion sautéed in 2 teaspoons olive oil

1 cup green salad with 1 tablespoon low-fat salad dressing

4 ounces wine *or* 1 slice whole grain bread

SNACK

1 cup hot chocolate (heat 1 cup fat-free milk, 2 teaspoons cocoa powder, 1½ tablespoons sugar, and ¼ teaspoon vanilla extract)

Note: Save 1 serving of the black beans and rice for tomorrow's dinner.

Daily Analysis
Calories: 1,579
Protein: 78 grams
Carbohydrate: 229 grams
Fat: 38 grams
Cholesterol: 113 milligrams
Sodium: 1,922 milligrams
Fiber: 43 grams

Exchanges
Carbs: 15 (9 bread/ starch, 3 fruit, 2 milk, 4 vegetable)
Lean Meats: 4
Fats: 4

GET YOURSELF MOVING

It's Friday night—go dancing! Or hold a dance party at home. Put on your favorite station or CD and cut a rug, with or without a partner.

TAKE A TRANQUILITY BREAK

Knock off early today and go to the movies—something no one but you wants to see.

Saturday

BREAKFAST

1 serving Banana-Stuffed Cinnamon French Toast (page 79)

SNACK

1 cup grapes

LUNCH

1 serving Greek Pita Pizzas (page 322)

1 cup spinach salad with 2 tablespoons Cool Buttermilk Dressing (page 191) or low-fat salad dressing

SNACK

1 sliced pear with 1 ounce string cheese

DINNER

3 ounces grilled pork chop

1 serving Black Beans and Rice

1 cup roasted asparagus, carrots, and red bell pepper

SNACK

1 cup fat-free milk

2 Oatmeal Cookies with Cherries (page 330)

Note: Save four cookies for next week's menus.

Daily Analysis
Calories: 1,470
Protein: 76 grams
Carbohydrate: 219 grams
Fat: 54 grams
Cholesterol: 70 milligrams
Sodium: 2,305 milligrams
Fiber: 31 grams

Exchanges
Carbs: 15 (9 bread/ starch, 3 fruit, 1 milk, 5 vegetable)
Lean Meats: 4
Fats: 2

GET YOURSELF MOVING

The playground at the local elementary school should be empty today. Swing on the swings, or hop on the seesaw with a friend or your partner.

TAKE A TRANQUILITY BREAK

Write on a sheet of paper: "In my life, I'm grateful for . . ." Take 2 minutes to write down everything you can think of.

Week 3

Sunday

BREAKFAST

1 serving Double Tomato and Turkey Bacon Omelette (page 72)

2 pieces whole grain toast spread with 1 teaspoon trans free margarine

NO SNACK

LUNCH

1½ cups minestrone soup

½ chicken salad sandwich: 1 ounce chicken, 2 teaspoons low-fat mayonnaise, 2 teaspoons minced onion and celery; add greens and sliced tomato

Raw veggie plate: 1 cup baby carrots, cauliflower, and broccoli with ¼ cup salsa

SNACK

1 serving Chocolate Malted Milkshake (page 101)

DINNER

1 serving Tuscan Tuna Cakes (page 229)

1 small baked potato with 1 tablespoon low-fat sour cream

Large tossed salad with 1 tablespoon Roasted Garlic Vinaigrette (page 190) or low-fat salad dressing

SNACK

1 serving Minted Honey-Lime Fruit Salad (page 85)

Note: Save 1 serving Minted Honey-Lime Fruit Salad for tomorrow evening's snack.

Daily Analysis

Calories: 1,592
Protein: 98 grams
Carbohydrate: 201 grams
Fat: 49 grams
Cholesterol: 358 milligrams
Sodium: 3,145 milligrams
Fiber: 21 grams

Exchanges

Carbs: 13 (8 bread/starch, 2 fruit, 2 milk, 3 vegetable)
Lean Meats: 8
Fats: 3

GET YOURSELF MOVING

Get outside for some fresh air and yard work. Make raking leaves or puttering in the garden a family affair.

TAKE A TRANQUILITY BREAK

Dreading work tomorrow? Make a paper airplane (you remember how, don't you?). Sail it across the room. Tell yourself, "I'm going to sail through this week."

Monday

BREAKFAST

1 serving "Baked" Stuffed Pears (page 86)

Note: To save time, prepare the night before.

1 cup fat-free milk

SNACK

1 piece whole grain toast with 1 tablespoon nut butter

LUNCH

Fruit and cottage cheese plate: Arrange ½ cup low-fat cottage cheese and 1 cup sliced fresh fruit on a bed of lettuce.

1 serving whole grain crackers

SNACK

3 cups air-popped popcorn

DINNER

3 ounces baked chicken breast

1 serving Macaroni and Cheese (page 227)

Tossed greens and cucumber salad with 1 table-spoon Roasted Garlic Vinaigrette (page 190) or low-fat salad dressing

SNACK

1 serving Minted-Honey Lime Fruit Salad

Note: Save ½ serving of the pears for tomorrow's snack.

Daily Analysis
Calories: 1,415
Protein: 80 grams
Carbohydrate: 204 grams
Fat: 37 grams
Cholesterol: 112 milligrams
Sodium: 1,424 milligrams
Fiber: 20 grams

Exchanges
Carbs: 14 (6 bread/starch, 6 fruit, 1 milk, 2 vegetable)
Lean Meats: 5
Fats: 2

GET YOURSELF MOVING

Today, move the printer and fax machine away from your desk, so you have to get up to use them. Or walk to a distant printer or fax.

TAKE A TRANQUILITY BREAK

Try to sit and stand straight today. Sitting straight promotes circulation, increases oxygen levels in your blood, and helps relieve muscle tension, all of which promote relaxation.

Tuesday

BREAKFAST

½ whole grain bagel

1 tablespoon low-fat cream cheese

1 ounce Canadian bacon

SNACK

½ serving "Baked" Stuffed Pears

LUNCH

1 serving Turkey Picadillo Sandwiches (page 151)

SNACK

2 Oatmeal Cookies with Cherries

Herb tea

DINNER

1 cup whole grain pasta with meatballs (2 ounces meat)

½ cup marinara sauce

1 cup greens sautéed in 1 teaspoon olive oil and garlic

1 cup steamed cauliflower

SNACK

1 cup fat-free plain or low-fat vanilla yogurt mixed with 1 cup berries

Daily Analysis

Calories: 1,490
Protein: 71 grams
Carbohydrate: 203 grams
Fat: 47 grams
Cholesterol: 129 milligrams
Sodium: 2,465 milligrams
Fiber: 35 grams

Exchanges

Carbs: 14 (9 bread/starch, 3 fruit, 1 milk, 5 vegetable)
Lean Meats: 4
Fats: 3

GET YOURSELF MOVING

Today is Do-It-Yourself Day. Carry your groceries to your car, instead of letting the bag boy do it. Walk into the coffee shop for your cup o' joe rather than hitting the drive-through.

TAKE A TRANQUILITY BREAK

Close your eyes for 10 seconds and pray. Release your stress to a higher power.

Wednesday

BREAKFAST

1 serving high-fiber cereal (mix in 1 tablespoon ground flaxseed)

1 cup fat-free milk or soymilk

SNACK

¼ cup low-fat cottage cheese (flavor with artificial sweetener and cinnamon, if you like)

½ serving whole grain crackers

LUNCH

2 servings Grapefruit, Mango, and Avocado Salad with Sherry Dressing (page 170)

1 slice dark rye toast

SNACK

1 ounce Spicy Glazed Pecans (page 93)

DINNER

3 ounces lean ground beef on a whole grain roll

1 serving Cajun-Spiced Oven Fries (page 224)

Tossed greens with 1 tablespoon Roasted Garlic Vinaigrette (page 190) or low-fat salad dressing

SNACK

2 Oatmeal Cookies with Cherries

1 cup fat-free milk

Note: Save ½ serving of the pecans for tomorrow's breakfast and 1 serving of the avocado salad for tomorrow's lunch.

Daily Analysis
Calories: 1,678
Protein: 82 grams
Carbohydrate: 191 grams
Fat: 70 grams
Cholesterol: 117 milligrams
Sodium: 2,402 milligrams
Fiber: 49 grams

Exchanges
Carbs: 13 (8 bread/ starch, 2 fruit, 2 milk, 4 vegetable)
Lean Meats: 4
Fats: 7

GET YOURSELF MOVING

If you work out in front of the TV, pick up the pace during each commercial break. Or pick a character on your favorite sitcom and speed up every time he or she is on-screen.

TAKE A TRANQUILITY BREAK

Muscles tighten during the course of the day, especially when we're under stress. Every hour, stretch to loosen your muscles—and your mind.

Thursday

BREAKFAST

1 cup fat-free plain or low-fat vanilla yogurt; mix with 1 tablespoon ground flaxseed and ½ cup mixed fruit; top with ½ serving Spicy Glazed Pecans (page 93)

SNACK

Open-faced egg-salad sandwich: Mash 1 hard-cooked egg; mix in 1 teaspoon low-fat mayonnaise and 1 tablespoon diced celery. Arrange on 1 piece whole grain toast or ½ whole grain English muffin.

LUNCH

1 serving Lentil Soup with Spinach (page 112)

1 serving Grapefruit, Mango, and Avocado Salad with Sherry Dressing

SNACK

1 apple

DINNER

1 serving Shrimp-Coconut Curry (page 302)

1 cup steamed broccoli or asparagus

SNACK

½ cup low-fat pudding

Daily Analysis
Calories: 1,583
Protein: 93 grams
Carbohydrate: 195 grams
Fat: 54 grams
Cholesterol: 484 milligrams
Sodium: 1,950 milligrams
Fiber: 43 grams

Exchanges
Carbs: 13 (7 bread/starch, 3 fruit, 2 milk, 3 vegetable)
Lean Meats: 6
Fats: 6

GET YOURSELF MOVING

Waiting around? Take a 5-minute stroll. If you're sitting down or standing in line, squeeze, then relax your abdominal muscles.

TAKE A TRANQUILITY BREAK

Your walking, your talking, your driving—take it down a notch. Slowing down can slow down blood flow and panic devices in your brain.

Friday

BREAKFAST

1 cup oat bran hot cereal: Mix in 1 tablespoon ground flaxseed, and top with 2 tablespoons fat-free plain or low-fat vanilla yogurt.

¼ cup blueberries

SNACK

1 cup sliced pineapple with ¼ cup low-fat lemon or plain yogurt

LUNCH

Mozzarella wrap with roasted tomatoes or peppers: On 1 whole grain tortilla, arrange 2 ounces part-skim mozzarella cheese, ½ cup roasted tomato or sliced pepper, 2 teaspoons pesto, and spinach leaves. Roll into a sandwich.

SNACK

2 teaspoons nut butter on 2 large celery stalks; top each stalk with a few raisins, if desired

DINNER

1 serving Grilled Chicken and Broccoli Rabe with Garlic-Parsley Sauce (page 256)

1 cup fat-free milk

SNACK

1 ounce whole grain tortilla chips

¼ cup salsa

¼ cup mashed avocado

Daily Analysis
Calories: 1,391
Protein: 94 grams
Carbohydrate: 150 grams
Fat: 54 grams
Cholesterol: 155 milligrams
Sodium: 2,206 milligrams
Fiber: 31 grams

Exchanges
Carbs: 10 (5 bread/ starch, 2 fruit, 2 milk, 3 vegetable)
Lean Meats: 6
Fats: 5

GET YOURSELF MOVING

When you watch TV tonight, get off the couch and walk up and down the stairs during every commercial break.

TAKE A TRANQUILITY BREAK

Shake off some steam! Hold your hands in front of you and shake them vigorously for 10 seconds. (Do this in private, so people don't think you've lost it.)

Saturday

BREAKFAST

1 serving Banana-Stuffed Cinnamon French Toast (page 79)

SNACK

1 cup raw baby carrots and cherry tomatoes dipped in 1 tablespoon low-fat salad dressing

LUNCH

6 ounces tomato soup made with fat-free milk or soymilk

1 grilled ham and cheese sandwich on 2 slices whole grain bread: 1 ounce low-fat cheese, 1 ounce ham, and 1 teaspoon canola or olive oil for grilling

SNACK

1 pear or 1 cup grapes

DINNER

1 serving Turkey and Bean Chili (page 270)

1 piece cornbread (2" square)

1 cup fat-free milk

SNACK

⅔ cup high-fiber cereal with ½ cup fat-free milk

Daily Analysis
Calories: 1,558
Protein: 78 grams
Carbohydrate: 259 grams
Fat: 32 grams
Cholesterol: 149 milligrams
Sodium: 3,493 milligrams
Fiber: 37 grams

Exchanges
Carbs: 17 (8 bread/ starch, 4 fruit, 3 milk, 5 vegetable)
Lean Meats: 4
Fats: 3

GET YOURSELF MOVING

It's Saturday; grab your partner or a friend and go dancing. Ballroom, country line, swing—all are great ways to get off the couch and have some fun on your feet.

TAKE A TRANQUILITY BREAK

Try a technique called "palming": Rub your hands together until they're warm, then cup them over your closed eyes for 5 seconds while you breathe deeply.

HEARTY, SUGAR-BALANCING BREAKFASTS

FAST SUPER FAST FAST PREP

DOUBLE TOMATO AND TURKEY BACON OMELETTE

Egg protein is one of the most complete and digestible of all proteins. With 6 grams of protein in each egg, it can help balance your blood sugar. *Photo on page 121.*

Prep time: 15 minutes • Cook time: 6 minutes • Stand time: 15 minutes

6 sun-dried tomato halves

2 plum tomatoes (2 ounces), quartered lengthwise and thinly sliced

2 thin strips turkey bacon, cooked and crumbled

2 tablespoons crumbled ricotta salata cheese or goat cheese

2 large eggs

3 egg whites

1 tablespoon water

2 tablespoons chopped chives or scallions

¼ teaspoon salt

¼ teaspoon freshly ground black pepper

1 teaspoon olive oil

Place the sun-dried tomatoes in a small dish. Add boiling water to cover and let stand for 15 minutes, or until softened. Drain the tomatoes and chop. In a small bowl, combine the sun-dried and plum tomatoes, bacon, and ricotta. In a medium bowl, whisk together the eggs, egg whites, water, chives or scallions, salt, and pepper until slightly frothy.

Heat ½ teaspoon oil in a 10" nonstick skillet over medium heat. Add half of the egg mixture (a scant ½ cup) and cook for 2 minutes, occasionally lifting the edges of the egg mixture with a spatula and tilting the pan, allowing the uncooked mixture to flow underneath.

When the eggs are almost set, spoon half of the tomato mixture down the center of the egg. Loosen the edges of the omelette with a spatula and fold the two sides over the filling. Slide out onto a warm plate. Repeat with the remaining oil and egg and tomato mixtures.

Makes 2 servings

Per serving: 215 calories, 17 g protein, 8 g carbohydrates, 13 g fat, 205 mg cholesterol, 800 mg sodium, 2 g dietary fiber
Diet Exchanges: 2 vegetable, 2 meat, 2 fat
Carb Choices: ½

SWISS AND TURKEY BACON STRATAS

This delicious dish will keep you immune to the midmorning munchies.

Prep time: 25 minutes • Cook time: 45 minutes • Stand time: 20 minutes to 12 hours

1 small red onion, chopped

½ green bell pepper, chopped

½ red bell pepper, chopped

2 slices extra-lean turkey bacon, chopped (cut crosswise into ¼"-wide strips)

4 slices multigrain bread (4 ounces), cut into ½" cubes

⅓ cup shredded reduced-fat Swiss cheese

2 large eggs

2 large egg whites

1¾ cups 1% milk

1 tablespoon Dijon mustard

¼ teaspoon freshly ground black pepper

Heat a nonstick skillet over medium heat and coat with cooking spray. Add the onion and bell peppers. Cook, stirring occasionally, for 8 minutes, or until the vegetables are almost tender. Stir in the bacon and cook for 2 minutes longer. Remove from the heat and stir in the bread cubes.

Coat a 7" × 11" baking dish or four 2-cup casserole dishes with cooking spray and set on a baking sheet. Spoon the vegetable mixture into the baking dish or casserole cups, dividing evenly. Sprinkle on the cheese, dividing evenly.

In a medium bowl, whisk together the eggs, egg whites, milk, mustard, and black pepper. Ladle into the baking dish or casserole cups, dividing evenly. Let stand for at least 20 minutes, or cover and refrigerate for up to 12 hours.

Preheat the oven to 375°F. Bake the stratas for 35 minutes, or until a knife inserted in the center comes out clean. Let stand for 10 minutes and serve hot.

Makes 4 servings

Per serving: 203 calories, 16 g protein, 22 g carbohydrates, 6 g fat, 120 mg cholesterol, 410 mg sodium, 2 g dietary fiber
Diet Exchanges: 1 vegetable, 1 bread, 2 meat, 1 fat
Carb Choices: 1½

ZUCCHINI AND DILL FRITTATA

Zucchini holds the honor of being one of the lowest-calorie foods in existence at 14 calories per ½-cup serving. This summer-fresh dish still tastes like an indulgence, perfect for weekend brunches. *Photo on page 122.*

Prep time: 10 minutes • Cook time: 14 minutes

2 **teaspoons butter**

2 **cups finely chopped zucchini (one 8-ounce zucchini)**

2 **large scallions, thinly sliced**

4 **eggs**

6 **egg whites**

1 **tablespoon water**

2 **tablespoons chopped fresh dill**

¼ **teaspoon freshly ground black pepper**

3 **tablespoons grated Parmesan cheese**

Preheat the broiler. Heat a 10" nonstick skillet over medium heat. Add the butter and zucchini. Cook for 5 minutes, stirring occasionally. Stir in the scallions and cook for 3 minutes more, or until the zucchini is just tender.

Meanwhile, in a medium bowl, whisk together the eggs, egg whites, water, dill, pepper, and 2 table-spoons of the cheese. Add to the skillet and cook for 5 minutes, occasionally lifting the edges of the egg mixture with a spatula and tilting the pan, allowing the uncooked mixture to flow underneath. (The eggs will be set on the bottom but will still be moist on the top.) Remove from the heat and sprinkle on the remaining 1 tablespoon cheese.

Wrap the skillet handle with a double thickness of foil. Broil 4" from the heat for 1 to 2 minutes, or until the eggs are set on the top. Cut into quarters and serve immediately.

Makes 4 servings

Per serving: 148 calories, 14 g protein, 4 g carbohydrates, 8 g fat, 220 mg cholesterol, 220 mg sodium, 1 g dietary fiber
Diet Exchanges: 2 meat, 1 fat
Carb Choices: 0

FRUIT AND SPICE CUT OATMEAL

Oats are an excellent source of fiber and one of the easiest foods to prepare. Cook them in milk instead of water, if you prefer a creamier texture. Here we suggest adding the oats to boiled water, which gives them a firm, slightly coarse texture. *Photo on page 123.*

Prep time: 10 minutes ● Cook time: 30 minutes

2¼ cups water

¾ cup steel-cut oats

⅛ teaspoon salt

1 large tart cooking apple (8 ounces), cored and chopped

¼ cup chopped dates or dried figs

3 tablespoons honey

1 teaspoon pumpkin pie spice

½ teaspoon ground ginger

1% milk (optional)

In a medium saucepan, bring the water to a boil. Stir in the oats and salt and bring to a bare simmer. Cook for 15 minutes, stirring occasionally.

Stir in the apple, dates or figs, honey, pie spice, and ginger. Return to a bare simmer and cook, covered, for 15 minutes longer, or until the oats are tender but still have a slight bite to them. Spoon into bowls and stir in the milk or drizzle it over the top, if using.

Makes 4 servings

Per serving: 223 calories, 4 g protein, 50 g carbohydrates, 2 g fat, 0 mg cholesterol, 100 mg sodium, 6 g dietary fiber
Diet Exchanges: 1 fruit, 2 bread
Carb Choices: 3

CARROT CAKE PANCAKES WITH MAPLE–CREAM CHEESE SPREAD

Natural sweetness makes breakfast taste like a piece of cake—but with a respectable amount of fiber, you shouldn't feel guilty.

Prep time: 25 minutes • Cook time: 15 minutes

SPREAD

- 3 ounces Neufchâtel cheese, at room temperature
- 2 tablespoons maple syrup + additional for serving
- 1/4 teaspoon ground cinnamon

PANCAKES

- 1/4 cup walnuts, halved
- 1 cup shredded carrot
- 1 1/2 cups whole grain pastry flour
- 3/4 cup unbleached or all-purpose flour
- 2 teaspoons baking powder
- 1 1/4 teaspoons ground cinnamon
- 1/4 teaspoon ground allspice
- 1/4 teaspoon salt
- 1 1/2 cups soymilk
- 1/3 cup packed brown sugar
- 3 egg whites
- 2 tablespoons canola oil

To make the spread: In a medium bowl, stir together the Neufchâtel, maple syrup, and cinnamon until blended. Set aside.

To make the pancakes: Preheat the oven to 300°F. Spread the walnuts on a baking sheet and toast just until fragrant, 5 minutes or longer. Chop the nuts and set aside.

Meanwhile, place the carrot in a small microwaveable bowl. Cover loosely with plastic wrap and microwave on high power for 1 minute, or until just tender. Set aside to cool.

In a large bowl, whisk together the whole grain flour, all-purpose flour, baking powder, cinnamon, allspice, salt, and walnuts until blended. Make a well in the center of the flour mixture. Add the milk, sugar, egg whites, and oil and whisk the ingredients together until blended. Add the cooled carrot and stir just until blended.

Preheat a large nonstick skillet or griddle over medium-high heat and coat with cooking spray. Ladle ¼ cup batter for each pancake and cook for 2 minutes, or until bubbles form on the surface. Flip with a spatula and cook for 1 minute longer, or until cooked through. (Keep warm in the preheated oven, if needed.) To serve, spoon a rounded teaspoon of the maple cream cheese spread on each pancake and drizzle with additional maple syrup, if you wish.

Makes 12 to 14 pancakes, ½ cup maple cream cheese spread

Per pancake: 171 calories, 5 g protein, 25 g carbohydrates, 7 g fat, 5 mg cholesterol, 180 mg sodium, 2 g dietary fiber
Diet Exchanges: 2 bread, 1 meat, 1 fat
Carb Choices: 2

PANCAKE AND WAFFLE TOPPINGS

Pancakes are an American classic. Try this simple fruit topping to jazz up your plain pancakes and waffles and enjoy a naturally sweet start to your morning.

APPLE TOPPING

    3 cups thinly sliced peeled apples

    2 tablespoons apple or white grape juice

    2 tablespoons honey

    ⅛ teaspoon ground nutmeg

In a medium saucepan over low heat, add the apples, juice, honey, and nutmeg. Cook, stirring occasionally, for 3 minutes. Cover the pan and cook for 5 minutes, or until the fruit is softened. Cool slightly before serving.

Note: This topping can be reheated on top of the stove or in the microwave. Try peaches instead of apples, too.

Makes 2 cups. Per ½ cup: 85 calories, 0.2 g protein, 22 g carbohydrates, 0.3 g fat, 0 mg cholesterol, 1 mg sodium, 1.9 g dietary fiber

BERRY SAUCE

    2 ¼ cups fresh or frozen mixed berries

    2 tablespoons water

    2 tablespoons honey

    ¼ teaspoon freshly grated citrus rind (optional)

In a small saucepan over low heat, combine the berries, water, honey, and rind, if using. Cook, stirring occasionally, for 8 minutes, or until the berry juices are released.

Puree in a food processor or blender. Pass through a sieve to remove the seeds.

Return the mixture to the saucepan. Cook over medium heat for 3 minutes, or until the sauce is reduced to about 1 cup. Cool.

Makes 1 cup. Per ¼ cup: 78 calories, 0.5 g protein, 20 g carbohydrates, 0.3 g fat, 0 mg cholesterol, 5 mg sodium, 2.2 g dietary fiber

SWEET POTATO PANCAKES

How sweet it is! These pancakes are not only delicious, but they are also low in calories and long on flavor.

Prep time: 20 minutes ● Cook time: 20 minutes

2   **sweet potatoes (1 pound), peeled and shredded**

1   **large tart cooking apple (8 ounces), peeled, cored, and shredded**

2   **scallions, chopped**

2   **tablespoons chopped fresh dill**

3   **tablespoons whole grain pastry flour**

³⁄₄   **teaspoon salt**

2   **egg whites**

1¹⁄₂   **teaspoons olive oil**

¹⁄₄   **cup unsweetened applesauce**

2   **tablespoons reduced-fat sour cream**

In a large bowl, stir together the potatoes, apple, scallions, dill, flour, salt, and egg whites. Coat a 10" skillet with cooking spray and heat over medium-low heat. Add ³⁄₄ teaspoon of the oil and swirl in the pan to coat. For each pancake, drop ¹⁄₂ cup of the sweet potato mixture into the skillet, making 4 pancakes at a time, flattening each with a spatula to a 4" round. Cook for 10 minutes, or until golden brown, turning with a spatula halfway through the cooking. Place on a baking sheet and keep warm in a preheated 300°F oven. Repeat with the remaining oil and sweet potato mixture.

Top the pancakes with the applesauce and sour cream.

Makes 8 to 10 pancakes

Per pancake: 77 calories, 2 g protein, 16 g carbohydrates, 1 g fat, 0 mg cholesterol, 250 mg sodium, 2 g dietary fiber
Diet Exchanges: 1 bread
Carb Choices: 1

BANANA-STUFFED CINNAMON FRENCH TOAST

Bananas lend an incredibly creamy, satisfying texture to this French toast dish, and they also help keep each serving virtually fat-free.

Prep time: 20 minutes • Cook time: 5 minutes

FILLING

1 ripe banana, thinly sliced

2 tablespoons Neufchâtel cheese

1 tablespoon confectioners' sugar

1 teaspoon grated lemon zest

2 pinches of ground nutmeg

FRENCH TOAST

8 thin slices whole wheat cinnamon-raisin bread

1 cup 1% milk

1 egg

1 egg white

3/4 teaspoon vanilla extract

Confectioners' sugar, for dusting

1/4 cup sugar-free pancake syrup

To make the filling: Mash 2 rounded tablespoons banana slices in a small bowl with the back of a spoon. (You should have about 2 tablespoons mashed.) Stir in the Neufchâtel, sugar, lemon zest, and nutmeg until smooth.

To make the French toast: Spread 4 slices of the bread with the banana filling, dividing evenly. Top with the remaining banana slices and bread slices to make 4 sandwiches. Whisk together the milk, egg, egg white, and vanilla in a shallow dish or pie plate until blended. Dip the sandwiches into the egg mixture, turning them over with a spatula to coat both sides.

Meanwhile, heat a large nonstick frying pan or griddle over medium-low heat and coat with cooking spray. (A drop of water should sizzle when dropped on the griddle.) Add the sandwiches and cook for 4 to 5 minutes, or until golden brown on both sides, turning with a spatula halfway through the cooking. (To keep warm, place the French toast sandwiches on a baking sheet in a preheated 250°F oven.) Dust with confectioners' sugar. Drizzle with sugar-free pancake syrup and serve hot.

Makes 4 servings

Per serving: 259 calories, 11 g protein, 41 g carbohydrates, 6 g fat, 40 mg cholesterol, 290 mg sodium, 3 g dietary fiber
Diet Exchanges: 1 milk, 1 fruit, 1 bread, 1 meat, 1 fat
Carb Choices: 3

COCOA-ESPRESSO WAFFLES

These chocolaty treats pack a healthy wallop of fiber and monounsaturated fats. They'll keep you smiling for hours. *Photo on page 124.*

Prep time: 20 minutes • Cook time: 15 minutes

1 ½ cups whole grain pastry flour

½ cup unsweetened cocoa powder

2 teaspoons baking powder

¼ teaspoon baking soda

1 cup 1% milk

½ cup packed brown sugar

2 teaspoons espresso powder

3 tablespoons light olive oil

3 egg whites

⅛ teaspoon salt

2 tablespoons mini chocolate chips (optional)

Maple syrup

Whisk together the flour, cocoa powder, baking powder, and baking soda in a large bowl until combined. Make a well in the center of the flour mixture and add the milk, sugar, espresso powder, and oil. Whisk the ingredients together until blended.

Preheat a waffle iron for 4 minutes, or according to the manufacturer's instructions. (A drop of water should sizzle and bounce when dropped on the iron.) Meanwhile, beat the egg whites and salt with an electric mixer at high speed just until they form soft peaks. Fold the whites into the chocolate batter in 3 additions, folding in the chocolate chips with the last addition of whites. Fold just until the mixture is combined.

Coat the heated waffle grids with cooking spray right before using. Add enough batter to almost cover the waffle grids (¾ cup) and cook for 3 to 4 minutes. Repeat with the remaining batter. (To keep warm, place a single layer of waffles on a foil-lined baking sheet in a preheated 250°F oven.) Serve with maple syrup.

Makes 5 round waffles

Per waffle: 235 calories, 10 g protein, 29 g carbohydrates, 10 g fat, 0 mg cholesterol, 400 mg sodium, 5 g dietary fiber
Diet Exchanges: 2 bread, 1 meat, 2 fat
Carb Choices: 2

PEANUT BUTTER AND BANANA STREUSEL MUFFINS

FAST PREP

Peanut butter is a powerhouse of nutrition! It not only contains fiber and protein to help balance your blood sugar, it also is an excellent source of monounsaturated fats.

Photo on page 125.

Prep time: 15 minutes • Cook time: 16 minutes

STREUSEL

3 tablespoons whole grain pastry flour

3 tablespoons packed brown sugar

1 tablespoon butter, melted

1 teaspoon honey

MUFFINS

2 cups whole grain pastry flour

2 teaspoons baking powder

1 teaspoon ground cinnamon

½ teaspoon salt

½ cup pureed ripe banana (about 1 medium banana)

½ cup unsweetened applesauce

⅓ cup peanut butter

½ cup packed brown sugar

1 egg

¾ cup 1% milk

1 teaspoon vanilla extract

Preheat the oven to 400°F. Coat a 12-cup muffin pan with cooking spray.

To make the streusel: In a small bowl, stir together the flour, sugar, butter, and honey with a spoon until the mixture forms wet crumbs.

To make the muffins: In a medium bowl, whisk together the flour, baking powder, cinnamon, and salt until combined. In a large bowl, whisk together the banana, applesauce, peanut butter, sugar, and egg until blended. Whisk the milk and vanilla into the banana mixture until combined.

Stir the flour mixture into the banana mixture with a spoon, just until blended. Do not overmix. Spoon the batter into the prepared muffin cups, dividing evenly. Crumble the streusel mixture on top of the muffin batter, dividing evenly.

Bake for 16 to 18 minutes, or until a wooden pick inserted in the center of a muffin comes out clean. Remove from the pan and serve warm.

Makes 18

Per muffin: 93 calories, 3 g protein, 13 g carbohydrates, 4 g fat, 15 mg cholesterol, 150 mg sodium, 2 g dietary fiber
Diet Exchanges: 1 bread, 1 fat
Carb Choices: 1

WHOLE GRAIN IRISH SODA BREAD

Using high-protein flours such as whole wheat and oat will make baked goods sturdy and dense. This bread is sweet and delicious.

Prep time: 15 minutes • Cook time: 40 minutes

⅓ cup golden raisins	1 teaspoon baking soda
⅓ cup dried currants	2 teaspoons caraway seeds (optional)
2 tablespoons apple juice or sherry	½ teaspoon salt
2 tablespoons butter	1⅓ cups buttermilk
2½ cups whole grain flour	1 egg
¾ cup + 1½ tablespoons oat flour	1 egg white
2 teaspoons baking powder	¼ cup packed brown sugar

Preheat the oven to 375°F. Coat a 9" springform pan or a 9" × 1" cake pan with cooking spray. Combine the raisins, currants, apple juice or sherry, and butter in a microwaveable dish. Cover loosely with plastic wrap and microwave on high power for 1 minute. Stir and set aside to cool.

In a large bowl, toss together the whole grain flour, the ¾ cup oat flour, baking powder, baking soda, caraway seeds (if using), and salt. In a medium bowl, whisk together the buttermilk, egg, egg white, and sugar until blended. Stir the raisin mixture into the egg mixture and then stir into the flour mixture just until combined. Do not overmix.

Pour into the prepared pan and spread to mound slightly in the center. Sprinkle the remaining 1½ tablespoons oat flour over the top. Slash a large X on the top of the bread using a sharp, flour-dipped knife.

Bake for 40 minutes, or until golden brown and a wooden pick inserted in the center comes out clean. Transfer to a rack to cool for at least 15 minutes. Cut into 16 wedges and serve warm or at room temperature.

Makes 16 servings

Per serving: 114 calories, 4 g protein, 20 g carbohydrates, 2 g fat, 20 mg cholesterol, 240 mg sodium, 2 g dietary fiber
Diet Exchanges: ½ fruit, 1 bread
Carb Choices: 1½

APRICOT-GINGER BUTTERMILK SCONES

Dried apricots lend a tangy sweetness and a nice kick of fiber to these breakfast treats.

Photo on page 126.

Prep time: 20 minutes • Cook time: 15 minutes

1 ¾ cups whole grain pastry flour

2 teaspoons baking powder

¼ teaspoon baking soda

¼ cup chopped dried apricots (about 7 small whole apricots)

2 tablespoons chopped crystallized ginger

½ cup buttermilk

1 egg

3 tablespoons butter, melted

1 teaspoon grated fresh ginger

1 teaspoon grated lemon peel

3 ½ tablespoons brown sugar

Honey

Preheat the oven to 400°F. Coat a baking sheet with cooking spray.

In a large bowl, stir together the flour, baking powder, baking soda, apricots, and crystallized ginger. In a medium bowl, whisk together the buttermilk, egg, butter, fresh ginger, lemon peel, and 3 tablespoons of the sugar until blended. Make a well in the center of the flour mixture and add the buttermilk mixture. Stir together just until combined. Do not overmix.

Sprinkle a sheet of plastic wrap lightly with flour. Scrape the dough onto the plastic and spread roughly into a 7" circle. Sprinkle the top of the dough lightly with flour and pat until smooth. Invert the round onto the baking sheet and score the top of the pastry into 8 wedges, using a sharp, flour-dipped knife. Spoon the remaining ½ tablespoon sugar into a sieve and sprinkle evenly over the top.

Bake for 15 to 17 minutes, or until golden. Cool on the baking sheet on a rack for 10 minutes. Cut into 8 wedges and serve with honey.

Makes 8 servings

Per serving: 138 calories, 4 g protein, 20 g carbohydrates, 5 g fat, 40 mg cholesterol, 190 mg sodium, 2 g dietary fiber
Diet Exchanges: 1 bread, 1 fat
Carb Choices: 1

BREAKFAST FRUIT CRISP

This crisp proves that high-fiber foods don't have to be dry and boring.
The peaches, raspberries, and oatmeal are a perfect trio of flavors.

Prep time: 15 minutes • Cook time: 23 minutes

FRUIT

1 pound frozen peaches (4 cups)	¼ teaspoon pumpkin pie spice
2 tablespoons whole grain pastry flour	1 tablespoon lemon juice
¼ cup packed brown sugar	1 cup fresh or frozen raspberries, thawed

TOPPING

½ cup whole grain pastry flour	⅛ teaspoon salt
⅓ cup old-fashioned rolled oats	2 tablespoons butter, cut into small pieces
3 tablespoons packed brown sugar	2 tablespoons reduced-fat sour cream
¾ teaspoon pumpkin pie spice	

Preheat the oven to 400°F.

To make the fruit: In a microwaveable and ovenproof 9" baking dish or pie plate, toss together the peaches, flour, sugar, and pie spice. Drizzle the lemon juice on top. Microwave on high power for 8 minutes, stirring halfway through the cooking. Stir in the raspberries, and spread the fruit until it is level.

To make the topping: In a medium bowl, combine the flour, oats, sugar, pie spice, and salt. Cut in the butter until the mixture has the texture of wet sand. Stir in the sour cream until combined, and crumble the topping evenly over the fruit. Bake for 15 minutes, or until the topping is browned and the fruit is bubbly.

Makes 4 servings

Per serving: 316 calories, 5 g protein, 62 g carbohydrates, 8 g fat, 20 mg cholesterol, 110 mg sodium, 8 g dietary fiber
Diet Exchanges: 1 ½ fruit, 2 ½ bread, 1 fat
Carb Choices: 4

MINTED HONEY-LIME FRUIT SALAD

FAST

This refreshing, low-calorie breakfast dish delivers a sweet early-morning kick of fiber.

Photo on page 127.

Prep time: 20 minutes

1 teaspoon grated lime peel	½ small honeydew, cubed
2 tablespoons lime juice	½ cantaloupe, cubed
3–4 tablespoons honey (see note)	1 pint fresh strawberries, halved and hulled
3 tablespoons chopped fresh mint	2 cups fresh pineapple or mango cubes

In a large bowl, stir together the lime peel, juice, honey, and mint until combined. Add the honeydew, cantaloupe, strawberries, and pineapple or mango. Toss to combine.

Note: Depending on the sweetness of the fruit, start with 3 tablespoons honey, adding more honey if needed.

Makes 8 servings

Per serving: 92 calories, 1 g protein, 24 g carbohydrates, 0 g fat, 0 mg cholesterol, 30 mg sodium, 2 g dietary fiber
Diet Exchanges: 2 fruit
Carb Choices: 2

"BAKED" STUFFED PEARS

Enjoy baked pears without ever turning on the oven! The smooth, rich texture of the sauce is loaded with flavor.

Prep time: 15 minutes • Cook time: 8 minutes

⅓ **cup dried cranberries**

3 **tablespoons orange juice**

2 **tablespoons honey**

4 **Anjou or Bosc pears, halved lengthwise and cored**

¼ **cup chopped walnuts**

1 **teaspoon vanilla extract**

¼ **teaspoon ground cinnamon**

⅛ **teaspoon grated nutmeg**

¼ **cup reduced-fat sour cream**

In a small microwaveable bowl, combine the cranberries, 1 tablespoon of the orange juice, and 1 tablespoon of the honey. Cover loosely with plastic wrap and microwave on high power for 1 minute. Set aside.

In a microwaveable 10" round baking dish or pie plate, arrange the pears in a spoke fashion, cut side up. Drizzle with the remaining 2 tablespoons orange juice and cover loosely with plastic wrap. Microwave on high power for 5 to 7 minutes. (The pears should be almost fork-tender.)

Meanwhile, combine the walnuts, vanilla, cinnamon, and nutmeg with the cranberries. Uncover the pears and spoon the cranberry mixture into the hollows, dividing evenly. Cover loosely with plastic wrap. Microwave on high power for 2 to 3 minutes longer, or until the pears are fork tender.

Stir together the sour cream and the remaining 1 tablespoon honey. Drizzle the mixture on the pears.

Makes 4 servings

Per serving: 240 calories, 3 g protein, 44 g carbohydrates, 7 g fat, 5 mg cholesterol, 10 mg sodium, 5 g dietary fiber
Diet Exchanges: 2 fruit, 1 bread, 1 fat
Carb Choices: 3

LEMON-BLUEBERRY CLAFOUTI

FAST
PREP

This refreshing breakfast is a great alternative to the more traditional favorites like omelettes and scrambled eggs.

Prep time: 10 minutes • Cook time: 30 minutes

2 **cups fresh or frozen blueberries (see note)**	1 **teaspoon vanilla extract**
4 **eggs**	3 **teaspoons grated lemon peel**
¾ **cup 1% milk**	**Pinch of salt**
3 **tablespoons honey**	½ **cup whole grain pastry flour**
2 **tablespoons butter, melted**	

Preheat the oven to 350°F. Coat a 9" pie plate with cooking spray. Scatter the blueberries in the pie plate and set aside.

In a bowl, whisk together the eggs, milk, honey, butter, vanilla, lemon peel, and salt. Stir in the flour until blended. Pour the batter over the blueberries.

Bake for 30 to 35 minutes, or just until the clafouti is set in the center. Serve hot.

Note: If using frozen blueberries, thaw and drain on paper towels before using.

Makes 6 servings

Per serving: 183 calories, 7 g protein, 23 g carbohydrates, 8 g fat, 155 mg cholesterol, 100 mg sodium, 2 g dietary fiber
Diet Exchanges: ½ fruit, 1 bread, ½ meat, 1 fat
Carb Choices: 1½

HEALTHY NIBBLES: SNACKS AND BEVERAGES

FAST   SUPER FAST   FAST PREP

ROASTED RED PEPPER HUMMUS WITH CILANTRO

Chickpeas are the main attraction in this Middle Eastern spread.
Just $1/2$ cup of this tasty snack delivers 7 grams of fiber.

Prep time: 20 minutes • Cook time: 15 minutes • Stand time: 10 minutes

2 red bell peppers	**2** tablespoons lemon juice
4 large cloves garlic, unpeeled	**1** tablespoon mild cayenne pepper sauce
1 can (15 $1/2$ ounces) chickpeas, rinsed and drained	$1/4$ cup chopped fresh cilantro
2 tablespoons tahini	**Assorted vegetable sticks, for dipping**

Preheat the broiler. Place the peppers on a foil-lined baking sheet. Wrap the garlic in foil and place on the sheet. Broil the peppers 6" from the heat for 15 to 20 minutes, turning until charred on all sides. Broil the garlic for 15 minutes. Place the peppers in a sealed bag and let stand for 10 minutes.

Meanwhile, when it's cool enough to handle, peel the garlic and finely chop in a food processor. When the peppers are cool enough to handle, peel, core, and seed them. (You should have 1 cup of roasted peppers.) Add the peppers, chickpeas, tahini, lemon juice, and pepper sauce to the processor and blend until smooth. Add the cilantro and process just until combined. For best flavor, store refrigerated for at least 4 hours or up to 3 days. Serve with vegetable sticks or use as a spread for wraps or sandwiches.

Makes 4 servings (2 cups)

Per serving: 174 calories, 7 g protein, 27 g carbohydrates, 5 g fat, 0 mg cholesterol, 260 mg sodium, 6 g dietary fiber
Diet Exchanges: 1 vegetable, 1 $1/2$ bread, 1 fat
Carb Choices: 2

ORANGE-DIJON MUSTARD DIP

SUPER
FAST

Dress up your vegetables or pretzels with this low-fat, low-calorie dip. The sweet and tangy flavor will win high praise from family and guests.

Prep time: 10 minutes

¼ **cup Dijon mustard**

2 **tablespoons frozen orange juice concentrate, thawed**

¼ **cup plain yogurt**

2 **tablespoons reduced-fat sour cream**

½ **teaspoon white wine vinegar**

Mini whole wheat pretzels, for dipping

Assorted vegetable sticks, for dipping

In a medium bowl, stir together the mustard, orange juice concentrate, yogurt, sour cream, and vinegar until smooth. (Can be made ahead and refrigerated up to 4 days in advance.) Serve as a dip, along with pretzels and vegetable sticks.

Makes 4 servings (1 cup)

Per serving: 45 calories, 2 g protein, 4 g carbohydrates, 3 g fat, 5 mg cholesterol, 390 mg sodium, 0 g dietary fiber
Diet Exchanges: ½ fat
Carb Choices: 0

MUSTARD-GLAZED SNACK MIX

An eclectic combination of wholesome munchables and flavorful spices makes this mix perfect for packed lunches, late-night snacks, or party dishes. *Photo on page 128.*

Prep time: 15 minutes • Cook time: 31 minutes

4 cups bite-size whole grain cereal squares	3 tablespoons honey
1 cup broken whole wheat pretzel sticks (approximately 1" lengths)	2 tablespoons butter, cut into 4 pieces
½ cup unsalted almonds or peanuts	1 tablespoon Worcestershire sauce
3 tablespoons yellow mustard	⅛ teaspoon ground red pepper

Preheat the oven to 325°F. Line a jelly-roll pan with foil and coat with cooking spray. Toss together the cereal, pretzels, and nuts in a large bowl and set aside.

Place the mustard, honey, butter, Worcestershire sauce, and red pepper in a medium microwaveable bowl. Cover with waxed paper and microwave on high power for 45 to 60 seconds, or just until the butter is melted. Stir together until smooth. Drizzle about one-third of the mustard mixture over the cereal mixture and toss, using a large spoon, until evenly coated. Repeat with the remaining mustard mixture. Spread the coated cereal mixture in a single layer on the prepared jelly-roll pan.

Bake for 30 to 35 minutes, stirring halfway through, until evenly toasted. Set the pan on a rack to cool to room temperature, and store in an airtight container for up to 2 weeks.

Makes 12 servings (6 cups)

Per serving: 161 calories, 4 g protein, 28 g carbohydrates, 6 g fat, 5 mg cholesterol, 200 mg sodium, 4 g dietary fiber
Diet Exchanges: 2 bread, 1 fat
Carb Choices: 2

SPICY GLAZED PECANS

FAST PREP

We've given these buttery rich nuts a thin coat of sweetness, so they are an ideal way to remedy a sweet tooth. Plus, pecans are an outstanding source of monounsaturated fats.
Photo on page 128.

Prep time: 10 minutes • Cook time: 25 minutes

2 **cups pecans**	¼ **teaspoon ground cinnamon**
1 **tablespoon brown sugar**	¼ **teaspoon ground red pepper**
1 **teaspoon ground ginger**	¼ **teaspoon salt**
¼ **teaspoon ground allspice**	1½ **tablespoons butter, melted**

Preheat the oven to 300°F. Line a jelly-roll pan with foil and coat with cooking spray. Place the pecans on the pan in a single layer. Bake for 5 minutes. (Do not turn off the oven.)

Meanwhile, in a small dish, stir together the sugar, ginger, allspice, cinnamon, red pepper, and salt. Place the warm pecans in a medium bowl and toss with the butter until well coated. Add the sugar mixture and stir until the nuts are coated. Spread the nuts on the foil-lined baking sheet in a single layer. Sprinkle any remaining sugar over the nuts.

Bake for 20 minutes, or until the nuts are toasted. Set the pan on a rack to cool completely. Store the nuts in an airtight container for up to 2 weeks.

Makes 12 servings (2 cups)

Per serving: 151 calories, 2 g protein, 4 g carbohydrates, 15 g fat, 5 mg cholesterol, 60 mg sodium, 2 g dietary fiber
Diet Exchanges: 3 fat
Carb Choices: 0

CAESAR SALAD SPEARS

Here's a great alternative to the traditional sandwich—crisp romaine wrapped around a delicious high-protein mix of chicken and cheese.

Prep time: 20 minutes

2 **cloves garlic, peeled**	¼ **cup chopped celery**
1 **tablespoon light mayonnaise**	3 **tablespoons grated Parmesan cheese**
1 **tablespoon reduced-fat sour cream**	8 **outer romaine leaves**
1 **tablespoon lemon juice**	¼ **cup Caesar-flavored croutons**
1 **cup chopped cooked chicken breast**	

Place the garlic in a small custard cup and add 1 tablespoon water. Microwave on high power for 1 minute, or until the garlic softens. Flatten the garlic by crushing it with the side of a knife and finely chop. Place the garlic in a medium bowl. Stir in the mayonnaise, sour cream, and lemon juice until blended. Add the chicken, celery, and 2 tablespoons of the cheese and stir until combined.

Arrange the romaine leaves on a serving plate. Spoon 2 tablespoons of the chicken mixture down the center of each leaf. Cut the croutons, if necessary, into approximately ½" pieces. Sprinkle the croutons over the chicken, and top with the remaining 1 tablespoon cheese. Serve or cover and chill for up to 3 hours.

Makes 8 servings

Per serving: 56 calories, 7 g protein, 2 g carbohydrates, 2 g fat, 20 mg cholesterol, 85 mg sodium, 0 g dietary fiber
Diet Exchanges: 1 meat, ½ fat
Carb Choices: 0

SUPER-CREAMY DEVILED EGGS

FAST PREP

We've given this picnic favorite a healthy makeover. Stuffed with buttery beans, these eggs are just as creamy and satisfying as the standard version but with substantially less saturated fat. *Photo on page 129.*

Prep time: 20 minutes • Cook time: 12 minutes • Chill time: 1 hour

6 **large eggs**

$\frac{1}{3}$ **cup canned butter beans or white kidney beans, rinsed and drained**

$1\frac{1}{2}$ **tablespoons light mayonnaise**

$\frac{1}{2}$ **teaspoon mustard powder**

$\frac{1}{4}$ **teaspoon freshly ground black pepper**

$\frac{1}{4}$ **cup finely chopped celery**

$\frac{1}{4}$ **cup shredded carrots**

1 **tablespoon thinly sliced chives or scallions**

Place the eggs in a saucepan and cover with cold water. Bring to a boil over high heat. Reduce the heat to low and simmer slowly for 12 minutes. Cool under cold running water. Shell by tapping the eggs against the side of the pan and gently removing the shells.

Cut the eggs lengthwise in half. Place 4 whole yolks in the bowl of a mini food processor and discard the remaining 2 yolks. Add the butter beans or kidney beans, mayonnaise, mustard, and pepper. Blend the mixture until smooth. Add the celery, carrots, and chives or scallions. Process using pulses, just until the vegetables are incorporated.

Spoon the filling into the hollows of the whites, mounding to fill. Place the egg halves on a platter, cover with plastic, and refrigerate at least 1 hour. (Can be made up to 1 day in advance.) Serve cold.

Makes 6 servings

Per serving: 100 calories, 7 g protein, 4 g carbohydrates, 6 g fat, 215 mg cholesterol, 120 mg sodium, 1 g dietary fiber
Diet Exchanges: 1 meat, 1 fat
Carb Choices: 0

FRESH SPRING ROLLS

Spring rolls are traditionally served on the first day of the Chinese New Year and are smaller and more delicate than egg rolls. We've loaded ours with a medley of colorful ingredients.

Prep time: 40 minutes • Chill time: Up to 6 hours

DIPPING SAUCE

2 tablespoons lime juice

2 tablespoons Oriental fish sauce

1 tablespoon white wine or rice wine vinegar

2 tablespoons sugar

1 small clove garlic, finely chopped

2 teaspoons ketchup

$\frac{1}{8} - \frac{1}{4}$ teaspoon cayenne pepper

SPRING ROLLS

2 small carrots, shredded

2 scallions, finely chopped

24 deveined medium shrimp, cooked and peeled

24 fresh mint leaves

1 cup thinly sliced English cucumber, cut into half-rounds

8 sprigs fresh cilantro, thick stems removed

1 cup watercress, thick stems removed

3 tablespoons dry-roasted peanuts, coarsely chopped

8 8" round rice paper wrappers

To make the dipping sauce: In a small dish, stir together the lime juice, fish sauce, wine or vinegar, sugar, garlic, ketchup, and cayenne. Let stand at least 20 minutes for the flavors to blend.

To make the spring rolls: In a small bowl, toss together the carrots, scallions, and 1 tablespoon of the prepared dipping sauce. Arrange the shrimp, mint leaves, carrot mixture, cucumber, cilantro, watercress, and peanuts in piles in front of you on a board.

Fill a large pie plate with very warm tap water. Set a clean towel nearby. Add 1 rice paper wrapper at a time and soak each for 30 to 45 seconds, or until it begins to soften. Place them in a stack on the towel and let stand for 2 minutes, or until soft and pliable.

Layer the ingredients in a 4" line in the center of the rice paper, starting 3" up from the edge closest to you. Arrange 3 shrimp, 3 mint leaves, 1 rounded tablespoon shredded carrots, 1 rounded table-spoon cucumber, 1 sprig cilantro, 2 tablespoons watercress, and 1 teaspoon peanuts. Fold in the sides and roll up, envelope-style. Set seam side down on a plate. Repeat with the remaining ingre-dients. Cover and refrigerate for up to 6 hours in advance.

To serve, cut each roll in half on the diagonal and serve with the dipping sauce.

Makes 8 servings

Per serving: 166 calories, 8 g protein, 27 g carbohydrates, 3 g fat, 30 mg cholesterol, 590 mg sodium, 2 g dietary fiber
Diet Exchanges: 1 vegetable, 1 1/2 bread, 1 meat, 1/2 fat
Carb Choices: 2

HAM AND GRISSINI ROLL-UPS

This robust snack is a deli delight! Enjoy a delicious roll-up of ham and cheese dipped in a zesty mustard dressing.

Prep time: 15 minutes

2 slices (2 ounces) deli-baked ham

4 teaspoons reduced-fat Boursin cheese

2 teaspoons chopped fresh parsley

6 grissini or Italian breadsticks, cut in half with a serrated knife

1½ tablespoons reduced-fat sour cream

1 tablespoon grainy deli-style mustard

Arrange the ham slices on a cutting board. Trim to square off the ham slices, if needed, to 6" × 4½" rectangles. Spread each piece with 2 teaspoons of the cheese. Sprinkle each piece with 1 teaspoon of the parsley.

Cut the ham lengthwise into six ¾"-wide strips, using a pizza wheel or a sharp knife. Roll each strip of ham diagonally around a grissini half, pressing the cheese side to the grissini to adhere.

Stir together the sour cream and mustard until smooth, and use as a dip for the grissini.

Makes 4 servings (12 pieces total)

Per serving: 257 calories, 13 g protein, 43 g carbohydrates, 4 g fat, 10 mg cholesterol, 650 mg sodium, 2 g dietary fiber
Diet Exchanges: 3 bread, ½ meat, ½ fat
Carb Choices: 3

BUFFALO CHICKEN BITES

If buffalo wings make your knees grow weak, try this spicy version. These bites have the same feisty flavor, but they aren't laden with saturated fat. Napkins are a must!

Photo on page 130.

Prep time: 25 minutes ▪ **Cook time: 15 minutes**

BLUE CHEESE DRESSING

3 tablespoons (1 ¼ ounces) crumbled blue cheese

⅓ cup reduced-fat sour cream

2 teaspoons finely chopped green onion

½ teaspoon white wine vinegar

CHICKEN BITES

2 boneless, skinless chicken breast halves (10 ounces), cut into 1" cubes

1 scallion, finely chopped

2 ½ tablespoons mild cayenne pepper sauce

1 tablespoon butter, melted

3 ribs celery, cut into 2" sticks

1 cup baby carrots

To make the blue cheese dressing: In a small bowl, mash together the blue cheese and sour cream with the back of a spoon. Stir in the green onion and vinegar until blended. Set aside.

To make the chicken bites: Preheat the oven to 400°F. In a medium bowl, toss together the chicken cubes, scallion, and 1 tablespoon of the pepper sauce. Thread the chicken on twelve 6" bamboo skewers, using 2 pieces of chicken per skewer. Arrange on a foil-lined baking sheet. Bake for 15 minutes, or until cooked through.

Meanwhile, in a small bowl, toss together the remaining 1 ½ tablespoons pepper sauce and the butter. Arrange the cooked chicken skewers on one half of a serving platter in a single layer. Brush the chicken cubes with the pepper sauce. Place the celery and carrots on the platter and serve with the blue cheese dressing.

Makes 4 servings

Per serving: 200 calories, 20 g protein, 9 g carbohydrates, 9 g fat, 65 mg cholesterol, 260 mg sodium, 3 g dietary fiber
Diet Exchanges: 1 vegetable, 2 ½ meat, 1 ½ fat
Carb Choices: 1

MINI PITA PIZZAS WITH CARAMELIZED SHALLOTS

Our pita pizzas feature a sprinkling of pine nuts, which are extracted from certain kinds of pinecones. While these light and flavorful nuts are high in fat, most of it is mono-unsaturated. And just 1 ounce packs an impressive 4 grams of fiber.

Prep time: 25 minutes • Cook time: 16 minutes

6 sun-dried tomato halves	½ teaspoon sugar
1½ tablespoons pine nuts	1 teaspoon white wine vinegar
1½ teaspoons olive oil	¼ cup herbed goat cheese
4 large shallots (6 ounces), peeled and thinly sliced crosswise	12 mini whole wheat pitas (2" diameter)

Preheat the oven to 350°F. Place the tomatoes in a small bowl. Add boiling water to cover and let stand 15 minutes, or until softened. Drain well and finely chop. Meanwhile, cook the pine nuts in a small nonstick skillet over medium heat, stirring often, for 3 to 4 minutes, or until lightly toasted. Tip onto a plate and let cool.

Heat the oil in the skillet over medium heat. Add the shallots and cook for 5 minutes, stirring occasionally, or until the shallots are softened and golden. Add the sugar and cook for 2 minutes longer, or until shallots are golden brown, stirring frequently. Stir in the vinegar and chopped tomatoes and cook for 1 minute longer.

Spread 1 teaspoon of the cheese on each mini pita and arrange on a baking sheet. Spoon 1 rounded measuring teaspoon of the shallot mixture onto each pita and sprinkle the pine nuts on top, dividing evenly. Bake for 6 minutes, or until heated through.

To make ahead: The shallot mixture can be refrigerated for up to 2 days in advance. Assemble and bake the pizzas as needed.

Makes 6 servings

Per serving: 161 calories, 6 g protein, 28 g carbohydrates, 4 g fat, 0 mg cholesterol, 290 mg sodium, 4 g dietary fiber
Diet Exchanges: 2 bread, ½ fat
Carb Choices: 2

CHOCOLATE MALTED MILKSHAKE

SUPER FAST

We've made healthy improvements on this all-American classic by cutting the fat and jacking up the rich malted flavor.

Prep time: 10 minutes

¾ cup vanilla frozen yogurt

3 tablespoons malted milk powder

1½ tablespoons cocoa powder

½ teaspoon instant espresso coffee powder

1 cup soymilk or 1% milk

1 teaspoon vanilla extract

In a blender, combine the frozen yogurt, malted milk powder, cocoa, coffee powder, milk, and vanilla. Process until smooth. Pour into tall glasses and serve immediately.

Makes 2 servings (1 cup each)

Per serving: 257 calories, 8 g protein, 45 g carbohydrates, 7 g fat, 5 mg cholesterol, 140 mg sodium, 3 g dietary fiber
Diet Exchanges: 3 bread, ½ meat, 1 fat
Carb Choices: 3

STRAWBERRY-MANGO SMOOTHIE

Enjoy the fruity kick of this amazing blend. Both mangoes and strawberries are low in calories and high in fiber. When choosing ripe mangoes, look for yellow-green or reddish skin that yields to gentle pressure.

Prep time: 10 minutes

1 ½ cups cubed fresh (about 1) or frozen mango

2 cups fresh strawberries + 2 berries for garnish

1 tablespoon minced candied ginger

2 tablespoons honey

1 cup cold soymilk or 1% milk

Pinch of ground allspice

In a blender, combine the mango, strawberries, ginger, honey, soymilk or milk, and allspice. Process until smooth. Pour the mixture into 2 glasses and garnish with fresh strawberries.

Note: For a frozen smoothie, place the fruit on a baking sheet lined with waxed paper and freeze for 2 hours, or until almost firm. Use as directed in the recipe.

Makes 2 servings (1 ½ cups each)

Per serving: 191 calories, 4 g protein, 42 g carbohydrates, 3 g fat, 20 mg cholesterol, 42 mg sodium, 4 g dietary fiber
Diet Exchanges: 1 ½ fruit, 1 bread, ½ meat, ½ fat
Carb Choices: 3

GAZPACHO-VEGGIE TWISTER

Gazpacho is a cold, savory drink hailing from southern Spain. A dash of Worcestershire and Tabasco sauce give it a zesty flavor that's guaranteed to dazzle your tastebuds.

Prep time: 10 minutes

1 ¾ cups tomato juice or vegetable-tomato cocktail

2 small (about 4") pickling cucumbers (6 ounces), peeled and cubed

½ red bell pepper, peeled and cubed

½ rib celery, sliced

1 tablespoon lemon juice

2 teaspoons Worcestershire sauce

1 teaspoon green Tabasco sauce, or 6 drops of regular Tabasco

Cucumber spears and lemon wedges (optional)

In a blender, combine the tomato juice or vegetable-tomato cocktail, cucumbers, bell pepper, celery, lemon juice, Worcestershire sauce, and Tabasco sauce. Process for 1 to 2 minutes, or until smooth. Serve over ice. Garnish with cucumber spears and lemon wedges, if you wish.

Makes 2 servings (1½ cups each)

Per serving: 69 calories, 3 g protein, 14 g carbohydrates, 0 g fat, 0 mg cholesterol, 830 mg sodium, 2 g dietary fiber
Diet Exchanges: 2 ½ vegetable
Carb Choices: 1

ALCOHOL-FREE SANGRIA

Chase away the heat with this refreshing cooler. Zesty orange slices and apple wedges float invitingly in this beautiful drink.

Prep time: 20 minutes • Chill time: 4 hours

3   cups Concord grape juice

2   cups orange juice

¼   cup lemon juice

2   tablespoons lime juice

1   orange, ends trimmed, sliced into half rounds

1   apple, cored and cut into thin wedges

In a 2-quart pitcher, stir together the grape, orange, lemon, and lime juices. Stir in the orange and apple wedges and refrigerate, covered, for 4 to 48 hours. Serve the sangria in tall glasses and spoon in some of the fruit.

Note: For a reduced-alcohol version, combine this sangria with an equal amount of dry red wine.

Makes 8 servings (8 cups)

Per serving: 101 calories, 1 g protein, 25 g carbohydrates, 0 g fat, 10 mg cholesterol, 25 mg sodium, 1 g dietary fiber
Diet Exchanges: 1 fruit, 1 bread
Carb Choices: 2

CRANBERRY-GINGER SPICED CIDER

You'll warm to this soothing cider. Accented with a festive mix of cranberries and ginger, it's the perfect drink for lounging by the fire or making a celebratory toast.

Prep time: 15 minutes • Cook time: 30 minutes

¾ cup fresh or frozen cranberries

4 slices fresh ginger, cut into matchsticks
  (2 tablespoons)

6 whole cloves

3 3" cinnamon sticks + 8 additional for garnish

8 cups apple cider

⅓ cup honey

Brandy or applejack (optional)

Cut a 7" square from a double layer of cheesecloth. Place the cranberries, ginger, cloves, and 3 cinnamon sticks in the center of the cheesecloth. Gather up the edges of the cheesecloth and tie with kitchen string. Place in a large saucepan, along with the cider and honey. Bring to a bare simmer, cover, and cook for 30 minutes, or until flavored through.

Place the cheesecloth bag in a strainer set over the pan, and press with the back of a spoon to extract the liquids. Discard the bag. Ladle the cider into mugs and serve with a cinnamon stick and a jigger of brandy or applejack, if you wish.

Makes 8 servings (1 cup each)

Per serving: 168 calories, 0 g protein, 43 g carbohydrates, 0 g fat, 0 mg cholesterol, 25 mg sodium, 0 g dietary fiber
Diet Exchanges: 2 fruit, 1 bread
Carb Choices: 3

HEARTY SOUPS AND SANDWICHES

FAST   SUPER FAST   FAST PREP

ONION AND ROASTED GARLIC SOUP

Roasted garlic lends a mellow, nutty flavor to this traditional soup. Topped with melted cheese, it's the perfect dish for a cozy winter evening.

Prep time: 15 minutes • Cook time: 1 hour 40 minutes

ROASTED GARLIC PASTE

1 **large head garlic**

SOUP

2 **tablespoons olive oil**

6 **cups sliced onions**

¼ **teaspoon salt**

1 **bay leaf**

¼ **teaspoon dried thyme, crumbled**

¼ **teaspoon dried rosemary, crumbled**

¼ **teaspoon freshly ground black pepper**

3 **cups fat-free beef broth**

1 **cup water**

¼ **cup dry sherry (optional)**

4 **small slices crusty whole grain bread, toasted (cut to fit the shape of your bowls)**

¼ **cup shredded low-fat Jarlsberg cheese**

3 **tablespoons freshly grated Parmesan cheese**

To make the roasted garlic paste: Preheat the oven to 400°F. Cut a thin slice from the top of the garlic to expose the cloves. Place the head cut side up on a large piece of foil. Seal the top and sides of the foil tightly. Place in the oven and roast for 45 to 60 minutes, or until the cloves are very soft and lightly browned. Remove and set aside until cool enough to handle. Squeeze the cloves into a medium bowl. With the back of a large metal spoon, mash the garlic to a smooth paste. Set aside.

To make the soup: Heat the oil in a heavy large saucepan or Dutch oven over medium-low heat. Add 4 cups of the onions and sprinkle with the salt. Cook, stirring often, for 20 to 25 minutes, or until the onions are very tender and lightly browned. Stir in the bay leaf, thyme, rosemary, pepper, and the remaining 2 cups onions. Cook, stirring often, 6 minutes longer, or just until the onions have softened slightly.

Add the broth, water, and sherry, if using. Increase the heat, cover, and bring to a boil. Lower the heat and let simmer, covered, for 20 minutes. Stir in the roasted garlic paste, cover, and let simmer for 10 minutes longer. Remove from the heat. Discard the bay leaf.

Preheat the broiler. Place 4 broilerproof onion soup crocks on a jelly-roll pan. Ladle the soup evenly into the bowls and place a slice of toast on top of each. Sprinkle evenly with the Jarlsberg and Parmesan. Broil about 6" from the heat source for 2 minutes, or until the cheese is melted and bubbly. Serve at once.

Note: Start the roasted garlic before you begin slicing and cooking the onions. You could also roast it a day before and keep it tightly wrapped in a small bowl in the refrigerator.

Makes 4 main-dish servings (5 cups)

Per serving: 269 calories, 13 g protein, 36 g carbohydrates, 9 g fat, 5 mg cholesterol, 490 mg sodium, 6 g dietary fiber
Diet Exchanges: 3 vegetable, 1 bread, 1 meat, 1 ½ fat
Carb Choices: 2

ITALIAN COUNTRY SOUP WITH PESTO

Wheat berries are whole, unprocessed kernels and can usually be found in natural food stores. Their level of fiber gives this dish extra blood sugar balancing power.

Prep time: 15 minutes • Cook time: 2 hours 20 minutes

½ cup wheat berries, rinsed

4 cups water

⅛ teaspoon salt

5 cups chicken or vegetable broth

3 cups coarsely chopped cabbage

1 medium sweet potato (about 8 ounces), peeled and cut into 1" chunks

2 large carrots, cut into thick slices (1 ½ cups)

1 large parsnip, peeled and cut into thick slices

1 large onion, coarsely chopped

½ teaspoon freshly ground black pepper

1 can (14 ½ ounces) diced tomatoes, drained

1 zucchini, halved lengthwise and cut into ½"-thick slices

½ cup prepared pesto

Place the wheat berries, 3 cups of the water, and the salt in a heavy medium saucepan and bring to a boil over high heat. Reduce the heat to low, cover, and simmer, checking a few times to make sure the water hasn't boiled away, for 2 to 2 ½ hours, or until the wheat berries are very tender. Drain and cool or refrigerate until ready to use.

Place the broth, cabbage, sweet potato, carrots, parsnip, onion, pepper, and the remaining 1 cup water in a Dutch oven. Cover and bring to a boil over high heat. Reduce the heat to low and simmer, covered, for 10 minutes.

Add the tomatoes and zucchini. Cover and simmer for 10 minutes longer, or until the vegetables are tender. Stir in the wheat berries, heat through, and remove from the heat.

Stir the pesto into the soup or add pesto to individual servings.

Note: The wheat berries may be cooked up to 2 days ahead and kept refrigerated. For a vegetarian soup, use vegetable broth.

Makes 6 main-dish servings (12 cups)

Per serving: 292 calories, 10 g protein, 43 g carbohydrates, 11 g fat, 5 mg cholesterol, 1,160 mg sodium, 8 g dietary fiber
Diet Exchanges: 3 vegetable, 1 ½ bread, ½ meat, 2 fat
Carb Choices: 3

TOMATO AND ORANGE SOUP

FAST PREP

The vibrant assortment of vegetables in this colorful soup also contains the antioxidants you need to boost your immunity and keep your heart strong and healthy. *Photo on page 136.*

Prep time: 20 minutes • Cook time: 30 minutes

2 tablespoons olive oil	1/8 teaspoon crushed red-pepper flakes
1 large onion, chopped	4 3" strips orange peel, removed with a vegetable peeler
1 1/2 cups chopped fennel bulb	1 can (28 ounces) crushed tomatoes
1 large carrot, chopped	2 cups chicken broth
1 small red bell pepper, chopped	1/2 cup orange juice
3 cloves garlic, minced	8 small slices whole grain bread or 8 thin slices of whole grain baguette, toasted
1/4 teaspoon dried thyme, crumbled	
1/4 teaspoon salt	
1/4 teaspoon freshly ground black pepper	

In a Dutch oven, warm the oil over medium-low heat. Stir in the onion, fennel, carrot, bell pepper, and garlic. Sprinkle with the thyme, salt, black pepper, and red-pepper flakes. Cover and cook, stirring often, for 12 minutes, or until the vegetables are tender. Stir in the orange peel.

Stir in the tomatoes and the broth. Increase the heat, cover, and bring to a boil. Lower the heat and simmer, covered, for 15 minutes. Remove the orange peel. Remove from the heat and stir in the orange juice. Serve the soup with toast.

Makes 6 to 8 side-dish servings (8 cups)

Per serving: 227 calories, 8 g protein, 37 g carbohydrates, 7 g fat, 0 mg cholesterol, 820 mg sodium, 7 g dietary fiber
Diet Exchanges: 3 vegetable, 1 bread, 1 fat
Carb Choices: 2

LENTIL SOUP WITH SPINACH

Lentils are an excellent source of protein. They satisfy your appetite just as well as beef but have only trace amounts of saturated fat.

Prep time: 10 minutes • Cook time: 36 minutes

1 tablespoon olive oil	1 ⅓ cups (8 ounces) lentils, sorted and rinsed
1 ½ teaspoons whole cumin seeds	5 cups water
1 large onion, chopped	1 can (14 ½ ounces) diced tomatoes
4 cloves garlic, minced	2 cups packed shredded fresh spinach
½ teaspoon ground coriander	½ teaspoon salt
½ teaspoon freshly ground black pepper	8 ounces fat-free plain yogurt
1 teaspoon paprika	

Place the oil and cumin seeds in a Dutch oven or heavy large saucepan over medium heat. Cook, stirring, for 2 to 3 minutes, or until fragrant. Stir in the onion, garlic, coriander, and pepper and cook, stirring often, for 4 to 6 minutes, or until the onions and garlic are tender. Stir in the paprika.

Add the lentils and water. Cover and bring to a boil. Reduce the heat to low and simmer, covered, for 30 to 35 minutes, or until the lentils are very tender.

Stir in the diced tomatoes, spinach, and salt. Increase the heat and simmer, uncovered, for 5 minutes longer. Serve with a swirl of yogurt.

Makes 4 main-dish servings (7 ½ cups)

Per serving: 303 calories, 21 g protein, 50 g carbohydrates, 4 g fat, 0 mg cholesterol, 490 mg sodium, 21 g dietary fiber
Diet Exchanges: 2 vegetable, 2 bread, 2 meat, ½ fat
Carb Choices: 3

COLD CUCUMBER AND MINT SOUP

Perfect for a summer day, this refreshing soup is loaded with calcium.

Prep time: 20 minutes • Chill time: 2 hours

2 cups 1" chunks hothouse cucumber, peeled	⅛ teaspoon celery seed
2 cups fat-free plain yogurt	¼ teaspoon salt
1 cup buttermilk	¼ teaspoon freshly ground black pepper
⅓ cup chopped sweet white onion	½ cup coarsely chopped red bell pepper
¼ cup chopped fresh mint	½ cup coarsely chopped tomato
2 cloves garlic, crushed through a press	1 hard-cooked egg, chopped

Place the cucumber in a food processor and pulse to chop finely, but don't puree. Transfer to a large bowl.

Stir in the yogurt, buttermilk, onion, mint, garlic, celery seed, salt, and black pepper. Cover and refrigerate for at least 2 hours.

To serve, ladle into chilled, small bowls and top each with a heaping tablespoon of bell pepper and tomato, and sprinkle with some of the egg.

Makes 6 first-course servings (4 ½ cups)

Per serving: 78 calories, 6 g protein, 12 g carbohydrates, 1 g fat, 35 mg cholesterol, 200 mg sodium, 1 g dietary fiber
Diet Exchanges: 1 milk, 1 vegetable
Carb Choices: 1

CHILLED BERRY AND RED WINE SOUP

This elegant soup is the perfect way to start a summer dinner party. The lightly toasted almonds add a nutty crunch to complement the sweet, ripe fruit.

Prep time: 25 minutes • Cook time: 3 minutes • Chill time: 1 hour

2   **tablespoons sugar**

1   **tablespoon seedless raspberry or strawberry reduced-sugar spread**

4   **cups (1 pound) whole strawberries**

1¼   **cups fresh raspberries**

½   **cup dry red wine (optional)**

3   **tablespoons frozen apple juice concentrate**

Pinch of ground cinnamon

Pinch of allspice

¼   **cup sliced unblanched almonds**

½   **cup fat-free plain yogurt**

¾   **cup fresh blueberries**

In a large bowl, stir the sugar and berry spread until blended. Hull the strawberries and cut all but 1 cup into thick slices. Add the sliced strawberries and ¾ cup of the raspberries to the sugar mixture. Stir the combined berries until coated, then stir in the red wine (if using), apple juice concentrate, cinnamon, and allspice. Cover and refrigerate for 1 hour.

Cook the almonds in a small nonstick skillet over medium heat, stirring often, for 3 to 4 minutes, or until lightly toasted. Tip onto a plate and let cool.

Puree the soup, in batches if necessary, in a food processor. Return to the bowl. Whisk in the yogurt. Add the blueberries to the soup with the reserved 1 cup whole strawberries and the remaining ½ cup raspberries. Ladle into bowls and sprinkle with the almonds.

Makes 8 first-course servings (4 cups)

Per serving: 86 calories, 2 g protein, 17 g carbohydrates, 2 g fat, 0 mg cholesterol, 10 mg sodium, 3 g dietary fiber
Diet Exchanges: 1 fruit, ½ fat
Carb Choices: 1

GREEN VEGETABLE AND QUINOA SOUP

FAST PREP

Quinoa figures prominently in South American cuisine. It contains more protein than any other grain. You can find it in health food stores and some grocery stores.

Prep time: 15 minutes • Cook time: 35 minutes

½ cup quinoa	2 cups chopped, peeled hothouse cucumber
1 cup water	½ teaspoon dried thyme, crumbled
⅛ teaspoon + ¼ teaspoon salt	½ teaspoon dried rosemary, crumbled
1 tablespoon olive oil	¼ teaspoon freshly ground black pepper
1 large leek, halved lengthwise, well washed, and cut into ½" slices	4 cups chicken broth
1 large onion, coarsely chopped	2 cups frozen peas
1 cup chopped celery	1 cup grated zucchini
2 cloves garlic, minced	

Place the quinoa in a fine-mesh strainer and rinse under cold running water for 2 minutes. Transfer to a heavy medium saucepan. Add the water and the ⅛ teaspoon salt and bring to a boil over high heat. Reduce the heat to low, cover, and simmer for 10 to 15 minutes, or until the quinoa is tender, the water is absorbed, and some of the grains start to uncoil. Remove from the heat and set aside, covered.

Meanwhile, heat the oil in a Dutch oven over medium heat. Add the leek, onion, celery, and garlic, and cook, stirring often, for 5 minutes, or until the vegetables begin to shrink down.

Add the cucumber, thyme, rosemary, pepper, and the ¼ teaspoon salt and stir well. Lower the heat, cover, and cook, stirring occasionally, for 10 minutes, or until the vegetables are very tender.

Add the broth and the cooked quinoa. Cover and bring to a boil over high heat. Reduce the heat to low and simmer, covered, for 5 minutes. Stir in the peas and zucchini. Cover and simmer for 5 to 7 minutes longer, or until the peas are heated through and the zucchini is tender.

Makes 8 first-course servings or 4 main-dish servings (10 cups)

Per serving: 131 calories, 5 g protein, 20 g carbohydrates, 4 g fat, 0 mg cholesterol, 680 mg sodium, 4 g dietary fiber
Diet Exchanges: 1 vegetable, 1 bread, ½ fat
Carb Choices: 1

POTATO AND VEGETABLE SOUP

Potatoes are the world's number-one vegetable crop. In this hearty dish, they are paired with an assortment of fresh vegetables, but they still take center stage.

Prep time: 25 minutes • Cook time: 35 minutes

1 ³/₄ **pounds baking potatoes, peeled and cut into chunks**

1 **large onion, sliced**

2 **ribs celery with leaves, sliced**

5 **cups chicken broth**

2 **cups water**

¹/₂ **teaspoon dried thyme, crumbled**

2 **tablespoons olive oil**

3 **cups sliced cremini or baby portobello mushrooms**

1 **large leek, halved lengthwise, well washed, and cut into ¹/₂" slices**

2 **large carrots, cut into ¹/₄" slices**

2 **cups small broccoli florets**

1 **medium yellow summer squash, sliced lengthwise and cut into ¹/₄" slices**

¹/₂ **teaspoon salt**

¹/₄ **teaspoon freshly ground black pepper**

1 **cup 1% milk**

Place the potatoes, onion, celery, broth, water, and thyme in a Dutch oven. Cover and bring to a boil over high heat.

Reduce the heat to low and simmer, covered, for 20 to 25 minutes, or until the potatoes and celery are very tender. In a food processor, puree the potatoes and celery to a smooth consistency.

Meanwhile, in a heavy large, deep skillet, heat the oil over medium heat. Add the mushrooms, leek, carrots, broccoli, and squash. Sprinkle with salt and pepper, mix well, and reduce the heat to low. Cover and cook, stirring occasionally, for 10 minutes, or until the vegetables are nearly tender.

Add the vegetables and milk to the potato mixture. Stir to blend, and bring to a simmer over medium-high heat. Cook, stirring often, for 5 minutes, or until the vegetables are very tender.

Makes 6 main-dish servings (14 cups)

Per serving: 239 calories, 10 g protein, 41 g carbohydrates, 7 g fat, 0 mg cholesterol, 1,090 mg sodium, 7 g dietary fiber
Diet Exchanges: 3 vegetable, 1 ¹/₂ bread, ¹/₂ meat, 1 fat
Carb Choices: 3

SPICY CORN AND SWEET POTATO CHOWDER

Interestingly, sweet potatoes are not botanically related to the potato. They are actually members of the morning glory family. With a respectable amount of protein and high levels of fiber and complex carbohydrates, sweet potatoes are a key ingredient in a blood sugar balancing diet.

Prep time: 20 minutes • Cook time: 27 minutes

1   tablespoon olive oil

1   large onion, coarsely chopped

1   red bell pepper, coarsely chopped

2   ribs celery, chopped

¼   teaspoon salt

¼   teaspoon freshly ground black pepper

1 ½   teaspoons ground cumin

¼   teaspoon dried oregano

1   large sweet potato (1 pound), peeled and cut into ½" chunks

1   package (10 ounces) frozen corn

4   cups chicken broth

½   cup medium-spicy salsa + extra for serving

½   ripe avocado, peeled and chopped

½   cup coarsely chopped fresh cilantro (optional)

In a Dutch oven, warm the oil over medium-low heat. Add the onion, bell pepper, celery, salt, and black pepper. Cover and cook, stirring often, for 10 minutes, or until tender. Stir in the cumin and oregano.

Add the sweet potato, corn, and broth. Cover, increase the heat, and bring to a boil. Lower the heat and simmer, covered, for 12 minutes, or until the sweet potato is tender. Stir in the salsa and simmer, uncovered, for 5 minutes longer.

Ladle into bowls and top each with some of the avocado, cilantro (if using), and extra salsa, if you wish.

Makes 8 first-course servings (9 cups)

Per serving: 161 calories, 4 g protein, 30 g carbohydrates, 5 g fat, 0 mg cholesterol, 680 mg sodium, 5 g dietary fiber
Diet Exchanges: 1 vegetable, 1 ½ bread, 1 fat
Carb Choices: 2

MAPLE SQUASH SOUP WITH APPLE

There are numerous varieties of winter squash to choose from, all of them tantalizing in this rich, buttery soup. Pumpkin, acorn, butternut, and Hubbard are just a few, and all contain rich sources of fiber and complex carbohydrates.

Prep time: 8 minutes • Cook time: 23 minutes

1 **tablespoon olive oil**	1/8 **teaspoon freshly ground black pepper**
1 **large onion, coarsely chopped**	1 **package (12 ounces) frozen winter squash, thawed**
2 **large Granny Smith apples (1 pound), peeled, cored, and cut into chunks**	2 1/2 **cups chicken broth**
1/4 **teaspoon ground cinnamon**	3/4 **cup 1% milk**
1/8 **teaspoon ground cumin**	1/4 **cup pure maple syrup**
1/8 **teaspoon salt**	1 **chopped apple**

In a Dutch oven, heat the oil over medium heat. Add the onion and apples and cook, stirring often, for 8 minutes, or until tender. Stir in the cinnamon, cumin, salt, and pepper.

Add the squash and broth. Cover and bring to a boil over high heat. Reduce the heat to low and simmer, covered, stirring occasionally, for 15 minutes.

Puree the soup in batches in a food processor or blender. Return to the saucepan and stir in the milk and maple syrup. Bring to a boil over medium heat, stirring often. Allow it to cool slightly, ladle into bowls, and garnish each with a little chopped apple.

Makes 6 first-course servings (6 cups)

Per serving: 180 calories, 3 g protein, 37 g carbohydrates, 4 g fat, 0 mg cholesterol, 500 mg sodium, 7 g dietary fiber
Diet Exchanges: 1 fruit, 1 vegetable, 1 bread, 1/2 fat
Carb Choices: 2

PEPPER STEAK SOUP

FAST
PREP

With only 25 percent of calories from fat, top round is one of the healthiest cuts of beef you can buy. The protein in this hearty soup will help keep those salty/crunchy cravings at bay.
Photo on page 131.

Prep time: 20 minutes • Cook time: 25 minutes

12 ounces well-trimmed lean boneless beef top round	1 tablespoon olive oil
½ teaspoon salt	1 medium sweet white onion, halved and thinly sliced
½ teaspoon coarsely ground black pepper	2 green bell peppers, cut into strips
4 cups fat-free beef broth	4 cloves garlic, minced
½ cup dry red wine (optional)	3 tablespoons water
½ cup tomato sauce	1½ cups halved cherry tomatoes
¼ teaspoon dried thyme	

Thinly slice the beef on the diagonal into ¼"-thick slices. Cut large pieces in half. Sprinkle with ¼ teaspoon of the salt and the black pepper. Set aside.

In a large saucepan, stir together the beef broth, wine (if using), tomato sauce, and thyme. Cover and bring to a boil over high heat. Reduce the heat to low and simmer, covered, for 10 minutes.

Meanwhile, in a large nonstick skillet, warm the oil over medium-high heat until hot but not smoking. Add half the beef slices and cook, turning once, for 2 minutes, or until browned. Transfer to a clean bowl. Cook the remaining beef.

Add the onion, bell peppers, garlic, and the remaining ¼ teaspoon salt to the skillet. Toss to mix well and add 2 tablespoons of the water. Lower the heat to medium and cook, stirring often, for 10 minutes, or until the vegetables are tender. If the pan gets dry, add the remaining 1 tablespoon water. Add the tomatoes and cook, stirring often, for 5 minutes, or until softened.

Add the beef and any juices and the vegetables to the broth mixture. Warm through but don't boil.

Makes 4 main-dish servings (8 to 10 cups)

Per serving: 230 calories, 26 g protein, 15 g carbohydrates, 7 g fat, 50 mg cholesterol, 670 mg sodium, 3 g dietary fiber
Diet Exchanges: 2 vegetable, 3 ½ meat, 1 fat
Carb Choices: 1

BEEF BARLEY SOUP WITH MUSHROOMS

Barley has a robust, slightly pungent taste that complements beef and mushrooms in this soup quite beautifully.

Prep time: 25 minutes • Cook time: 1 hour 40 minutes

1 tablespoon olive oil

1 pound well-trimmed lean boneless beef top round, cut into ¾" cubes

2 medium onions, halved and thinly sliced

3 cloves garlic, minced

¾ teaspoon salt

¼ teaspoon freshly ground black pepper

½ teaspoon dried thyme, crumbled

10 ounces cremini or baby portobello mushrooms, sliced

2 ribs celery with some leaves, thinly sliced

2 medium carrots, sliced

1 medium parsnip, halved lengthwise and sliced

3 cups water

3 ½ cups fat-free beef broth

½ cup pearl barley

Chopped fresh parsley or dill (optional)

Heat the oil in a Dutch oven or a heavy large saucepan over medium heat. Add the beef cubes. Lightly brown the beef until the liquid evaporates. Add the onions and garlic and cook for 3 to 5 minutes, or until the onions soften. Add the salt, pepper, and thyme and cook for 1 minute. Add the mushrooms and cook for 3 minutes, or until the mushrooms begin to soften. Add the celery, carrots, and parsnip and stir for 2 minutes. Add the water and the broth and simmer for 45 minutes. Stir in the barley and simmer for 45 minutes longer, or until the barley is soft. Sprinkle with fresh parsley or dill, if using.

Makes 4 main-dish servings (8 cups)

Per serving: 462 calories, 52 g protein, 39 g carbohydrates, 11 g fat, 100 mg cholesterol, 670 mg sodium, 9 g dietary fiber
Diet Exchanges: 2 vegetable, 2 bread, 7 meat, 1 ½ fat
Carb Choices: 3

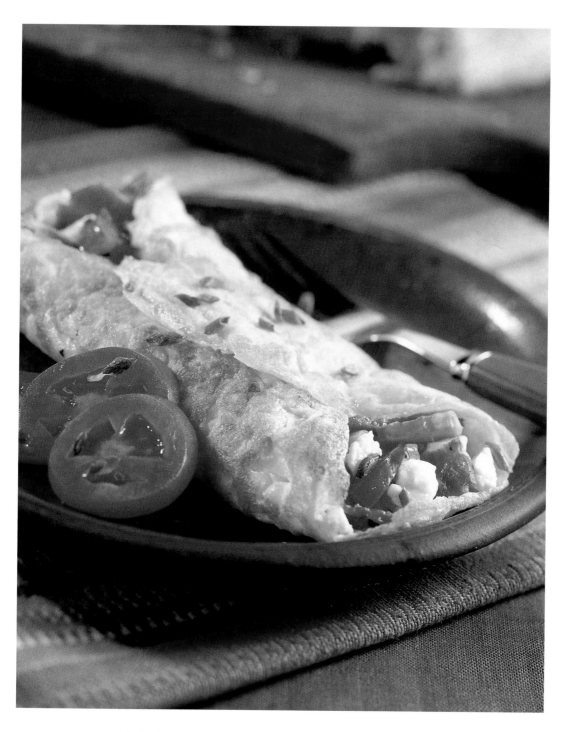

DOUBLE TOMATO AND TURKEY BACON OMELETTE

Recipe on page 72

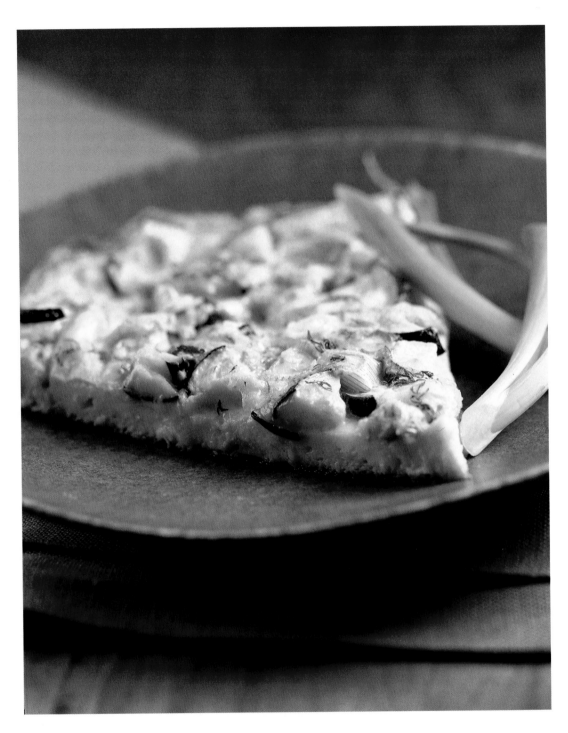

ZUCCHINI AND DILL FRITTATA
Recipe on page 74

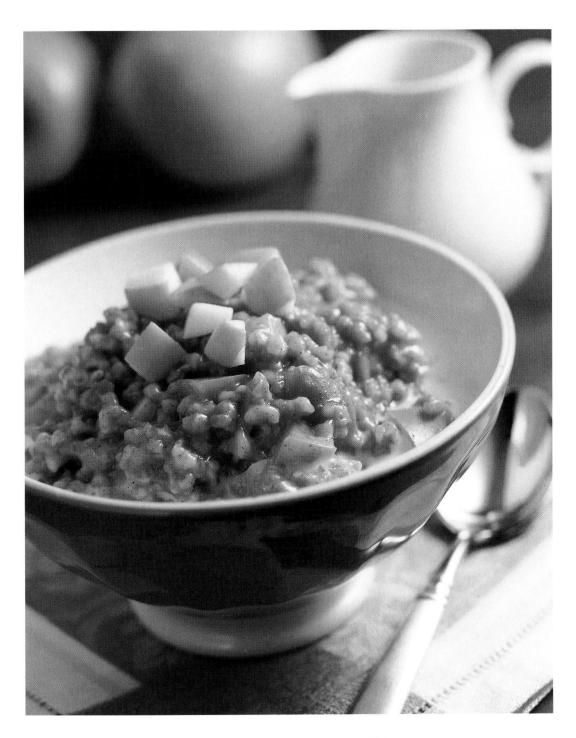

FRUIT AND SPICE CUT OATMEAL

Recipe on page 75

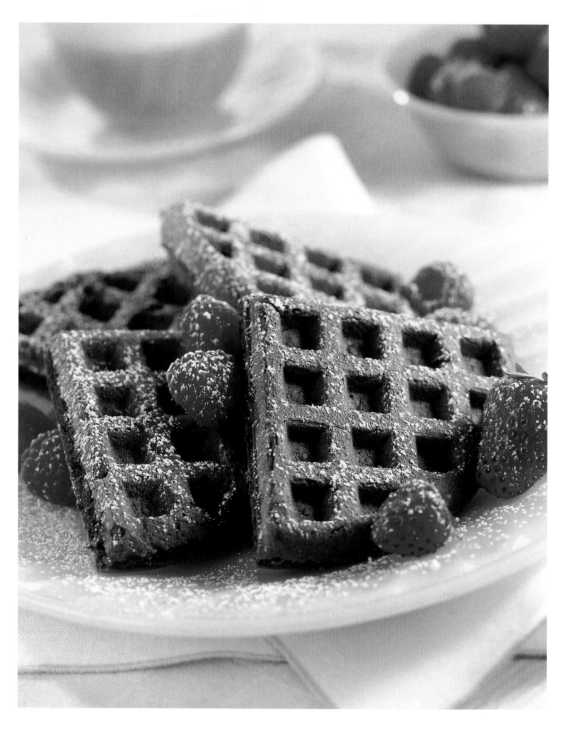

COCOA-ESPRESSO WAFFLES

Recipe on page 80

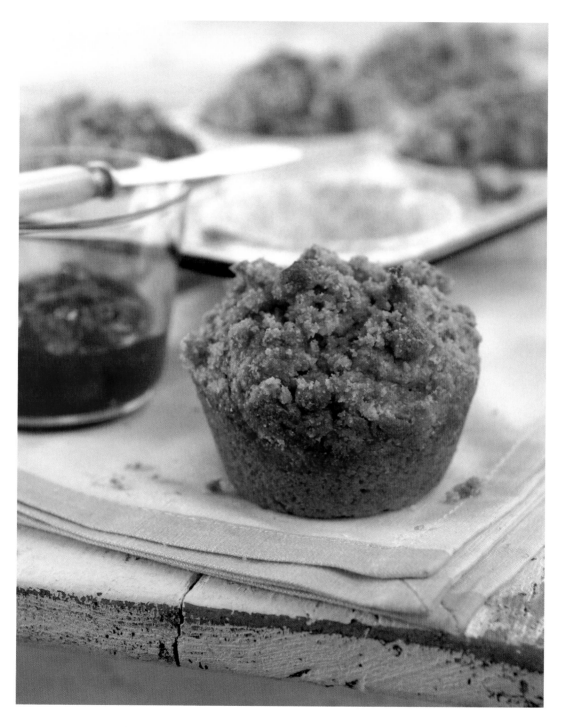

PEANUT BUTTER AND BANANA STREUSEL MUFFINS

Recipe on page 81

125

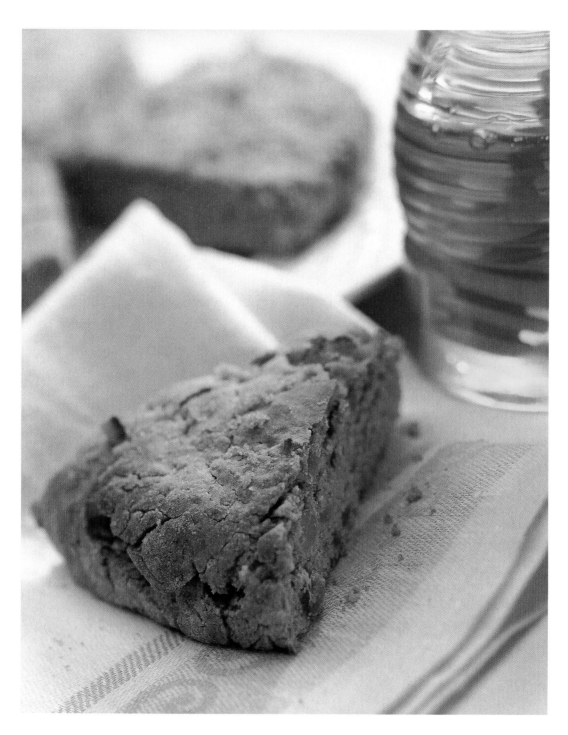

APRICOT-GINGER BUTTERMILK SCONES

Recipe on page 83

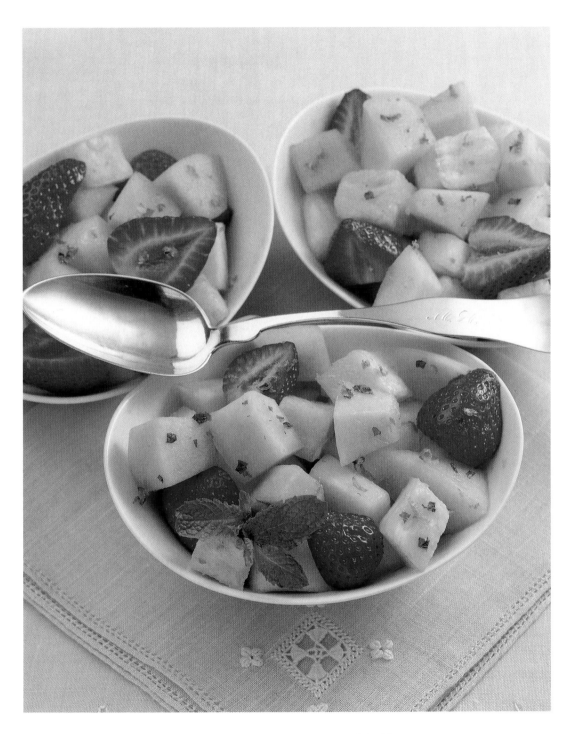

MINTED HONEY-LIME FRUIT SALAD

Recipe on page 85

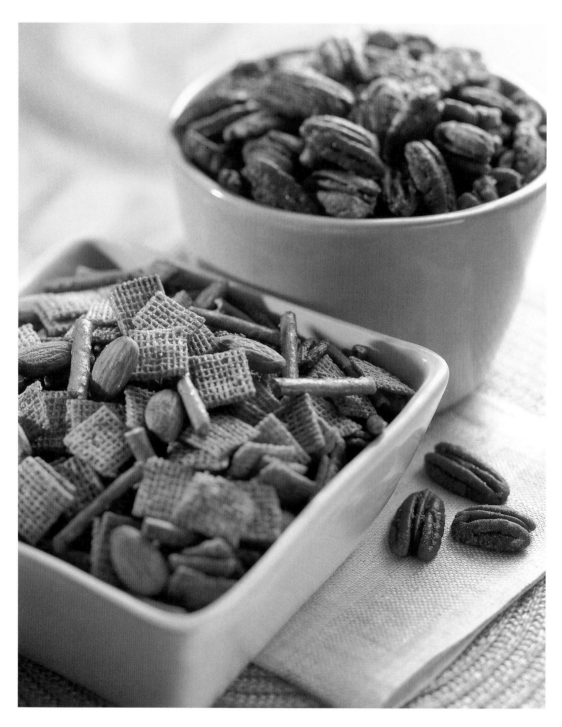

MUSTARD-GLAZED SNACK MIX *(FRONT)* AND SPICY GLAZED PECANS *(BACK)*

Recipes on pages 92 and 93

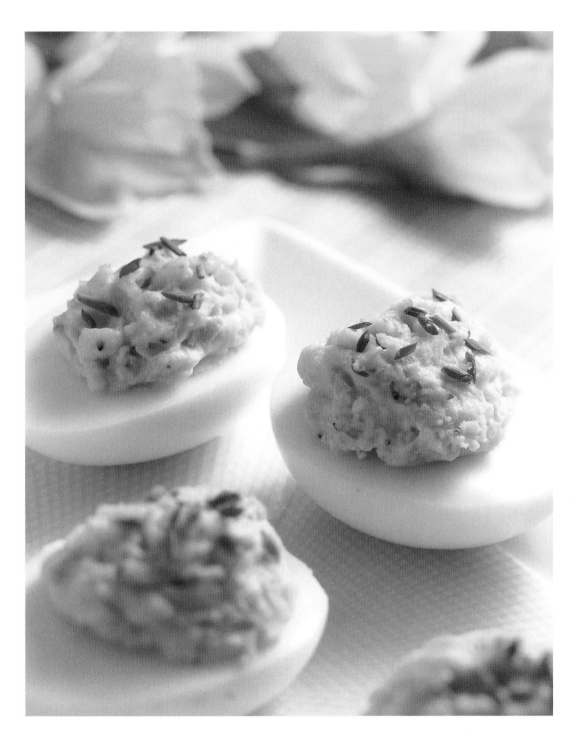

SUPER-CREAMY DEVILED EGGS

Recipe on page 95

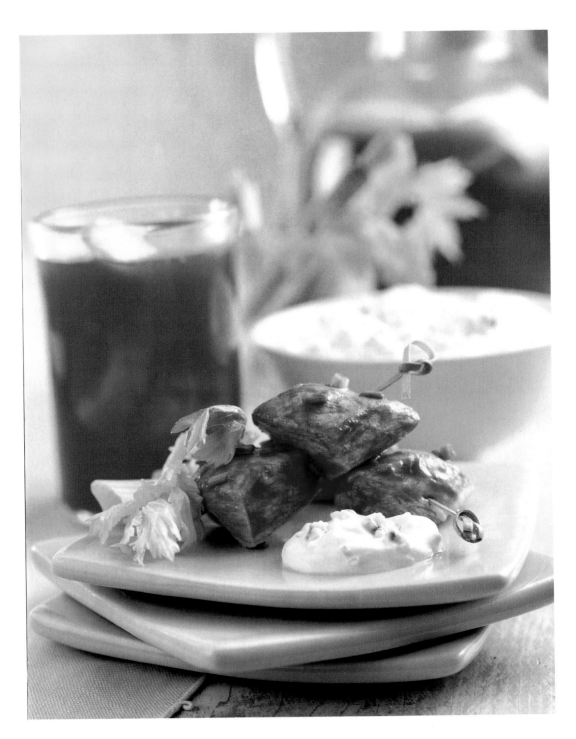

BUFFALO CHICKEN BITES

Recipe on page 99

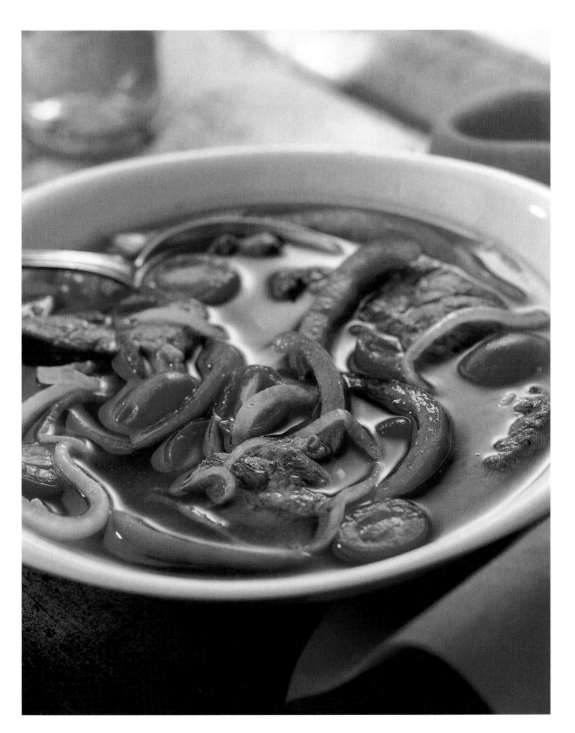

PEPPER STEAK SOUP

Recipe on page 119

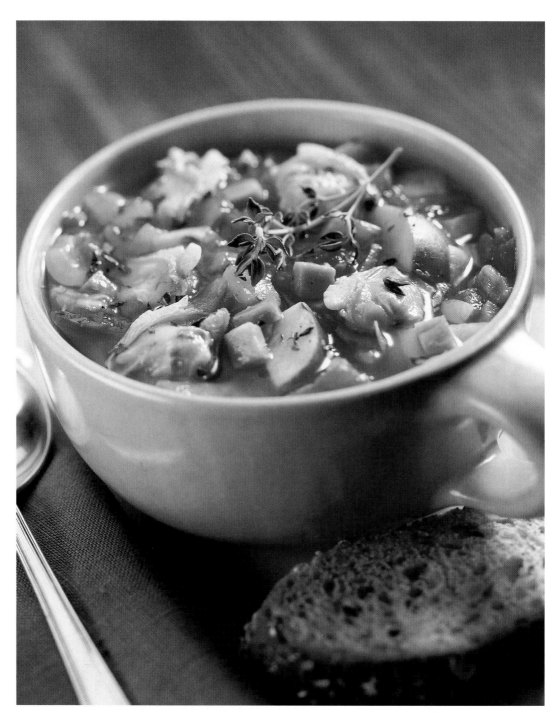

CONFETTI CLAM SOUP

Recipe on page 141

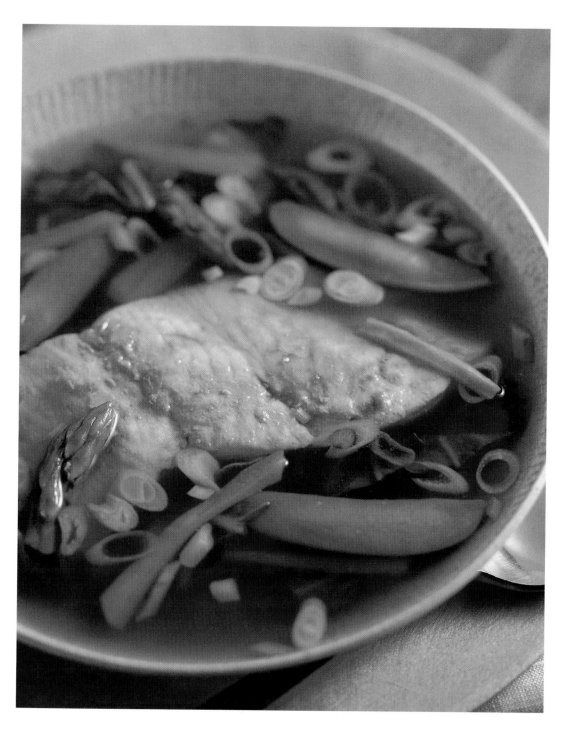

MISO SOUP WITH ASPARAGUS AND BROILED SALMON
Recipe on page 144

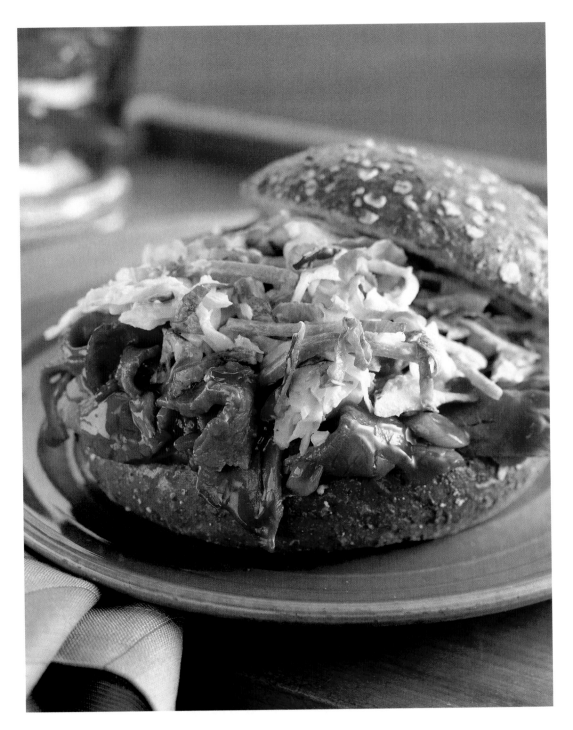

SHAVED BARBECUE BEEF SANDWICHES WITH SPICY SLAW

Recipe on page 147

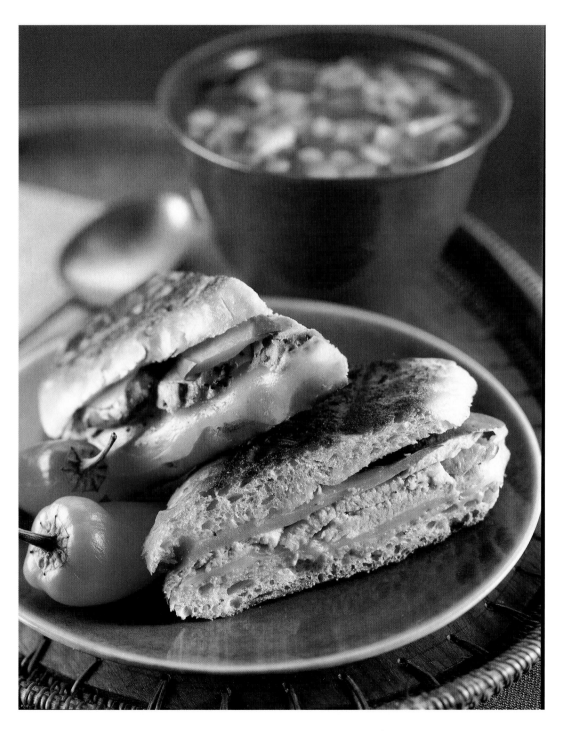

CUBANO PANINI *(FRONT)* AND LATIN CHICKEN AND RICE SOUP *(BACK)*

Recipes on pages 148 and 138

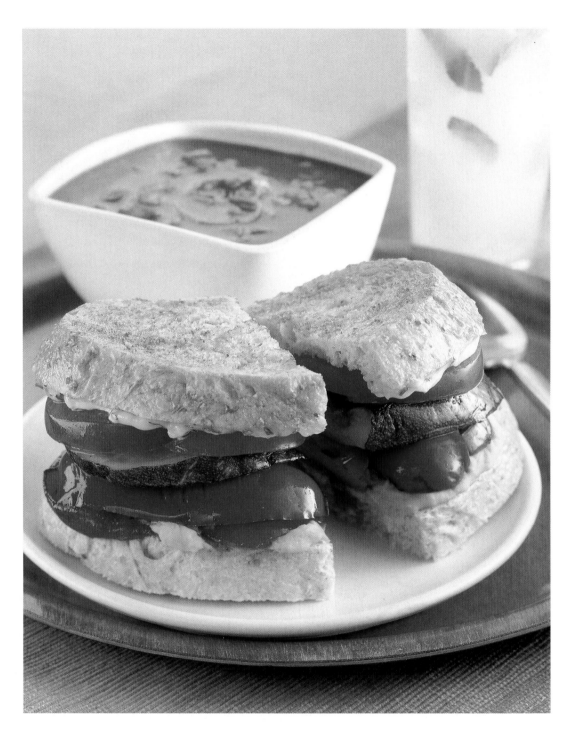

GRILLED VEGETABLE SANDWICHES *(FRONT)* AND TOMATO AND ORANGE SOUP *(BACK)*

Recipes on pages 154 and 111

CHICKEN AND VEGETABLE SOUP

Making high-protein, low-fat meals part of your diet will keep you from overeating. It helps to prevent those blood sugar hikes that send you to the snack machine. Chicken is an excellent way to keep your appetite steady and predictable.

Prep time: 20 minutes • Cook time: 45 minutes

4 **skinless, bone-in chicken breast halves, well trimmed (about 2 pounds)**

2 **large cloves garlic, minced**

1 **tablespoon chopped fresh thyme**

½ **teaspoon salt**

¼ **teaspoon freshly ground black pepper**

5 **cups chicken broth**

1 **cup water**

3 **medium carrots, cut into chunks (1 ½ cups)**

2 **medium white turnips, peeled and cut into wedges**

3 **ribs celery with leaves, cut into 1" pieces**

2 **medium onions, cut into wedges**

½ **cup chopped fresh flat-leaf parsley**

With kitchen shears, cut the chicken breasts in half crosswise. In a cup, mix the garlic, thyme, ¼ teaspoon of the salt, and the pepper. Rub the mixture all over the chicken and place the chicken in a Dutch oven.

Add the broth, water, carrots, turnips, celery, onions, and the remaining ¼ teaspoon salt. Cover and bring to a boil over high heat. Reduce the heat to low and simmer, covered, for 45 minutes, or until the vegetables are tender and the chicken is no longer pink.

Stir in the parsley and ladle into deep soup bowls.

Makes 4 to 6 main-dish servings (12 cups)

Per serving: 323 calories, 48 g protein, 21 g carbohydrates, 5 g fat, 105 mg cholesterol, 1,490 mg sodium, 5 g dietary fiber
Diet Exchanges: 4 vegetable, 6 meat, ½ fat
Carb Choices: 1

LATIN CHICKEN AND RICE SOUP

Brown rice is the entire grain with only the outer husk removed. With the whole grain intact, you get more nutritious fiber than you would from the white, stripped-down version. You also get a nuttier, chewier texture. *Photo on page 135.*

Prep time: 20 minutes • Cook time: 47 minutes

½ cup brown rice

1 pound trimmed boneless, skinless chicken breast halves, cut into 1" chunks

1 tablespoon chili powder

½ teaspoon salt

½ teaspoon freshly ground black pepper

2 tablespoons olive oil

2 large onions, halved and cut into thick slices

4 cloves garlic, minced

5 cups chicken broth

4 large carrots, cut into thick slices

1 can (15 ½ ounces) chickpeas, rinsed and drained

1 ripe avocado, halved, pitted, peeled, and cut into chunks

2 teaspoons grated lime peel

¼ cup lime juice

In a heavy medium saucepan, cook the rice according to package directions. Remove from the heat and set aside, covered.

Meanwhile, in a medium bowl, mix the chicken, 1 ½ teaspoons of the chili powder, ¼ teaspoon salt, and ¼ teaspoon pepper. Cover and set aside.

Heat the oil in a Dutch oven over medium-high heat. Add the onions and garlic and cook, stirring often, for 8 minutes, or until tender and light golden. Stir in the remaining 1 ½ teaspoons chili powder, ¼ teaspoon salt, and ¼ teaspoon pepper. Cook, stirring, for 1 minute.

Add the broth, carrots, and 2 cups water. Cover and bring to a boil. Reduce the heat to medium and simmer, covered, for 5 minutes, or until the carrots are tender.

Add the chickpeas and chicken. Lower the heat, cover, and simmer, stirring once or twice, for 8 minutes, or until the chicken is no longer pink. Stir in the rice, cover, and cook for 2 minutes longer.

Remove from the heat and stir in the avocado, lime peel, and lime juice. Serve immediately.

Note: You can cook the rice a day or so ahead. If not serving the soup right away, or if you're freezing it, leave out the avocado, lime peel, and lime juice. Add these ingredients right before serving so their flavors remain fresh.

Makes 6 main-dish servings (14 cups)

Per serving: 333 calories, 25 g protein, 32 g carbohydrates, 12 g fat, 45 mg cholesterol, 1,260 mg sodium, 8 g dietary fiber
Diet Exchanges: 2 vegetable, 1 bread, 3 meat, 2 fat
Carb Choices: 2

WHITE BEAN AND SQUASH SOUP WITH SAUSAGE AND SAGE

Beans are a dieter's best friend since they are packed with fiber and are digested slowly.

Prep time: 40 minutes • Cook time: 1 hour 25 minutes • Stand time: Overnight

1 ½ cups Great Northern or navy beans, sorted and rinsed

4 cups water

2 cups chicken broth

8 cloves garlic, peeled

2 sprigs fresh sage + 1 tablespoon chopped

½ teaspoon freshly ground black pepper

2 cups ½" pieces peeled and seeded butternut squash

1 medium leek, halved lengthwise, well washed, and cut into ½" slices

2 ribs celery, sliced

¼ teaspoon salt

1 teaspoon olive oil

2 links (8 ounces) Italian-style sweet or hot turkey sausage, sliced

¼ cup freshly grated Parmesan cheese

Place the beans in a Dutch oven. Add water to cover by 2". Cover and let soak overnight. Drain and rinse and return to the pot.

Add the 4 cups water, the broth, garlic, sage sprigs, and pepper. Cover and bring to a boil over high heat. Reduce the heat to low and simmer, covered, stirring occasionally, for 1 hour, or until the beans are very tender.

Discard the sage sprigs. With a spoon, mash the garlic cloves against the side of the pot.

Add the squash, leek, celery, and salt to the beans, increase the heat, and bring to a boil. Lower the heat, cover, and simmer for 10 minutes.

Meanwhile, in a medium nonstick skillet, heat the oil over medium heat. Add the sausages and cook, turning often, for 5 minutes, or until cooked through. Drain on paper towels.

Add the sausages and chopped sage to the soup. Simmer, uncovered, for 10 minutes, or until the vegetables are tender and the soup is lightly thickened. Ladle into bowls and top with some cheese.

Makes 6 main-dish servings (10 cups)

Per serving: 377 calories, 20 g protein, 42 g carbohydrates, 15 g fat, 30 mg cholesterol, 800 mg sodium, 15 g dietary fiber
Diet Exchanges: 2 vegetable, 2 bread, 2 meat, 2 fat
Carb Choices: 3

CONFETTI CLAM SOUP

The omega-3 fatty acids in shellfish have a number of benefits, not the least of which may be a reduced risk of depression. If feeling blue triggers your appetite, try a bowl of this colorful soup! *Photo on page 132.*

Prep time: 30 minutes • Cook time: 45 minutes

4   teaspoons olive oil

1   large onion, chopped

2   ribs celery, coarsely chopped

2   large red and/or yellow bell peppers, coarsely chopped

½   teaspoon freshly ground black pepper

3   ounces Canadian bacon, chopped

3   cloves garlic, minced

4   teaspoons chopped fresh thyme

3   cups chicken broth

12   ounces new potatoes, cut into ½" chunks

1   can (14 ½ ounces) diced tomatoes, drained

½   cup dry white wine (optional)

1½   cups water

2   dozen littleneck clams, well scrubbed

Heat the oil in a Dutch oven over medium heat. Add the onion, celery, bell peppers, and black pepper. Stir well, cover, and cook, stirring occasionally, for 12 to 14 minutes, or until the vegetables are tender.

Stir in the Canadian bacon, garlic, and thyme. Increase the heat to medium-high and cook and stir for 5 minutes, or until all the juices have evaporated.

Add the broth and potatoes, cover, and bring to a boil. Reduce the heat to medium-low and simmer, covered, for 10 minutes, or until the potatoes are tender. Stir in the tomatoes and wine (if using), cover, and simmer for 5 minutes longer. Remove from the heat.

In a covered medium skillet, bring the water to a boil over high heat. Add the clams. Reduce the heat to medium, cover, and cook, stirring often, for 8 to 10 minutes, or until the clams open.

With tongs, transfer the clams to a bowl, discarding those that don't open. Line a fine-mesh strainer with dampened paper towels. Pour the clam broth through the strainer into a glass measure, leaving any sand behind. Add the broth to the soup. Reheat if necessary.

Remove the clams from their shells and chop coarsely. Add the clams to the soup, reheat briefly, and ladle into bowls.

Makes 6 first-course servings (9 ½ cups without clams)

Per serving: 169 calories, 14 g protein, 20 g carbohydrates, 5 g fat, 25 mg cholesterol, 770 mg sodium, 4 g dietary fiber
Diet Exchanges: 2 vegetable, 1 ½ meat, 1 fat
Carb Choices: 3

ASIAN NOODLE AND MUSHROOM SOUP

Noodles are a traditional breakfast food in many parts of Asia. This hearty soup
is so satisfying, you may be tempted to eat it any time of day as well.

Prep time: 25 minutes • Cook time: 40 minutes

12	ounces pork tenderloin, well trimmed	3	cups (8 ounces) thinly sliced mushrooms
1/8	teaspoon salt	2	large carrots, thinly sliced on an angle (1 1/3 cups)
1	tablespoon Asian chili sauce or chili-and-garlic sauce	4	cups chicken broth
3	ounces soba noodles or whole wheat spaghetti	3	cups shredded romaine lettuce (1 romaine heart)
1	tablespoon olive or peanut oil	1/3	cup diagonally sliced scallions
3	cloves garlic, slivered	1/3	cup roughly chopped fresh cilantro
1	teaspoon minced peeled fresh ginger	2	teaspoons reduced-sodium soy sauce

Preheat the broiler. Line a small baking pan or the bottom of a broiler pan with foil. Coat the foil
with cooking spray. Place the pork in the prepared pan, sprinkle with the salt, and spread with the
chili sauce. (Wash your hands if they come in contact with the chili sauce, which is hot.)

Broil the pork 7" to 8" from the heat source, turning several times (and averting your face from the
spicy fumes), for 18 to 20 minutes, or until charred in spots, cooked to medium doneness (155°F on
an instant-read thermometer), and the juices run clear. Remove the pork from the heat and set
aside to rest. (It doesn't matter if it gets cold, as it will reheat in the hot soup.)

Meanwhile, bring a covered medium saucepan of water to a boil over high heat. Add the soba
noodles or spaghetti and cook, stirring often, for 5 minutes, or according to package directions,
until tender. Drain the noodles, return to the pot, and cover to keep warm.

In a Dutch oven, warm the oil over medium heat. Add the garlic and ginger and cook, stirring, for 1 minute, or until fragrant. Add the mushrooms and carrots and stir-fry for 8 minutes, or until the vegetables are softened.

Stir in the broth, increase the heat, cover, and bring to a boil. Reduce the heat and simmer, covered, to blend the flavors, for 5 minutes, or until the noodles are cooked. Stir in the lettuce, scallions, cilantro, soy sauce, and the soba noodles, and remove from the heat.

Cut the pork into thin, diagonal slices and arrange the slices in 4 large soup bowls, pouring any pork juices over it. Ladle the soup over the pork.

Note: Keep the kitchen fan on while broiling the pork. You could also barbecue the pork tenderloin, which will take about the same amount of time.

Makes 4 main-dish servings (8 cups of broth and vegetables, not measured with the pork)

Per serving: 292 calories, 26 g protein, 26 g carbohydrates, 9 g fat, 55 mg cholesterol, 1,410 mg sodium, 4 g dietary fiber
Diet Exchanges: 2 vegetable, 1 bread, 3 meat, 1 fat
Carb Choices: 2

MISO SOUP WITH ASPARAGUS AND BROILED SALMON

Miso, or bean paste, is a culinary mainstay in Japan. It comes in an assortment of colors and flavors, and it is a great source of protein. *Photo on page 133.*

Prep time: 20 minutes • Cook time: 25 minutes

4   3-ounce salmon fillets, skinned

2   tablespoons miso paste

1   tablespoon reduced-sodium soy sauce

1   tablespoon canola oil

2   cloves garlic, minced

1½ teaspoons minced peeled fresh ginger

2   tablespoons shao-hsing cooking wine or dry sherry, optional (see note)

3   cups vegetable broth

2   cups ¼" slices bok choy (halve wide stems lengthwise and slice crosswise)

1   cup sugar snap peas, stringed

1   cup 1"-pieces asparagus

2   carrots, cut into matchsticks

½   cup diagonally sliced scallions

Place the salmon in a pie plate. Mix 1 tablespoon of the miso paste and the soy sauce in a cup and spread over the top of the salmon. Set aside.

Preheat the broiler. Line a broiler pan with foil. Coat the broiler-pan rack with cooking spray.

Place the oil, garlic, and ginger in a heavy large saucepan and cook over medium heat, stirring, for 1 to 2 minutes, or until fragrant.

Add the shao-hsing or sherry (if using) and vegetable broth, increase the heat, cover, and bring to a boil. Reduce the heat to medium. Add the bok choy, peas, asparagus, and carrots. Cover and cook for 5 to 6 minutes, or until crisp-tender. Add the scallions and remove from the heat. Stir in the remaining 1 tablespoon miso and cover to keep warm.

After adding the vegetables to the broth, begin to cook the salmon. Broil the salmon 5" from the heat source for 8 to 10 minutes, or until browned and just opaque in the thickest part.

Transfer the salmon to soup bowls, ladle the soup on top, and serve immediately.

Note: Shao-hsing cooking wine is found in any Asian grocery and many large supermarkets. It's also inexpensive.

Makes 4 main-dish servings (4 ¾ cups soup without salmon)

Per serving: 280 calories, 22 g protein, 18 g carbohydrates, 13 g fat, 50 mg cholesterol, 1,120 mg sodium, 4 g dietary fiber
Diet Exchanges: 2 vegetable, ½ bread, 2 ½ meat, 1 fat
Carb Choices: 1

MADRAS SPLIT PEA SOUP

Peas turn this recipe into a powerhouse of fiber and complex carbohydrates! This spice-laden soup digests slowly, so you'll be well satisfied for hours.

Prep time: 20 minutes • Cook time: 1 hour 10 minutes

SOUP

2 tablespoons olive oil	3/4 teaspoon freshly ground black pepper
1 large onion, coarsely chopped	1 1/2 cups green split peas, sorted and rinsed
3 cloves garlic, minced	1 quart chicken broth
2 1/2 teaspoons ground cumin	2 large carrots, sliced
1 teaspoon ground coriander	1 1/2 cups frozen cut spinach (from a bag)
1 teaspoon ground ginger	1/2 teaspoon salt
1 teaspoon ground turmeric	

RAITA

8 ounces fat-free plain yogurt	1 tablespoon chopped fresh mint or 1/2 teaspoon dried

To make the soup: Warm the oil in a Dutch oven over medium heat. Add the onion and garlic and cook, stirring often, for 5 minutes, or until tender. Add the cumin, coriander, ginger, turmeric, and pepper and cook, stirring, for 1 minute.

Add the split peas and broth. Increase the heat, cover, and bring to a boil. Reduce the heat to low and simmer, covered, for 40 minutes, or until the split peas are very tender.

Add the carrots, spinach, and salt. Cover and cook, stirring occasionally, for 15 minutes longer, or until the vegetables are tender.

To make the raita: Meanwhile, mix the yogurt and mint in a small bowl. Cover and refrigerate until serving.

Ladle the soup into bowls and top each with some of the raita.

Makes 4 main-dish servings (6 cups soup, 1 1/4 cups raita)

Per serving: 419 calories, 24 g protein, 62 g carbohydrates, 10 g fat, 0 mg cholesterol, 1,410 mg sodium, 14 g dietary fiber
Diet Exchanges: 2 vegetable, 3 bread, 2 meat, 1 1/2 fat
Carb Choices: 4

VERY CLASSY BLACK BEAN SOUP

Sometimes called turtle beans, black beans are sweet flavored, with black skin and creamy colored flesh. At 6 grams of fiber per half-cup, black beans can help you cut calories by blocking the digestion of some fats.

Prep time: 30 minutes • Cook time: 45 minutes

2 tablespoons olive oil

2 large onions, chopped

6 cloves garlic, minced

1/2 serrano chile pepper, seeded and minced, or 1 jalapeño chile pepper, minced, with the seeds (wear plastic gloves when handling)

3 cans (15 1/2 ounces each) black beans, rinsed and drained

4 cups water

1/2 teaspoon salt

1/2 teaspoon freshly ground black pepper

2 tablespoons medium-dry sherry (optional)

2 hard-cooked eggs, coarsely chopped

1/3 cup chopped sweet onion

Lemon slices

In a Dutch oven, heat the oil over medium heat. Add the onions, garlic, and chile pepper. Cook, stirring often, for 7 minutes, or until light golden.

Stir in the beans, water, salt, pepper, and sherry (if using). Cover and bring to a boil over high heat. Reduce the heat to low and simmer, covered, for 30 minutes to blend the flavors.

With a potato masher, mash the soup in the pot to a chunky, thick texture.

Ladle the soup into bowls and garnish each with some chopped egg and onion and a lemon slice.

Makes 4 main-dish or 6 first-course servings (7 cups)

Per serving: 200 calories, 8 g protein, 26 g carbohydrates, 9 g fat, 95 mg cholesterol, 680 mg sodium, 7 g dietary fiber
Diet Exchanges: 2 vegetable, 1 bread, 1/2 meat, 1 1/2 fat
Carb Choices: 2

SHAVED BARBECUE BEEF SANDWICHES WITH SPICY SLAW

FAST

This robust sandwich is loaded with all the right flavors—tangy barbecue sauce and juicy beef topped with a generous amount of creamy homemade coleslaw. A perfect combination! *Photo on page 134.*

Prep time: 15 minutes • Cook time: 5 minutes

- **⅓ cup smoky barbecue sauce + additional for serving**
- **1 scallion, thinly sliced**
- **12 ounces sliced roast beef, cut into 2" × ½" strips**
- **2 tablespoons reduced-fat sour cream**
- **2 tablespoons light mayonnaise**

- **1 tablespoon prepared horseradish**
- **2 teaspoons white wine vinegar**
- **1 teaspoon honey**
- **1 teaspoon jalapeño pepper sauce**
- **3 cups shredded cabbage and carrot coleslaw mix**
- **4 soft whole wheat rolls or sandwich buns**

In a small saucepan, bring the barbecue sauce and scallion to a simmer. Stir in the beef and bring to a bare simmer. Cover, remove from the heat, and set aside.

In a medium bowl, stir together the sour cream, mayonnaise, horseradish, vinegar, honey, and pepper sauce until blended. Toss in the coleslaw until evenly coated with the dressing.

Open up the rolls and spoon the beef mixture on the roll bottoms, dividing evenly. Spoon the slaw over the beef, dividing evenly, and cover with the roll tops. Serve with additional barbecue sauce, if you wish.

Makes 4 servings

Per serving: 319 calories, 22 g protein, 42 g carbohydrates, 8 g fat, 45 mg cholesterol, 1,350 mg sodium, 5 g dietary fiber
Diet Exchanges: 1 vegetable, 2 bread, 2 ½ meat, 1 fat
Carb Choices: 3

CUBANO PANINI

This is the healthier, more satisfying version of a traditional Cuban sandwich that is typically made with full-fat cheese and roast pork. You get the same delicious flavor and high-quality protein but with less of the saturated fat. *Photo on page 135.*

Prep time: 30 minutes • Cook time: 41 minutes

¾ **pound pork tenderloin, trimmed of all visible fat**

1 **teaspoon olive oil**

½ **teaspoon garlic salt**

⅛ **teaspoon freshly ground black pepper**

1 **multigrain baguette (8 ounces), cut into 4 sections and then each halved lengthwise**

2 **tablespoons prepared yellow mustard**

4 **ounces low-fat Swiss cheese**

4 **ounces dill pickle sandwich toppers**

Preheat the oven to 425°F. Coat a wire rack with cooking spray and place on a shallow baking pan.

Rub the pork tenderloin with the olive oil. Sprinkle with the garlic salt and pepper. Roast for 30 to 35 minutes, or until a meat thermometer inserted into the center of the pork registers 155°F and the juices run clear. Cool the pork for 15 minutes.

Thinly slice the meat against the grain. Spread the cut side of the bottom half of the bread with the mustard. Top each with the cheese, pork, and an overlapping layer of pickle slices. Top with the remaining bread halves.

Heat a large nonstick skillet over medium heat. Add the sandwiches top side down and place another heavy skillet on top of the sandwiches, pressing down slightly to help flatten. Cook for 6 minutes. Turn the sandwiches over and replace the second skillet on top. Cook for 5 to 6 minutes, or until the cheese melts and the sandwiches are flat and heated through. Remove from the pan and cut each sandwich in half on a sharp angle. Serve immediately.

Makes 4 servings

Per serving: 415 calories, 31 g protein, 45 g carbohydrates, 12 g fat, 65 mg cholesterol, 1,130 mg sodium, 4 g dietary fiber
Diet Exchanges: 3 bread, 4 meat, 1 ½ fat
Carb Choices: 3

GRILLED HAM, PEAR, AND GORGONZOLA SANDWICHES

FAST

Gorgonzola is one of Italy's greatest cheeses. Its pungent flavor is the perfect accompaniment to the sweetness of pear and the saltiness of lean ham.

Prep time: 15 minutes ● Cook time: 1 minute

8   slices multigrain bread, toasted

2   tablespoons sun-dried tomato–flavored light mayonnaise

1   cup baby arugula or watercress sprigs

8   thin slices lean, low-sodium baked ham

1   ripe red Bartlett pear, quartered, cored, and cut into thin wedges

¼   cup crumbled Gorgonzola cheese

Preheat the broiler. Place 4 slices of bread on a baking sheet. Spread with the mayonnaise and mound the arugula or watercress on top, dividing evenly. Cover with 2 slices of ham on each sandwich. Arrange the pear wedges on top, and sprinkle on the cheese.

Place under the broiler for 1 to 2 minutes, or until the cheese is melted. Top with the remaining toast slices. Cut on the diagonal and serve warm.

Makes 4 servings

Per serving: 259 calories, 14 g protein, 34 g carbohydrates, 9 g fat, 25 mg cholesterol, 800 mg sodium, 5 g dietary fiber
Diet Exchanges: ½ fruit, 2 bread, 1 meat, 1 fat
Carb Choices: 2

SOUTHWESTERN SMOKED TURKEY WRAPS

Turkey breast wins the blue ribbon when it comes to cold cuts. It contains trace amounts of saturated fat and has few calories, yet it's just as satisfying as those high-fat deli meats.

Prep time: 25 minutes • Cook time: 10 minutes

1 tablespoon olive oil

2 onions, thinly sliced

1 jalapeño chile pepper, seeded and minced (wear plastic gloves when handling)

¼ teaspoon chili powder

¼ teaspoon dried oregano

1 pound deli-sliced smoked turkey breast

4 spinach-flavored tortillas (8" diameter)

½ cup prepared cranberry sauce

1 small bunch arugula, trimmed and washed (about 1 cup)

Heat a medium nonstick skillet over medium heat and add the oil. Add the onions, pepper, chili powder, and oregano. Cook, stirring occasionally, for 10 to 12 minutes, or until the onions are golden and tender. Remove from the heat and cool for 10 minutes.

Place ¼ pound turkey down the center of each tortilla. Top with 2 tablespoons cranberry sauce, 2 tablespoons onion mixture, and ¼ cup loosely packed arugula leaves. With the filling facing you horizontally, fold the bottom of the tortilla up over the filling. Fold in the 2 sides and then roll the bottom over the filling and tidy-up the sides to form a neat package.

Makes 4 servings

Per serving: 331 calories, 26 g protein, 39 g carbohydrates, 9 g fat, 45 mg cholesterol, 1,120 mg sodium, 4 g dietary fiber
Diet Exchanges: ½ fruit, 1 ½ vegetable, 1 bread, 3 meat, 1 ½ fat
Carb Choices: 3

TURKEY PICADILLO SANDWICHES

The mix of sweet and savory flavors in this sandwich, combined with a kick of fiber, will stay with you longer so you won't be vulnerable to between-meal snacking.

Prep time: 30 minutes • Cook time: 31 minutes

1 teaspoon olive oil	3 tablespoons balsamic vinegar
1 large onion, finely chopped	⅓ cup golden raisins, chopped
1 large red bell pepper, chopped	¼ cup pimiento-stuffed green olives, chopped
¾ pound ground turkey breast meat	
2 cloves garlic, chopped	¼ teaspoon salt
1 tablespoon chili powder	¼ teaspoon freshly ground black pepper
2 teaspoons ground cumin	4 soft whole wheat sandwich buns
¼ teaspoon ground cinnamon	
1 can (16 ounces) no-salt-added tomato sauce	

Heat a nonstick skillet over medium heat. Add the oil, onion, and bell pepper and cook for 10 minutes, or until softened, stirring occasionally. Increase the heat to medium-high and add the turkey. Cook for 5 minutes, or until browned and no longer pink in the center, breaking up the meat with a spoon.

Stir in the garlic, chili powder, cumin, and cinnamon and cook for 1 minute. Add the tomato sauce, vinegar, raisins, olives, salt, and black pepper. Bring to a simmer and cook for 15 minutes, or until thickened, stirring occasionally.

Spoon the meat mixture onto the bottom halves of the buns, dividing evenly. Cover with the bun tops.

Makes 4 servings

Per serving: 391 calories, 21 g protein, 53 g carbohydrates, 12 g fat, 65 mg cholesterol, 620 mg sodium, 8 g dietary fiber
Diet Exchanges: 1 fruit, 3 vegetable, 2 bread, 2 meat, ½ fat
Carb Choices: 4

SICILIAN TUNA ON WHOLE GRAIN BREAD

Tuna is a rich source of body-building protein and omega-3 fatty acids. This sandwich, brimming with the sunny flavor of lemon and loads of crunchy vegetables, provides a nice alternative to traditional mayo-laden tuna combinations.

Prep time: 10 minutes

1 **can (6 ounces) solid white tuna in water, drained**

3 **tablespoons finely chopped carrot**

3 **tablespoons finely chopped celery**

2 **tablespoons finely chopped red onion**

2 **tablespoons finely chopped parsley**

2 **teaspoons capers, drained**

2 $^{1}/_{2}$ **teaspoons olive oil**

1 $^{1}/_{2}$ **teaspoons lemon juice**

$^{1}/_{8}$ **teaspoon crushed fennel seeds**

$^{1}/_{8}$ **teaspoon salt**

$^{1}/_{8}$ **teaspoon freshly ground black pepper**

4 **slices multigrain bread**

In a medium bowl, combine the tuna, carrot, celery, onion, parsley, and capers. Mix well to combine. Stir in the olive oil, lemon juice, fennel seeds, salt, and pepper. Place 2 slices of the bread on a work surface and top each with half of the tuna mixture. Top with the remaining bread slices.

Note: Prepare the tuna and chopped vegetables the day before and refrigerate until ready to use. Before serving, stir in the capers, olive oil, lemon juice, fennel seeds, salt, and pepper.

Makes 2 servings

Per serving: 270 calories, 26 g protein, 29 g carbohydrates, 6 g fat, 35 mg cholesterol, 900 mg sodium, 5 g dietary fiber
Diet Exchanges: $^{1}/_{2}$ vegetable, 2 bread, 3 meat
Carb Choices: 2

LEMONY SHRIMP AND FENNEL SALAD SANDWICHES

Shrimp is America's favorite shellfish. It's a great source of low-calorie protein—only 84 calories for a 3-ounce serving. In this sandwich, it pairs particularly well with the light licorice flavors of fresh fennel.

Prep time: 15 minutes

¼ cup low-fat plain yogurt

1½ tablespoons light mayonnaise

1 tablespoon lemon juice

1 teaspoon grated lemon peel

¼ teaspoon sugar

¼ teaspoon salt

⅛ teaspoon hot red-pepper sauce

½ small fennel bulb, cored, trimmed, thinly sliced crosswise, and coarsely chopped into ¾" pieces

8 ounces medium shrimp, cooked

2 tablespoons chopped fennel fronds or parsley

2 tablespoons chopped peeled shallots or scallions

8 slices whole grain bread, toasted

8 soft lettuce leaves

In a medium bowl, whisk together the yogurt, mayonnaise, lemon juice, lemon peel, sugar, salt, and pepper sauce until blended. Add the fennel, shrimp, fennel fronds or parsley, and shallots or scallions to the bowl. Toss to combine.

Set 4 slices of bread on a cutting board. Top each with 2 lettuce leaves. Spoon the salad on top, dividing evenly and spreading level. Top with the remaining bread slices and cut on the diagonal.

Note: The salad can be made up to 6 hours in advance and kept refrigerated.

Makes 4 servings

Per serving: 238 calories, 19 g protein, 32 g carbohydrates, 5 g fat, 115 mg cholesterol, 650 mg sodium, 5 g dietary fiber
Diet Exchanges: ½ vegetable, 2 bread, 2 meat, ½ fat
Carb Choices: 2

GRILLED VEGETABLE SANDWICHES

This colorful assortment of vegetables, dressed with a splash of olive oil, makes for a sandwich sure to be on top of any menu. *Photo on page 136.*

Prep time: 20 minutes • Cook time: 16 minutes

¼ cup light mayonnaise

2 tablespoons chopped fresh basil

1 tablespoon jarred roasted garlic, chopped

2 teaspoons lemon juice

1 medium red onion, cut into 4 slices

1 large red bell pepper, cut into 8 slices

1 large zucchini, cut on an angle into 8 slices

2 teaspoons olive oil

¼ teaspoon salt

¼ teaspoon freshly ground black pepper

8 slices whole wheat sourdough bread

¾ cup prepared hummus

1 medium tomato, cut into 8 slices

In a small bowl, combine the mayonnaise, basil, garlic, and lemon juice. Set aside.

Coat a grill rack with cooking spray. Preheat the grill. Brush the onion, bell pepper, and zucchini with the olive oil. Sprinkle with salt and pepper.

Place the onion and peppers on the rack and grill for 10 to 12 minutes, turning once, or until the vegetables are well marked and tender. Place the zucchini slices on the rack and cook for 6 to 8 minutes, turning once, or until marked and tender.

Spread 4 slices of the bread with the hummus and place on a cutting board. Top each with an onion slice separated into rings, 2 bell pepper slices, 2 zucchini slices, and 2 tomato slices. Spread the remaining bread slices with the mayonnaise mixture and place on top of the tomatoes. Cut each sandwich in half to serve.

Note: The vegetables for this sandwich can be grilled the day before, then wrapped and stored in the refrigerator until ready to use.

Makes 4 servings

Per serving: 310 calories, 11 g protein, 45 g carbohydrates, 12 g fat, 5 mg cholesterol, 680 mg sodium, 9 g dietary fiber
Diet Exchanges: 1 ½ vegetable, 2 bread, 2 fat
Carb Choices: 3

ROASTED PEPPER AND SHALLOT PITAS WITH FETA

Sweet peppers are one of the most nutrient-dense vegetables you can buy. They are loaded with antioxidants, as are shallots, which are members of the onion family. Here they are gently caramelized to bring out even more of their natural sweetness.

Prep time: 30 minutes • Cook time: 15 minutes

4 red bell peppers, halved and cored

8 shallots, peeled (halved lengthwise if large)

¾ cup crumbled feta cheese

2 tablespoons chopped fresh basil

1 tablespoon chopped chives or scallions

1 tablespoon lemon juice

⅛ teaspoon salt

¼ teaspoon freshly ground black pepper

4 whole wheat pitas (6" diameter)

2 teaspoons chopped kalamata olives

Preheat the broiler. Line a baking sheet with foil.

Arrange the bell peppers skin side up on the baking sheet, nestling the shallots under the pepper halves. Broil for 8 minutes. Turn over the peppers and uncover the shallots. Broil for 4 to 6 minutes longer, or until softened and charred. Wrap up the vegetables in the foil and let stand for 10 minutes. Remove the peels from the peppers. Cut the peppers in half lengthwise and then cut crosswise into short strips. Slice the shallots.

Meanwhile, in a small bowl, stir together the feta, basil, chives or scallions, lemon juice, salt, and black pepper.

Spoon the feta mixture on the pitas, dividing evenly, and spread level. Top with the peppers, shallots, and olives, dividing evenly. Cut into quarters and serve warm or at room temperature.

Note: To serve warm, set the pitas on a baking sheet. Bake in a preheated 425°F oven for 4 minutes, or until heated through.

Makes 4 servings

Per serving: 304 calories, 12 g protein, 48 g carbohydrates, 9 g fat, 25 mg cholesterol, 810 mg sodium, 7 g dietary fiber
Diet Exchanges: 2 ½ vegetable, 2 bread, 1 ½ fat
Carb Choices: 3

CHICKPEA, FLAXSEED, AND OATMEAL BURGERS WITH TZATZIKI

These satisfying burgers put their distant fast-food cousins to shame! Chickpeas contain a whopping 7 grams of fiber per half-cup. Flaxseed (found in health food stores) is not only an excellent source of fiber but also a rich source of omega-3 fatty acids. Rolled oats will keep your blood sugar levels steady.

Prep time: 20 minutes • Cook time: 10 minutes

TZATZIKI

½ medium cucumber, peeled, seeded, grated, and squeezed dry

¼ cup fat-free plain yogurt

½ teaspoon minced garlic

⅛ teaspoon salt

⅛ teaspoon freshly ground black pepper

BURGERS

6 tablespoons flaxseed

1 can (15 ½ ounces) chickpeas, rinsed and drained

¼ cup rolled oats

2 cloves garlic

2 tablespoons water

¼ cup chopped fresh mint

2 tablespoons lemon juice

2 teaspoons ground cumin

1 teaspoon salt

⅛ teaspoon freshly ground black pepper

¼ cup panko bread crumbs

1 egg, lightly beaten

1 tablespoon olive oil

4 whole wheat hamburger buns

1 medium tomato, cut into 8 slices

½ cup alfalfa sprouts

To make the tzatziki: In a small bowl, combine the cucumber, yogurt, garlic, salt, and pepper. Cover and refrigerate while preparing the burgers.

To make the burgers: In a spice or coffee grinder, process 5 tablespoons of the flaxseed to a fine meal. In the bowl of a food processor, combine the chickpeas, oats, garlic, and water. Pulse until the mixture is coarsely chopped. Add the mint, lemon juice, cumin, salt, pepper, and flaxseed meal. Pulse the food processor until the mixture is just combined. Divide the mixture into 4 equal portions and shape each into a ½"-thick patty.

Combine the bread crumbs and remaining flaxseed on a plate. Dip the burgers in the egg, then dredge in the bread crumb mixture.

In a large nonstick skillet, heat the oil over medium-high heat. Add the burgers and cook for 5 to 6 minutes per side, or until golden.

On the bottom of each bun, place 2 tomato slices and 2 tablespoons alfalfa sprouts. Place the burgers on top of the sprouts and top each burger with a slightly rounded tablespoon of the tzatziki.

Makes 4 servings

Per serving: 408 calories, 15 g protein, 60 g carbohydrates, 14 g fat, 45 mg cholesterol, 1,220 mg sodium, 13 g dietary fiber
Diet Exchanges: ½ vegetable, 4 bread, ½ meat, 2 fat
Carb Choices: 4

FILL-YOU-UP

SALADS

(REALLY!)

FAST ■ SUPER FAST ■ FAST PREP

PERFECT TOMATO SALAD

Americans eat more nutrient-dense tomatoes, both fresh and processed, than any other vegetable or fruit. Pairing them with olive oil makes them even healthier. The mono-unsaturates in the oil will help your body absorb the red pigment in tomatoes called lycopene, a compound that may protect you from cancer and heart disease.

Prep time: 15 minutes • Stand time: 30 minutes

2 **pounds large red beefsteak or heirloom tomatoes**

1 **cup halved mixed yellow, red, and green cherry tomatoes or small pear tomatoes**

½–¾ **cup thinly sliced sweet white onion (optional)**

½ **teaspoon freshly ground black pepper**

¼ **teaspoon salt**

1 **tablespoon olive oil**

1 **tablespoon balsamic vinegar**

½ **cup loosely packed torn fresh basil (or small whole basil leaves)**

Rinse the large tomatoes and core them. Cut into thick slices and arrange on a large platter. Scatter the halved cherry or pear tomatoes and the onion slices (if using) over the tomato slices. Sprinkle with the pepper and salt.

In a cup, mix the oil and balsamic vinegar with a fork. Drizzle over the salad and sprinkle the basil over all. Cover with a sheet of waxed paper and let stand for 30 minutes before serving.

Makes 6 side-dish servings

Per serving: 61 calories, 2 g protein, 9 g carbohydrates, 3 g fat, 0 mg cholesterol, 115 mg sodium, 2 g dietary fiber
Diet Exchanges: 1 ½ vegetable, ½ fat
Carb Choices: 1

ROASTED BEET AND APPLE SALAD

The combination of beets and apples in this salad makes for a one-of-a-kind taste!

Prep time: 10 minutes ● Cook time: 1 hour 3 minutes

3/4 **pound medium beets, weighed without greens (see note)**

2 **tablespoons pecans**

5 **teaspoons balsamic vinegar**

1 **tablespoon olive oil**

1 **teaspoon chopped fresh rosemary**

1/2 **teaspoon Dijon mustard**

1/4 **teaspoon salt**

1/8 **teaspoon freshly ground black pepper**

1 **medium shallot, halved and thinly sliced**

3 **cups torn escarole, or 1 large bunch watercress, tough stems trimmed**

1 **medium Gala or Fuji apple (6 ounces), cored and cut into matchsticks**

Preheat the oven to 400°F.

Trim the tops from the beets, leaving 1/2" of the stems and the roots intact. Place the beets on a piece of foil. Fold the foil up and over the beets and fold the edges to seal. Place the foil packet directly on the oven rack and roast for 1 to 1 1/2 hours, or until the beets are tender. Remove from the oven, open the packet, and set aside until cool enough to handle. Peel the beets and cut into thin wedges.

Cook the pecans in a small nonstick skillet over medium heat, stirring often, for 3 to 4 minutes, or until lightly toasted. Tip onto a plate and let cool. Chop coarsely.

In a salad bowl, mix the vinegar, oil, rosemary, mustard, salt, and pepper with a fork. Stir in the shallot. Add the beets, escarole or watercress, apple, and the toasted pecans. Toss gently to mix.

Note: The beets can be cooked 1 or 2 days ahead.

Makes 4 side-dish servings

Per serving: 129 calories, 2 g protein, 18 g carbohydrates, 6 g fat, 0 mg cholesterol, 240 mg sodium, 5 g dietary fiber
Diet Exchanges: 1/2 fruit, 2 vegetable, 1 fat
Carb Choices: 1

SAUTÉED PEPPER SALAD WITH GOLDEN RAISINS AND PINE NUTS

Not many vegetables can live up to the fine nutritional profile of a sweet pepper. They are dense with the vitamins and minerals your body needs, including heart-healthy beta-carotene. This dish contains lots of monounsaturated fats, another nutrient your heart loves.

Prep time: 6 minutes • Cook time: 12 minutes • Stand time: 15 minutes

1 **tablespoon + 1 teaspoon olive oil**

1 **large red bell pepper, cut into thin strips**

1 **teaspoon brown sugar**

1/4 **teaspoon + 1/8 teaspoon salt**

1/4 **teaspoon freshly ground black pepper**

1 **tablespoon + 1 teaspoon balsamic vinegar**

2 **tablespoons orange juice**

2 **tablespoons golden raisins**

2 **tablespoons pine nuts or slivered almonds**

3 **cups arugula or baby spinach**

Heat 1 tablespoon oil in a large nonstick skillet over medium heat. Add the pepper and sprinkle with the brown sugar, 1/4 teaspoon salt, and 1/8 teaspoon of the pepper. Stir to mix well. Cook, stirring often, for 8 to 10 minutes, or until the pepper is very tender and lightly browned.

Add 1 tablespoon of the vinegar and let bubble for 30 seconds. Stir in the orange juice and raisins and transfer the pepper strips and any cooking juices to a small bowl. Cover loosely with a sheet of waxed paper and let stand for 15 to 25 minutes, or until at room temperature.

Meanwhile, cook the pine nuts or slivered almonds in a small nonstick skillet over medium heat, stirring often, for 3 to 4 minutes, or until lightly toasted. Tip onto a plate and let cool.

Place the arugula or spinach in a shallow serving bowl. Add the 1/8 teaspoon salt and the remaining 1 teaspoon oil, 1 teaspoon balsamic vinegar, and 1/8 teaspoon pepper. Toss to coat the leaves.

Spoon the pepper mixture over the arugula or baby spinach and sprinkle with the pine nuts or almonds.

Makes 4 side-dish or first-course servings

Per serving: 105 calories, 2 g protein, 11 g carbohydrates, 7 g fat, 0 mg cholesterol, 240 mg sodium, 1 g dietary fiber
Diet Exchanges: 1/2 fruit, 1 vegetable, 1 fat
Carb Choices: 1

ANTIPASTO SALAD

Enjoy the bright, summer-fresh flavors in this salad any time of year.

Prep time: 18 minutes • Stand time: 5 minutes

- 2 **tablespoons lemon juice**
- 1 **tablespoon + 1 teaspoon extra-virgin olive oil**
- 1 **small clove garlic, minced**
- ¼ **teaspoon salt**
- ¼ **teaspoon freshly ground black pepper**
- 1 **cup water-packed artichoke hearts, drained and rinsed, cut into quarters, tough outer leaves removed**
- ⅓ **cup thinly sliced red onion**
- 2 **cups baby arugula or baby spinach**
- 2 **cups torn escarole or romaine lettuce**
- 2 **medium plum tomatoes, cut into thin wedges**
- ½ **cup sliced celery hearts**
- ½ **cup sliced roasted red peppers**
- ¼ **cup coarsely chopped fresh basil**

In a small jar, place the lemon juice, oil, garlic, salt, and black pepper. Cover the jar with the lid and shake until blended.

Put the artichoke hearts and red onion in a small bowl and mix with 1 tablespoon of the dressing. Set aside for 5 to 10 minutes to blend the flavors.

To assemble, in a large bowl, combine the arugula or spinach, escarole or romaine, tomatoes, celery, and red peppers. Add the remaining dressing and toss until well coated. Arrange on a platter. Spoon the marinated artichokes over top and sprinkle with the basil.

Makes 4 side-dish servings

Per serving: 80 calories, 2 g protein, 9 g carbohydrates, 5 g fat, 0 mg cholesterol, 390 mg sodium, 3 g dietary fiber
Diet Exchanges: 1 ½ vegetable, 1 fat
Carb Choices: ½

WINTER SALAD WITH ROQUEFORT

Walnuts are a nutritional powerhouse. They not only contain compounds that may protect you from heart disease and cancer, but they are also rich in fiber and monounsaturated fats and have a smattering of omega-3s.

Prep time: 20 minutes • Cook time: 4 minutes

2   tablespoons walnuts

5   teaspoons cider vinegar

1   tablespoon walnut oil (see note)

2   teaspoons honey

1   teaspoon olive oil

1   teaspoon salt

¼   teaspoon freshly ground black pepper

¼   cup chopped red onion

3   cups torn romaine lettuce

½   cup finely shredded red cabbage

½   cup shredded carrot

1   medium Granny Smith, Gala, or Golden Delicious apple, cored and thinly sliced, slices cut in half

2   tablespoons crumbled Roquefort or blue cheese

Cook the walnuts in a small nonstick skillet over medium heat, stirring often, for 3 to 4 minutes, or until lightly toasted. Tip onto a plate and let cool. Chop coarsely.

In a salad bowl, mix the vinegar, walnut oil, honey, olive oil, salt, and pepper with a fork. Stir in the red onion.

Add the romaine, red cabbage, carrot, and apple and toss to mix well. Sprinkle with the cheese and the toasted walnuts.

Note: Walnut oil is very perishable and must be kept in the refrigerator. Let it come to room temperature before using.

Makes 4 side-dish servings

Per serving: 131 calories, 3 g protein, 13 g carbohydrates, 8 g fat, 5 mg cholesterol, 670 mg sodium, 3 g dietary fiber
Diet Exchanges: ½ fruit, 1 vegetable, 1 ½ fat
Carb Choices: 1

CURRIED SWEET POTATO SALAD

FAST PREP

Put an end to those erratic blood sugar levels. Sweet potatoes are rich in complex carbo-hydrates and fiber, which will help your body maintain stable stores of energy.

Photo on page 201.

Prep time: 20 minutes • Cook time: 14 minutes

2 **pounds sweet potatoes, peeled and cut into rough $^3/_4$" chunks**

3 **tablespoons pecans**

$^1/_2$ **cup fat-free plain yogurt**

2 **tablespoons light mayonnaise**

2 **tablespoons brown sugar**

$^1/_2$ **teaspoon curry powder**

$^1/_8$ **teaspoon salt**

1 **cup juice-packed canned pineapple tidbits, drained**

3 **scallions, sliced**

Place the sweet potatoes in a large saucepan and barely cover with cold water. Cover and bring to a boil over high heat. Reduce the heat to low, and simmer, covered, for 10 to 12 minutes, or until tender. Drain and let cool.

Meanwhile, cook the pecans in a small nonstick skillet over medium heat, stirring often, for 3 to 4 minutes, or until lightly toasted. Tip onto a plate and let cool. Chop coarsely.

In a salad bowl, whisk the yogurt, mayonnaise, sugar, curry powder, and salt until well blended. Add the pineapple, scallions, and sweet potatoes. Mix gently with a rubber spatula. Sprinkle with the toasted pecans and serve immediately, or cover and chill until ready to serve.

Makes 6 side-dish servings

Per serving: 241 calories, 4 g protein, 49 g carbohydrates, 4 g fat, 0 mg cholesterol, 125 mg sodium, 6 g dietary fiber
Diet Exchanges: $^1/_2$ fruit, 2 $^1/_2$ bread, $^1/_2$ fat
Carb Choices: 3

BROWN RICE AND MINTED CUCUMBER SALAD

Brown rice contains more fiber and complex carbohydrates than its paler cousin. It acts like a sponge, absorbing water as it makes its way through the intestinal tract, leaving you feeling full and satisfied.

Prep time: 20 minutes • **Cook time: 50 minutes** • **Stand time: 30 minutes**

1 **cup brown rice, preferably short-grain (see note)**	2 **cups chopped hothouse or kirby cucumbers, peeled (about ½ long cucumber)**
2½ **cups water**	1 **cup chopped radishes (about 6 radishes)**
4 **cardamom pods**	4 **scallions, chopped**
1 **bay leaf**	⅓ **cup coarsely chopped fresh mint**
1¼ **teaspoons salt**	½ **teaspoon freshly ground black pepper**
1½ **cups fat-free plain yogurt**	

Put the rice, water, cardamom pods, bay leaf, and ¾ teaspoon of the salt in a heavy medium saucepan. Bring to a boil over high heat. Reduce the heat to low, cover, and simmer for 50 to 60 minutes, or until the rice is tender and the water has been absorbed.

Transfer the rice to a bowl, cover with waxed paper, and refrigerate or let stand at room temperature for 30 minutes, or until cooled. Discard the cardamom pods and bay leaf.

Add the yogurt, cucumbers, radishes, scallions, mint, pepper, and the remaining ½ teaspoon salt to the rice. Stir to mix well. Serve immediately or cover and chill until ready to serve.

Note: You can use leftover rice for this recipe, in which case you'll need 3 cups. Otherwise, you can cook the rice earlier in the day or the day before.

Makes 6 side-dish servings

Per serving: 156 calories, 6 g protein, 32 g carbohydrates, 2 g fat, 0 mg cholesterol, 530 mg sodium, 2 g dietary fiber
Diet Exchanges: ½ milk, 1 vegetable, 1½ bread
Carb Choices: 2

BROCCOLI AND NAPA CABBAGE SALAD WITH MISO DRESSING

Perfect for a picnic, the bright, sweet flavors in this crunchy salad are pure refreshment.

Prep time: 15 minutes • Cook time: 10 minutes

1 tablespoon sesame seeds

2 cups small broccoli florets

1 ½ tablespoons mellow white miso

1 ½ tablespoons rice wine vinegar

1 tablespoon canola oil

2 teaspoons reduced-sodium soy sauce

1 teaspoon flax oil

¾ teaspoon finely grated peeled fresh ginger

½ teaspoon brown sugar

4 cups sliced napa cabbage or iceberg lettuce (1"-thick slices)

½ cup thinly sliced radishes

1 kirby cucumber, thinly sliced

2 scallions, thinly sliced

1 large carrot, peeled

In a small skillet, cook the sesame seeds over medium heat, tossing, for 2 minutes, until light golden. Tip out onto a plate and let cool.

Bring ½" water to a boil in a medium saucepan. Add the broccoli, cover, and cook, stirring several times, for 4 minutes, until crisp-tender. Drain and cool briefly under cold running water.

In a salad bowl, whisk together the miso, rice vinegar, canola oil, soy sauce, flax oil, ginger, and sugar, until well blended.

Add the cabbage or lettuce, radishes, cucumber, scallions, and broccoli. With a vegetable peeler, peel long, curly strands from the carrot, letting them drop into the salad bowl. Toss the salad to mix, sprinkle with the toasted sesame seeds, and serve.

Makes 4 servings

Per serving: 110 calories, 4 g protein, 12 g carbohydrates, 6 g fat, 0 mg cholesterol, 330 mg sodium, 5 g dietary fiber
Diet Exchanges: 2 vegetable, 1 fat
Carb Choices: 1

CANTALOUPE AND WATERCRESS SALAD WITH PICKLED ONIONS

Both cantaloupe and plums are succulent, low-calorie treats that are just as tempting as any sugary snack but with a kiss of fiber thrown in for good measure. *Photo on page 202.*

Prep time: 20 minutes

$\frac{1}{3}$ **cup coarsely chopped red onion**

$\frac{1}{4}$ **teaspoon grated lime peel**

2 **tablespoons lime juice**

$\frac{1}{8}$ **teaspoon salt**

1 **tablespoon olive oil**

2 **tablespoons honey**

$\frac{1}{4}$ **teaspoon freshly ground black pepper**

3 **cups $\frac{3}{4}$" chunks ripe cantaloupe**

2 **ripe plums, thinly sliced**

1 **bunch watercress, tough stems trimmed**

2 **tablespoons crumbled goat cheese or feta cheese**

2 **tablespoons sliced almonds or pumpkin seeds**

In a salad bowl, mix the onion, lime peel, lime juice, salt, oil, honey, and pepper with a fork. Stir to combine.

Add the cantaloupe, plums, watercress, cheese, and almonds or pumpkin seeds, and toss to mix. Serve immediately.

Makes 6 first-course servings

Per serving: 110 calories, 2 g protein, 18 g carbohydrates, 4 g fat, 0 mg cholesterol, 75 mg sodium, 2 g dietary fiber
Diet Exchanges: 1 fruit, 1 fat
Carb Choices: 1

ORANGE AND OLIVE SALAD

Everyone knows that oranges are an awesome source of vitamin C, but they are also bursting with fiber. One orange packs 3.1 grams of fiber. *Photo on page 203.*

Prep time: 20 minutes ● Stand time: 15 minutes

5 medium navel oranges (1 ½ cups sliced)

½ cup thinly sliced radishes (optional)

¼ cup thinly sliced red onion

6 kalamata olives, pitted and sliced

¼ teaspoon freshly ground black pepper

1 tablespoon olive oil

1 teaspoon balsamic vinegar

   Pinch of dried oregano

¼ teaspoon salt

With a sharp knife, peel the oranges, cutting off most, but not all, of the white pith. Cut the oranges in thin crosswise slices and arrange on a platter. Scatter the radishes (if using), red onion, and olives on top. Sprinkle with the pepper.

In a cup, mix the oil, vinegar, oregano, and salt with a fork. Spoon evenly over the oranges. Cover and let stand for at least 15 minutes before serving.

Makes 4 side-dish servings

Per serving: 140 calories, 1 g protein, 27 g carbohydrates, 5 g fat, 0 mg cholesterol, 238 mg sodium, 9 g dietary fiber
Diet Exchanges: 1 ½ fruit, ½ vegetable, 1 fat
Carb Choices: 2

GRAPEFRUIT, MANGO, AND AVOCADO SALAD WITH SHERRY DRESSING

Avocados are one of the best sources of monounsaturated fats you can buy. Just half of one of these buttery beauties delivers 9.7 grams! Mixing avocados with the fiber of mangoes and grapefruit gives you a tropical treat for your tastebuds.

Prep time: 20 minutes

1 tablespoon olive oil

1 tablespoon medium-dry sherry or sherry vinegar

1 ½ teaspoons red wine vinegar

¼ teaspoon salt

⅛ teaspoon freshly ground black pepper

1 large pink grapefruit

4 cups colorful mixed baby greens

1 cup sliced ripe avocado

1 cup sliced ripe mango

2 tablespoons chopped red onion

In a salad bowl, mix the oil, sherry or sherry vinegar, red wine vinegar, salt, and pepper with a fork.

With a serrated knife, peel the grapefruit, cutting off most, but not all, of the white pith. Working over a bowl, cut out the fruit from between the membranes. Add 1 ½ tablespoons of the grapefruit juice to the dressing and mix well.

Add the greens, avocado, mango, red onion, and the grapefruit sections to the dressing and toss gently to mix. Serve immediately.

Makes 4 first-course servings

Per serving: 129 calories, 2 g protein, 12 g carbohydrates, 9 g fat, 0 mg cholesterol, 220 mg sodium, 4 g dietary fiber
Diet Exchanges: ½ fruit, ½ vegetable, 2 fat
Carb Choices: 1

PINEAPPLE AND STRAWBERRIES WITH CILANTRO AND PEPPER

Pineapples and strawberries offer a fresh, delicious way to indulge your sweet tooth without the saturated fat and sugar found in many processed treats.

Prep time: 10 minutes • Stand time: 15 minutes • Chill time: 30 minutes

2   cups hulled and quartered fresh straw-
    berries

1   tablespoon packed brown sugar

4   cups ½" chunks fresh pineapple

¼   cup chopped fresh cilantro

¼   teaspoon ground cinnamon

⅛   teaspoon ground cumin

¼   teaspoon freshly ground black pepper

Mix the strawberries and sugar in a serving bowl. Let stand for 15 minutes to let the juices flow.

Add the pineapple, cilantro, cinnamon, cumin, and pepper to the strawberries and stir gently to mix. Cover and chill for at least 30 minutes, or until ready to serve.

Makes 6 to 8 side-dish servings

Per serving: 75 calories, 1 g protein, 19 g carbohydrates, 1 g fat, 0 mg cholesterol, 0 mg sodium, 3 g dietary fiber
Diet Exchanges: 1 fruit
Carb Choices: 1

SPINACH AND STRAWBERRY SALAD
WITH FRESH MOZZARELLA

This colorful salad is bursting with flavor. The smooth, creamy textures of fresh mozzarella and perfectly ripe avocados are the perfect match when paired with this sweet strawberry dressing.

Prep time: 18 minutes • Cook time: 5 minutes

3 tablespoons chopped whole or slivered almonds

2 cups hulled and sliced strawberries

2 tablespoons extra-virgin olive oil

2 tablespoons honey

1 tablespoon + 1 teaspoon balsamic vinegar

½ teaspoon salt

⅛ teaspoon freshly ground black pepper

1 bag (6 ounces) baby spinach

1 ripe medium mango, peeled and cut in small chunks

3 small balls fresh mozzarella (about 5 ounces total), cut in small chunks

1 ripe avocado, peeled and cut in small chunks

Cook the almonds in a small skillet over medium heat, tossing often, for 3 to 4 minutes, or until lightly toasted. Tip onto a plate and let cool.

Put ½ cup of the strawberries, the oil, honey, and balsamic vinegar in a food processor. Process until smooth. Scrape into a salad bowl and stir in the salt and pepper.

Add the spinach, mango, the toasted almonds, and the remaining 1 ½ cups strawberries to the dressing and toss to mix well. Sprinkle the mozzarella and avocado over the top.

Makes 4 main-dish servings

Per serving: 330 calories, 10 g protein, 26 g carbohydrates, 22 g fat, 30 mg cholesterol, 420 mg sodium, 6 g dietary fiber
Diet Exchanges: ½ fruit, 1 vegetable, ½ bread, 1 meat, 4 fat
Carb Choices: 2

A BIG FAT GREEK SALAD

With a nod to the heart-healthy cuisine enjoyed by our Mediterranean friends, this robust salad is loaded with monounsaturated fats and fiber. *Photo on page 204.*

Prep time: 20 minutes ● Stand time: 15 minutes

2 tablespoons olive oil	2 cups hothouse cucumber chunks
1 tablespoon lemon juice	½ cup thinly sliced red onion
1 tablespoon red wine vinegar	½ cup coarsely chopped fresh flat-leaf parsley
½ teaspoon dried oregano, crumbled	8 kalamata olives, pitted and sliced
½ teaspoon freshly ground black pepper	4 cups torn mixed dark-hued greens, such as escarole and romaine lettuce, or use all romaine
2 large red tomatoes (1 pound), cut into chunks	
1 can (15 ounces) chickpeas, rinsed and drained	4 ounces feta cheese, chopped

In a large salad bowl, mix the oil, lemon juice, vinegar, oregano, and pepper with a fork.

Add the tomatoes, chickpeas, cucumber, red onion, parsley, and olives. Toss to mix well. If you have time, let marinate for 15 minutes.

Add the greens and feta and toss again.

Makes 4 main-dish servings

Per serving: 338 calories, 12 g protein, 34 g carbohydrates, 16 g fat, 25 mg cholesterol, 690 mg sodium, 8 g dietary fiber
Diet Exchanges: 2 vegetable, 1 ½ bread, 3 fat
Carb Choices: 2

ROASTED POTATO AND GREEN BEAN SALAD
WITH OLIVE DRESSING

Roasted potatoes, crunchy beans, and zippy olive dressing share center stage in this summer-fresh salad that's sure to become a regular menu item.

Prep time: 18 minutes • Cook time: 35 minutes • Cooling time: 10 minutes

1 **pound small thin-skinned potatoes, quartered**

3 **tablespoons extra-virgin olive oil**

2 **large cloves garlic, minced**

2 **teaspoons Dijon mustard**

¼ **teaspoon salt**

½ **teaspoon freshly ground black pepper**

1 **pound fresh green beans, trimmed and halved**

3 **large eggs**

1 **tablespoon + 2 teaspoons red wine vinegar**

8 **kalamata olives, pitted and coarsely chopped**

½ **cup thinly sliced red onion**

3 **cups colorful mixed greens**

2 **medium tomatoes**

Preheat the oven to 425°F. Coat an 11" × 8" baking pan with olive oil cooking spray.

Place the potatoes in the prepared pan. Drizzle with 1 teaspoon of the oil, the garlic, mustard, ⅛ teaspoon of the salt, and ¼ teaspoon of the pepper. Toss to mix. Roast, turning several times, for 30 to 35 minutes, until the potatoes are tender and browned. Remove from the oven and let cool for 10 minutes.

Meanwhile, bring ½" water to a boil in a medium skillet. Add the beans. Cover and cook for 6 to 8 minutes, until tender. Drain and cool briefly under cold running water.

Place the eggs in a medium saucepan and cover with cold water. Bring to a boil over high heat. Reduce the heat to low and simmer slowly for 10 minutes. Cool under cold running water and shell.

In a small bowl, mix the vinegar, olives, and the remaining oil, $1/8$ teaspoon salt, and $1/4$ teaspoon pepper with a fork.

Put the green beans and red onion in a medium bowl and toss with 1 to 2 tablespoons of the dressing.

Arrange the greens on a large oval platter. Place a mound of potatoes on one side and a mound of green beans on the other side. Cut the eggs and tomatoes into wedges and arrange around the salad. Drizzle with the remaining dressing.

Makes 4 main-dish servings

Per serving: 340 calories, 10 g protein, 37 g carbohydrates, 17 g fat, 160 mg cholesterol, 380 mg sodium, 8 g dietary fiber
Diet Exchanges: 2 $1/2$ vegetable, 1 $1/2$ bread, 1 meat, 3 fat
Carb Choices: 2

DRESS FOR SUCCESS

On this plan, you can use any low-fat dressing you like, but Ann Fittante, MS, RD, recommends using dressings made with olive, canola, or flax oil. Unlike many bottled low-fat brands, these dressings are 100 percent healthy fats with no artery-clogging trans fats.

Flax oil is light and nutty tasting, so it's perfect for salad dressing. Plus, it's a rich source of omega-3 fatty acids.

Note: Flax oil is highly vulnerable to heat and light. To keep it fresh and tasty, store it in the refrigerator and use it in salad dressing or add it to cooked food. For cooking, use canola or olive oil.

FLAXSEED VINAIGRETTE

4 tablespoons flax oil

2 tablespoons balsamic or red wine vinegar

1 medium clove crushed garlic

Pinch of salt

Freshly ground pepper, rosemary, thyme, and other fresh or dried herbs to taste

In a small bowl, whisk together the oil, vinegar, garlic, salt, and spices. Each tablespoon contains about 70 calories and 8 grams of fat. To make a larger batch, use 1 cup flax oil, $1/2$ cup balsamic or red wine vinegar, 3 to 5 cloves of crushed garlic, and spices.

SPRING'S BEST SALAD

Salads don't have to be "rabbit food." This hearty mix of lean protein, fiber, and complex carbohydrates has the staying power to act as a real meal.

Prep time: 15 minutes • Cook time: 26 minutes

3 large eggs

½ pound small thin-skinned potatoes, scrubbed and quartered

2 pinches of salt

1 pound asparagus, tough stems trimmed, cut into 2" lengths

4 cups baby spinach

½ cup sliced radishes

½ cup halved grape tomatoes

1 knobby spring onion, or 3 scallions, thinly sliced

⅓ cup Herbed Mustard Vinaigrette (page 212) or Roasted Garlic Vinaigrette (page 214)

Freshly ground black pepper

Place the eggs in a small saucepan and cover with cold water. Bring to a boil over high heat. Reduce the heat to low and simmer slowly for 10 minutes. Cool under cold running water and shell.

Place the potatoes in a medium saucepan and add a pinch of salt. Barely cover with cold water, cover, and bring to a boil over high heat. Reduce the heat to medium and cook for 8 to 10 minutes, or until tender. Drain and cool briefly under cold running water.

Place 1" of water in the same medium saucepan and bring to a boil over high heat. Add a pinch of salt and the asparagus and cook, stirring often, for 3 to 4 minutes, or until bright green and crisp-tender. Drain and cool briefly under cold running water.

On a large platter, make a bed of the spinach. Cut the eggs into wedges. Place the eggs, potatoes, asparagus, radishes, and tomatoes in mounds. Sprinkle with the onion. Spoon the dressing over or serve on the side. Season to taste with the pepper.

Note: For a little more variety, try adding 1 can of flaked water-packed tuna, salmon, or some cooked and shelled medium shrimp.

Makes 4 main-dish servings

Per serving: 207 calories, 11 g protein, 21 g carbohydrates, 10 g fat, 160 mg cholesterol, 250 mg sodium, 6 g dietary fiber
Diet Exchanges: 2 vegetable, ½ bread, 1 meat, 1½ fat
Carb Choices: 1

CURRIED COUSCOUS SALAD

Couscous, a tiny pearl-like grain, is a staple in North African countries. Just a ½-cup serving of whole wheat couscous provides over 7 grams of protein, which will help you feel less tempted to snack. Some experts believe that combining protein with complex carbohydrates (like those found in beans) reduces cravings for sweets.

Prep time: 15 minutes • Cook time: 8 minutes • Stand time: 1 hour

1 ¼ cups reduced-sodium chicken or vegetable broth

1 small zucchini, coarsely chopped

1–2 teaspoons green curry paste

¼ teaspoon freshly ground black pepper

1 cup whole wheat couscous

⅓ cup chopped dried apricots

3 tablespoons golden raisins

3 tablespoons slivered almonds

1 can (15–16 ounces) small pink beans, chili beans, or red kidney beans, rinsed and drained

1 large tomato, chopped

½ cup coarsely chopped fresh flat-leaf parsley

¼ cup chopped red onion

¼ cup lime juice

2 tablespoons olive oil

Stir the broth, zucchini, curry paste, and pepper in a medium saucepan. Cover and bring to a boil over high heat. Stir in the couscous, apricots, and raisins. Remove from the heat and let stand, covered, for 10 minutes.

Meanwhile, cook the almonds in a small nonstick skillet over medium heat, stirring often, for 3 to 4 minutes, or until lightly toasted. Tip onto a plate and let cool.

Fluff the couscous with a fork. Transfer to a large bowl, cover with a sheet of waxed paper, and let stand for 20 minutes, until cooled.

Add the beans, tomato, parsley, red onion, lime juice, and oil to the couscous mixture and stir to blend well. Cover and let stand for 30 minutes or refrigerate until ready to serve. Sprinkle with the almonds just before serving.

Makes 4 main-dish servings, 6 to 8 side-dish servings

Per serving: 350 calories, 12 g protein, 57 g carbohydrates, 10 g fat, 0 mg cholesterol, 480 mg sodium, 11 g dietary fiber
Diet Exchanges: 2 bread, ½ meat, 2 fat
Carb Choices: 4

MIDDLE-EASTERN SALAD WITH CRISP PITA WEDGES

The whole grain in this salad will help balance your blood sugar for hours.

Prep time: 20 minutes • Cook time: 12 minutes • Cooling time: 10 minutes

2 medium whole wheat pitas (6" diameter)

¾ teaspoon dried oregano, crumbled

3 tablespoons pine nuts

1 tablespoon sesame seeds

¼ cup lemon juice

3 tablespoons extra-virgin olive oil

1 clove garlic, minced

½ teaspoon paprika

½ teaspoon salt

1 can (15 ounces) pink beans or pinto beans, rinsed and drained

4 scallions, sliced

4 cups sliced romaine lettuce

1 cup chopped red bell pepper

1 cup small radishes, quartered

1 cup cucumber chunks

¼ cup snipped fresh dill

Preheat the oven to 400°F.

With kitchen scissors, cut around the perimeter of each pita to make 2 rounds. Place the rounds rough side up on a baking sheet and sprinkle with ½ teaspoon of the oregano. Place the pine nuts and sesame seeds in a small baking pan or ovenproof skillet.

Bake the pita for 8 to 10 minutes, without turning, until crisp and toasted. Bake the pine nuts and sesame seeds for 4 to 5 minutes, stirring twice, until browned. Remove both from the oven. Leave the pita breads on the baking sheet. Tip the nuts and seeds into a bowl. Let both cool. When the pita is cooled, break into rough 1" chunks.

Meanwhile, in a large salad bowl, mix the lemon juice, oil, garlic, paprika, salt, and the remaining ¼ teaspoon oregano with a fork. Add the beans and scallions, and stir to mix well. Let stand 10 minutes to blend the flavors.

Add the romaine, bell pepper, radishes, cucumber, and dill to the beans. Toss to mix well. Add the toasted pitas, pine nuts, and sesame seeds, and toss again.

Makes 4 main-dish servings

Per serving: 340 calories, 10 g protein, 40 g carbohydrates, 16 g fat, 0 mg cholesterol, 710 mg sodium, 10 g dietary fiber
Diet Exchanges: ½ vegetable, 2 bread, 3 fat
Carb Choices: 3

MEXICAN SHRIMP AND AVOCADO SALAD

Shrimp are a great low-fat, high-protein delicacy with a touch of omega-3 fatty acids.

Prep time: 25 minutes • Cook time: 4 minutes • Stand time: 10 minutes

1 pound medium shrimp, thawed if frozen, peeled and deveined

½ teaspoon grated lime peel

3 tablespoons lime juice

1 teaspoon ground cumin

½ teaspoon salt

¼ teaspoon freshly ground black pepper

Cayenne pepper

1 pound red tomatoes (1 ½ cups), cut into ½" chunks

½ cup coarsely chopped sweet white onion

¼ cup + 2 tablespoons coarsely chopped fresh cilantro

2 tablespoons chopped pimiento-stuffed green olives

1–2 tablespoons minced fresh jalapeño pepper, with the seeds

2 tablespoons olive oil

1 ripe avocado, halved, pitted, peeled, and cut into chunks

4 cups mixed blend of greens

Place the shrimp in a medium bowl and add the lime peel, 1 tablespoon of the lime juice, ½ teaspoon of the cumin, ¼ teaspoon of the salt, the black pepper, and cayenne pepper to taste. Mix well, cover, and set aside while preparing the salad.

In another medium bowl, place the tomatoes, onion, the ¼ cup cilantro, the olives, jalapeño pepper (to taste), oil, and the remaining 2 tablespoons lime juice, ½ teaspoon cumin, and ¼ teaspoon salt. Mix well. Let stand for 10 to 15 minutes to blend the flavors. Add the avocado and mix gently.

Place the mixed greens in a large shallow bowl and mound the avocado mixture in the center.

Coat a medium nonstick skillet with cooking spray. Warm over medium-high heat. Add the shrimp and cook, turning often, for 4 minutes, or until just opaque in the thickest part.

Add the shrimp and any pan juices to the salad and sprinkle with the 2 tablespoons cilantro. Serve immediately.

Makes 4 main-dish servings

Per serving: 296 calories, 27 g protein, 15 g carbohydrates, 16 g fat, 170 mg cholesterol, 570 mg sodium, 7 g dietary fiber

Diet Exchanges: 2 vegetable, 3 meat, 3 fat

Carb Choices: 1

SESAME NOODLES WITH SALMON

All fish contain omega-3 fatty acids, but salmon earns top honors. The deeper the color, the more fatty acids it has. Chinook salmon has the most.

Prep time: 20 minutes • Cook time: 15 minutes

5 ounces soba or whole wheat noodles	1 teaspoon grated lemon peel
3 cups small broccoli florets	2 tablespoons creamy peanut butter
2 large carrots, cut into thin diagonal slices	2 tablespoons reduced-sodium soy sauce
2 teaspoons toasted sesame oil	2 tablespoons lemon juice
1 cup thinly sliced scallions	1½–2 teaspoons Asian chili-and-garlic sauce
1 tablespoon minced peeled fresh ginger	1½ cups julienne-cut hothouse cucumber
1 tablespoon minced garlic	
12 ounces skinned salmon fillet, cut crosswise into slices about 1½" long and ⅓" thick	

Bring a large covered pot of water to a boil over high heat.

Add the soba or whole wheat noodles and cook, stirring often, for 2 minutes. Add the broccoli and carrots and continue cooking, stirring occasionally, for 4 minutes longer, or until the noodles are tender and the vegetables crisp-tender. Scoop out and reserve about ½ cup cooking liquid. Drain the noodles and vegetables in a colander.

In a large nonstick skillet, stir the oil, scallions, ginger, and garlic. Cook over medium heat, stirring often, for 3 to 4 minutes, or until the scallions are wilted. Transfer half of the mixture to a large salad bowl, leaving the remaining half in the skillet.

Add the salmon to the skillet and sprinkle with the lemon peel. Cook, stirring gently with a spatula, for 4 to 5 minutes, or until just opaque in the thickest part. Remove from the heat.

With a whisk, mix the peanut butter, soy sauce, lemon juice, and chili sauce into the scallion mixture in the salad bowl. Gradually whisk in 3 to 4 tablespoons of the reserved pasta cooking liquid until creamy.

Add the noodles, vegetables, and cucumber to the peanut butter mixture and toss to mix well. Add the salmon and any pan juices and toss gently. Serve immediately or refrigerate for 1 to 2 hours, until ready to serve. If the salad is too dry, add a little more pasta cooking liquid.

Makes 4 main-dish servings

Per serving: 410 calories, 28 g protein, 42 g carbohydrates, 16 g fat, 50 mg cholesterol, 610 mg sodium, 5 g dietary fiber
Diet Exchanges: 2 vegetable, 2 bread, 3 meat, 2 fat
Carb Choices: 3

ROASTED CARROT AND CHICKEN SALAD WITH PISTACHIOS

Roasting is a great way to bring out any vegetable's natural sweetness. In this colorful salad, tender chunks of carrot are the perfect counterpoint to the lingering, nutty flavor of crunchy pistachios. *Photo on page 205.*

Prep time: 20 minutes • Cook time: 25 minutes

- 1 **pound large carrots, peeled and cut into ½" diagonal slices (2 cups)**
- 1 **tablespoon brown sugar**
- 2 **tablespoons extra-virgin olive oil**
- ½ **teaspoon salt**
- ½ **teaspoon freshly ground black pepper**
- 2 **boneless, skinless chicken-breast halves (6 ounces each), cut crosswise in thin slices**
- 4 **tablespoons snipped fresh chives or sliced scallion greens**

- 1 **tablespoon + 1 teaspoon cider vinegar**
- 1 **medium shallot, thinly sliced**
- 2 **cups baby arugula**
- 1 **bunch watercress, tough stems removed**
- 1½ **cups halved red seedless grapes**
- 2 **tablespoons unsalted shelled chopped pistachios**

Preheat the oven to 425°F. Coat an 11" × 9" baking pan and a rimmed baking sheet with olive oil cooking spray.

Place the carrots in the prepared baking pan. Sprinkle with the sugar, 1 teaspoon of the olive oil, and ⅛ teaspoon each of the salt and pepper. Toss to coat well. Roast, stirring several times, for 25 minutes, until the carrots are tender and lightly golden at the edges.

About 5 minutes before the carrots are done, place the chicken in a mound on the prepared baking sheet. Drizzle with 1 teaspoon of the oil, and sprinkle with 2 tablespoons of the chives, and ⅛ teaspoon each of the salt and pepper. Toss to mix. Arrange in a single layer. Roast, turning once, for 5 to 7 minutes, until cooked through. Remove carrots and chicken from the oven and let cool a few minutes.

Meanwhile, in a salad bowl, mix the vinegar, shallot, and the remaining oil, 2 tablespoons chives, and ¼ teaspoon each salt and pepper. Let stand 5 minutes or more to blend the flavors.

To finish the salad, add the arugula, watercress, and grapes to the dressing and toss to mix well. Spread out on a platter. Top with the carrots, the chicken and any juices, and sprinkle with the pistachios. Serve warm.

Makes 4 main-dish servings

Per serving: 310 calories, 23 g protein, 32 g carbohydrates, 10 g fat, 50 mg cholesterol, 450 mg sodium, 5 g dietary fiber
Diet Exchanges: 1 fruit, 2 vegetable, ½ bread, 3 meat, 2 fat
Carb Choices: 2

WARM CHICKEN AND CASHEW STIR-FRY SALAD

The amount of fat in one cashew seems sinful. Fortunately, most of it is the mono-unsaturated kind, which means these rich, delicious nuggets are still allowed.

Prep time: 25 minutes • Cook time: 14 minutes

12 ounces boneless, skinless chicken breast halves, cut into thin crosswise strips

4 tablespoons reduced-sodium soy sauce

¼–½ teaspoon crushed red-pepper flakes

3 tablespoons raw cashews

2 tablespoons olive or canola oil

5 cloves garlic, slivered

1½ tablespoons slivered peeled fresh ginger

1 large red bell pepper, cut into thin strips

2 medium carrots, cut into thin slices

4 scallions, diagonally sliced

½ cup orange juice

3 cups shredded iceberg lettuce

3 cups baby spinach

In a medium bowl, mix the chicken, 2 tablespoons of the soy sauce, and the red-pepper flakes, to taste. Cover and set aside.

Cook the cashews in a small nonstick skillet over medium heat, stirring often, for 3 to 4 minutes, or until lightly toasted. Tip onto a plate and let cool.

Heat 1 tablespoon of the oil in a large nonstick skillet over medium-high heat. Add the garlic and ginger and stir-fry for 1 to 2 minutes, or until fragrant and lightly golden. Add the chicken and stir-fry for 3 to 4 minutes, or until no longer pink. Transfer to a clean bowl.

Place the remaining 1 tablespoon oil in the same skillet and heat over medium-high heat. Add the bell pepper and carrots, and stir-fry for 3 minutes. Add the scallions and stir-fry for 2 minutes longer, or until the vegetables are crisp-tender. Return the chicken and any juices to the skillet. Add the orange juice and the remaining 2 tablespoons soy sauce. Bring to a boil, stirring. Let boil for 30 seconds; remove from the heat.

Mix the lettuce and spinach on a large, deep platter or in a wide, shallow bowl. Spoon the chicken mixture on top. Sprinkle with the cashews and serve immediately.

Makes 4 main-dish servings

Per serving: 286 calories, 24 g protein, 18 g carbohydrates, 11 g fat, 50 mg cholesterol, 670 mg sodium, 4 g dietary fiber
Diet Exchanges: 2 vegetable, 3 meat, 2 fat
Carb Choices: 1

CHICKEN AND ASPARAGUS SALAD
WITH TARRAGON DRESSING

Extra guests dropping by for lunch? Serve this lovely salad on a bed of greens, such as a mixture of watercress and Bibb lettuce, a toss of baby greens, or with sliced tomatoes.

Prep time: 12 minutes • **Cook time: 30 minutes**

2 **boneless, skinless chicken breast halves
    (6 ounces each)**

   Pinch of salt

2 **large eggs**

1 **pound asparagus, tough ends trimmed, cut
    into 1" pieces**

¼ **cup + 2 tablespoons light mayonnaise**

1 **teaspoon grated lemon zest**

1 **tablespoon lemon juice**

½ **teaspoon dried tarragon, crumbled**

½ **teaspoon grainy mustard**

½ **teaspoon freshly ground black pepper**

1 **cup roughly chopped cucumber**

1 **cup thinly sliced celery**

4 **scallions, thinly sliced**

2 **tablespoons coarsely chopped walnuts**

Place the chicken breasts in a medium skillet. Add water to just cover and salt. Cover and bring to a boil over high heat. Reduce the heat to low and simmer slowly, turning the chicken once, for 8 to 10 minutes, until cooked through. Transfer to a plate and let stand until cool enough to handle. Tear into pieces.

Meanwhile, place the eggs in a medium saucepan and cover with cold water. Bring to a boil over high heat. Reduce the heat to low and simmer slowly for 10 minutes. Cool under cold running water and shell. Remove the yolks and save for another use. Coarsely chop the whites.

In the same saucepan, bring ½" water to a boil over high heat. Add the asparagus and cook, stirring often, for 4 to 5 minutes, until crisp-tender. Drain and cool briefly under cold running water.

In a salad bowl, whisk the mayonnaise, lemon zest and juice, tarragon, mustard, pepper, and ½ teaspoon salt. Add the cucumber, celery, scallions, chicken, egg whites, and asparagus and mix gently with a rubber spatula. Sprinkle with the walnuts and serve.

Makes 4 servings

Per serving: 260 calories, 26 g protein, 9 g carbohydrates, 14 g fat, 165 mg cholesterol, 310 mg sodium, 3 g dietary fiber
Diet Exchanges: 1 vegetable, 3 ½ meat, 2 fat
Carb Choices: ½

PORK AND CORN SALAD WITH TOMATO-BASIL DRESSING

Salads with meats such as pork and chicken make great stand-alone dinners, combining all of the elements of a healthy meal into one bowl.

Prep time: 15 minutes • Cook time: 8 minutes

1 pork tenderloin (12 ounces), well trimmed, cut into ½"- thick slices, each slice halved crosswise

½ cup slivered fresh basil

2 tablespoons olive oil

2 cloves garlic, minced

½ teaspoon coarsely ground black pepper

½ teaspoon salt

6 ounces diced canned tomatoes

2 teaspoons red wine vinegar

1½ cups frozen corn kernels

2 cups chopped red bell pepper

3 tablespoons water

4 cups colorful mixed baby greens

Place the pork in a medium bowl. Add ¼ cup of the basil, 1 tablespoon of the oil, the garlic, pepper, and ¼ teaspoon of the salt. Toss to coat the pork well. Set aside while preparing the rest of the salad.

Place the diced tomatoes in a large salad bowl. Stir in the vinegar and the remaining ¼ cup basil, 1 tablespoon oil, and ¼ teaspoon salt.

Place the corn, bell pepper, and water in a large nonstick skillet. Cover and cook over medium-high heat, stirring often, for 3 to 4 minutes, or until the corn is tender. Stir into the tomato mixture.

Dry the skillet. Place the pork in the same skillet and cook over medium heat, turning often, for 5 minutes, or until just slightly pink in the thickest part.

Add the pork and any pan juices to the tomato-corn mixture. Add the mixed greens and toss to blend the ingredients and wilt the greens slightly. Serve immediately.

Makes 4 main-dish servings

Per serving: 258 calories, 22 g protein, 23 g carbohydrates, 10 g fat, 55 mg cholesterol, 460 mg sodium, 5 g dietary fiber
Diet Exchanges: 1 vegetable, 1 bread, 3 meat, 2 fat
Carb Choices: 2

THAI BEEF SALAD

FAST PREP

Did you know that beef can be just as low in saturated fat and as good for you as chicken? Choose cuts that have the word *loin* or *round* in the name and you have a high-protein meal that is just as healthy as chicken. *Photo on page 206.*

Prep time: 20 minutes • Cook time: 12 minutes • Stand time: 10 minutes

1 lean boneless beef top round steak (12 ounces), well-trimmed

½ teaspoon crushed red-pepper flakes

3 tablespoons lime juice

5 teaspoons fish sauce

2 tablespoons olive or canola oil

1 tablespoon sugar

1 clove garlic, crushed through a press

6 cups shredded mixed red and green leaf lettuce, romaine, or colorful, crisp mixed greens

1 cup sliced cucumber

½ cup thinly sliced sweet white onion

½ cup thinly sliced radishes

½ cup coarsely chopped fresh cilantro

¼ cup coarsely chopped fresh mint

Preheat the broiler. Line a broiler pan with foil. Coat the broiler-pan rack with cooking spray. Rub the steak on both sides with ¼ teaspoon of the red-pepper flakes.

Broil the steak 4" to 6" from the heat source, turning once, for 12 to 15 minutes, depending on thickness, or until an instant read thermometer inserted in the center registers 145°F for medium-rare. Transfer to a plate.

In a large salad bowl, mix the lime juice, fish sauce, oil, sugar, garlic, and the remaining ¼ teaspoon red-pepper flakes with a fork. Spoon 1 tablespoon of the dressing over the steak on the plate and let the steak stand for 10 minutes.

Add the lettuce or greens, cucumber, onion, radishes, cilantro, and mint to the remaining dressing and toss to mix well. Divide among the 4 plates.

Cut the steak into thin slices on an angle and arrange on top of the salads. Spoon the steak juices over the top.

Makes 4 main-dish servings

Per serving: 250 calories, 21 g protein, 11 g carbohydrates, 14 g fat, 35 mg cholesterol, 630 mg sodium, 2 g dietary fiber
Diet Exchanges: 1 vegetable, 3 meat, 2 fat
Carb Choices: 1

HERBED MUSTARD VINAIGRETTE

This is a good basic dressing that's delicious on mixed greens, steamed asparagus, and boiled potatoes. Change the flavor by adding minced shallot or garlic or substituting lemon juice for the vinegar.

Prep time: 8 minutes

¼ **cup vegetable broth**

2 **tablespoons chopped fresh parsley**

2 **tablespoons red wine vinegar**

4 **teaspoons Dijon mustard**

1½ **teaspoons chopped fresh thyme**

¼ **teaspoon salt**

⅛ **teaspoon freshly ground black pepper**

⅓ **cup olive oil**

Place the broth, parsley, vinegar, mustard, thyme, salt, and pepper in a medium bowl. Whisk until well blended. Whisk in the oil in a slow, steady stream. Transfer to a small jar and refrigerate until ready to serve.

Note: This dressing will keep for 4 to 5 days in the refrigerator.

Makes twelve 1-tablespoon servings (¾ cup)

Per serving: 59 calories, 0 g protein, 0 g carbohydrates, 6 g fat, 0 mg cholesterol, 100 mg sodium, 0 g dietary fiber
Diet Exchanges: 1 fat
Carb Choices: 0

RASPBERRY VINAIGRETTE

This vinaigrette is great on mixed baby greens tossed with a few fresh raspberries and some chunks of cantaloupe. It's also nice on fresh fruit salads.

Prep time: 7 minutes

½ cup frozen raspberries, thawed, juices reserved

1 teaspoon sugar

¼ cup raspberry no-sugar spread

2 tablespoons frozen white grape and raspberry juice concentrate

2 tablespoons red wine vinegar

2 tablespoons olive oil (not extra-virgin)

½ teaspoon salt

⅛ teaspoon freshly ground black pepper

In a medium bowl, with a whisk, mash the raspberries and any juices with the sugar.

Add the raspberry spread, juice concentrate, vinegar, oil, salt, and pepper and whisk until well blended. Transfer to a small jar and refrigerate until ready to serve.

Makes twelve 1-tablespoon servings (¾ cup)

Per serving: 34 calories, 0 g protein, 6 g carbohydrates, 1 g fat, 0 mg cholesterol, 60 mg sodium, 0 g dietary fiber
Diet Exchanges: ½ fat
Carb Choices: 0

ROASTED GARLIC VINAIGRETTE

Try this vinaigrette on Spring's Best Salad (page 176) or with arugula tossed with sliced ripe pears, toasted pecans, and goat cheese.

Prep time: 12 minutes • Cook time: 45 minutes

1 medium head garlic, roasted

3 tablespoons chicken or vegetable broth

2 tablespoons balsamic vinegar

¼ cup chopped fresh flat-leaf parsley

2 teaspoons chopped fresh rosemary (optional)

½ teaspoon salt

¼ teaspoon freshly ground black pepper

⅓ cup olive oil

Preheat the oven to 400°F.

Cut a thin slice from the top of the garlic to expose the cloves. Place the head cut side up on a large piece of foil. Seal the top and sides of the foil tightly. Place in the oven and roast for 45 to 60 minutes, or until the cloves are very soft and lightly browned. Remove from the oven, open the packet, and set aside until cool enough to handle.

Squeeze the cloves into a medium bowl. With the back of a large metal spoon, mash the garlic to a smooth paste.

Gradually whisk in the broth and vinegar. Whisk in the parsley, rosemary (if using), salt, and pepper. Then whisk in the oil in a slow, steady stream. Transfer to a small jar and refrigerate until ready to serve.

Note: The dressing thickens in the fridge. Let it come to room temperature before using.

Makes twelve 1-tablespoon servings (³/₄ cup)

Per serving: 64 calories, 0 g protein, 2 g carbohydrates, 6 g fat, 0 mg cholesterol, 115 mg sodium, 0 g dietary fiber
Diet Exchanges: 1 fat
Carb Choices: 0

COOL BUTTERMILK DRESSING

This dressing is delicious on crisp lettuces, tomato salads, or cucumber and onion salads with a few sliced beets added. It is also a tasty complement to oven-fried fish.

Prep time: 8 minutes

1 cup buttermilk	1 tablespoon lemon juice
¼ cup light mayonnaise	½ teaspoon grainy mustard
2 tablespoons snipped fresh dill	¼ teaspoon salt
1 clove garlic, crushed through a press	¼ teaspoon freshly ground black pepper
¼ teaspoon grated lemon peel	

In a medium bowl, whisk together the buttermilk, mayonnaise, dill, garlic, lemon peel, lemon juice, mustard, salt, and pepper until well blended. Transfer to a small jar and refrigerate until ready to serve.

Makes ten 2-tablespoon servings (1 ¼ cups)

Per serving: 25 calories, 1 g protein, 2 g carbohydrates, 1 g fat, 0 mg cholesterol, 120 mg sodium, 0 g dietary fiber
Diet Exchanges: 0
Carb Choices: 0

A FEW LESS THAN A THOUSAND ISLANDS DRESSING

This is a low-cal twist on a high-cal favorite. Serve it on iceberg lettuce wedges, sprinkled with shreds of red cabbage and carrots for fiber. It's also delicious with broiled shrimp.

Prep time: 5 minutes

½ **cup light mayonnaise**

¼ **cup fat-free sour cream**

¼ **cup medium-spicy chunky salsa**

2 **tablespoons dill pickle relish**

2 **tablespoons balsamic vinegar**

1 **tablespoon tomato paste**

⅛ **teaspoon salt**

⅛ **teaspoon freshly ground black pepper**

Place the mayonnaise, sour cream, salsa, relish, vinegar, tomato paste, salt, and pepper in a medium bowl. Whisk until blended. Transfer to a small jar and refrigerate until ready to serve.

Makes sixteen 1-tablespoon servings (1 cup)

Per serving: 24 calories, 0 g protein, 3 g carbohydrates, 1 g fat, 0 mg cholesterol, 105 mg sodium, 0 g dietary fiber
Diet Exchanges: 0
Carb Choices: 0

LEMONY YOGURT DRESSING

This tangy dressing is great on a salad of crisp romaine and watercress, on sliced ripe tomatoes with cucumbers, and on scallions. It can be spooned over avocado chunks, and it also makes an especially tasty dip for crisp raw vegetables.

Prep time: 7 minutes

²⁄₃ **cup fat-free plain yogurt**

3 **tablespoons olive oil**

¹⁄₂ **teaspoon grated lemon peel**

3 **tablespoons lemon juice**

1 **tablespoon chopped fresh mint**

1 **tablespoon chopped fresh cilantro**

1 **teaspoon honey**

¹⁄₄ **teaspoon dried oregano, crumbled**

¹⁄₂ **teaspoon salt**

¹⁄₈ **teaspoon freshly ground black pepper**

Place the yogurt, oil, lemon peel, lemon juice, mint, cilantro, honey, oregano, salt, and pepper in a medium bowl. Whisk until blended. Transfer to a small jar and refrigerate until ready to serve.

Makes eight 2-tablespoon servings (1 cup)

Per serving: 60 calories, 1 g protein, 3 g carbohydrates, 5 g fat, 0 mg cholesterol, 160 mg sodium, 0 g dietary fiber
Diet Exchanges: 1 fat
Carb Choices: 0

SIDE DISHES

FAST   SUPER FAST   FAST PREP

ROASTED ASPARAGUS AND CORN SUCCOTASH

The high-fiber vegetables in this salad guard against a plunging blood sugar level, so you aren't inclined to hunt out the nearest doughnut.

Prep time: 10 minutes • Cook time: 15 minutes

1 **pound asparagus, trimmed**

4 **teaspoons olive oil**

2 **teaspoons minced garlic**

1 **package (10 ounces) frozen baby lima beans, thawed**

1 **can (7 ounces) yellow corn kernels, drained**

1 **teaspoon chopped fresh oregano**

1 **cup cherry tomatoes, halved**

½ **teaspoon salt**

¼ **teaspoon freshly ground black pepper**

Preheat the oven to 400°F. Coat a baking sheet lightly with cooking spray.

Toss the asparagus with 1 teaspoon of the oil in a medium bowl and spread in a single layer on the baking sheet. Roast for 8 to 10 minutes, or until tender. Remove from the oven and cool for 5 minutes. Cut the asparagus into 1" lengths and reserve.

In a large nonstick skillet over medium-high heat, heat the remaining 3 teaspoons oil. Add the garlic and cook for 30 seconds. Add the lima beans, corn, and oregano. Cook, stirring occasionally, for 3 to 4 minutes, or until the lima beans are tender and the corn begins to brown slightly. Stir in the cherry tomatoes and cook for 2 to 3 minutes, or until the tomatoes begin to wilt. Add the asparagus, salt, and pepper and cook for 1 to 2 minutes, until hot.

Makes 4 servings

Per serving: 199 calories, 9 g protein, 31 g carbohydrates, 5 g fat, 0 mg cholesterol, 420 mg sodium, 8 g dietary fiber
Diet Exchanges: 1 ½ vegetable, 1½ bread, 1 fat
Carb Choices: 2

ANISE-SCENTED BALSAMIC BEETS

Whether you cook beets fresh or from the can, the nutrient value is virtually the same.

Photo on page 207.

Prep time: 15 minutes • Cook time: 45 minutes • Stand time: 30 minutes

1 pound beets (about 1 bunch), about 2" in diameter each, trimmed

1 cup orange juice

2 tablespoons balsamic vinegar

2 star anise pods

1 tablespoon sugar

1 medium bunch arugula (about 4 cups), trimmed and washed

1 tablespoon lemon juice

1 teaspoon grated lemon zest

1 tablespoon olive oil

¼ teaspoon salt

⅛ teaspoon freshly ground black pepper

Preheat the oven to 425°F.

Wrap the beets in aluminum foil and place directly on the oven rack. Roast for 45 minutes, or until a knife easily pierces the beets. Cool for 30 minutes, then peel and cut each beet into 8 wedges.

Meanwhile, in a medium saucepan over medium-high heat, combine the orange juice, vinegar, star anise, and sugar. Bring the mixture to a boil and cook for 12 to 14 minutes, or until reduced to about 2 ½ to 3 tablespoons of syrup. Discard the star anise pods, then toss the syrup with the beets.

Toss the arugula with the lemon juice, lemon zest, oil, salt, and pepper. Arrange over 4 serving plates. Divide the beets into 4 portions and place each on top of the arugula. Drizzle any remaining orange-balsamic syrup over each plate. Serve immediately.

Note: The beets and glaze in this recipe can be made up to 3 days in advance. Toss them, chilled, right before serving for a cool salad.

Makes 4 servings

Per serving: 130 calories, 3 g protein, 23 g carbohydrates, 4 g fat, 0 mg cholesterol, 240 mg sodium, 4 g dietary fiber
Diet Exchanges: ½ fruit, 2 vegetable, 1 fat
Carb Choices: 1

CORN ON THE COB WITH CHILE-MAPLE GLAZE

Chipotle chiles are actually jalapeño peppers. You can find them dry or canned in adobo sauce. Fiery peppers are said to increase metabolism and help burn calories.

Prep time: 10 minutes • Cook time: 25 minutes

⅓ **cup maple syrup**

2 **tablespoons butter**

2 **teaspoons lime juice**

1 **small chipotle chile pepper in adobo sauce, finely minced, about 1 teaspoon (see note)**

1 **teaspoon reduced-sodium soy sauce**

¼ **teaspoon ground cumin**

¼ **teaspoon salt**

4 **ears corn on the cob, husked**

1 **tablespoon chopped fresh cilantro (optional)**

Coat a grill rack with cooking spray. Preheat the grill.

In a medium saucepan, combine the maple syrup, butter, lime juice, pepper, soy sauce, cumin, and salt. Bring to a simmer over low heat and cook for 12 to 14 minutes, or until thick and syrupy.

Place the corn on the grill rack and grill for 2 minutes. Brush the corn with some of the syrup mixture and turn a quarter turn. Continue brushing and turning the corn every 2 minutes for 6 to 8 minutes longer, or until the corn is well marked and cooked through. Transfer the corn to a serving platter and brush with the remaining syrup. Sprinkle with the cilantro, if using, and serve immediately.

Note: Chile oil sticks to the skin, and water alone won't wash it away. After handling chiles, be sure to use soap and water to wash your hands.

Makes 4 servings

Per serving: 206 calories, 3 g protein, 38 g carbohydrates, 7 g fat, 15 mg cholesterol, 260 mg sodium, 2 g dietary fiber
Diet Exchanges: 2 ½ bread, 1 fat
Carb Choices: 3

SUMMER SQUASH AND TOMATO SKILLET SAUTÉ

Make the most of garden-fresh vegetables. This easy side dish is
perfect served with fish and beef.

Prep time: 8 minutes • Cook time: 10 minutes

1	tablespoon olive oil	3	large plum tomatoes, halved, cored, and sliced
2	cloves garlic, minced		
2	medium zucchini, halved and cut into thin half-moon slices	¼	teaspoon salt
			Pinch of freshly ground black pepper
1	medium yellow summer squash, halved and cut into thin half-moon slices	2–3	tablespoons chopped fresh basil or snipped fresh chives

In a large nonstick skillet, heat the oil over medium heat. Add the garlic and cook for 1 minute, stirring, until fragrant.

Add the zucchini and squash and toss to coat well with the oil. Cook for 5 minutes, stirring often, until they become tender. Stir in the tomatoes and sprinkle with the salt and pepper. Cover and cook for 3 to 4 minutes, stirring often, until the tomatoes are softened and begin to release their juices.

Sprinkle with the basil or chives and serve.

Makes 4 servings

Per serving: 60 calories, 2 g protein, 7 g carbohydrates, 3 ½ g fat, 0 mg cholesterol, 160 mg sodium, 2 g dietary fiber
Diet Exchanges: 1 vegetable, 1 fat
Carb Choices: ½

ROASTED RATATOUILLE

Ratatouille can be served hot or cold, as a side dish or appetizer. Either way, the roasting process in this recipe guarantees sweet results.

Prep time: 20 minutes • Cook time: 1 hour 10 minutes

1 eggplant (about 1 pound), trimmed, peeled, and cut into ½" pieces

1 medium zucchini (about 8 ounces), trimmed and cut into ½" pieces

1 medium onion, chopped

1 red bell pepper, seeded and cut into ½" pieces

½ medium fennel bulb, cored and thinly sliced

1 tablespoon olive oil

1 teaspoon chopped fresh thyme

½ teaspoon chopped fresh rosemary

1 can (15 ½" ounces) diced tomatoes

2 teaspoons minced garlic

1 ½ teaspoons chopped fresh oregano

½ teaspoon salt

¼ teaspoon freshly ground black pepper

1 tablespoon grated Parmesan cheese

Preheat the oven to 400°F. Coat a large roasting pan with cooking spray.

In a large bowl, combine the eggplant, zucchini, onion, bell pepper, and fennel. Toss with the oil, thyme, and rosemary. Spread the vegetables evenly in the pan. Roast, stirring occasionally, for 50 to 55 minutes, or until the vegetables are lightly browned and tender. Transfer the vegetables to a 9" square baking dish coated with cooking spray. Add the diced tomatoes (with juice), garlic, oregano, salt, and pepper. Mix well to combine. Sprinkle the top with cheese. Bake for 20 to 22 minutes, or until the sauce thickens and the top is bubbly.

Makes 4 servings

Per serving: 129 calories, 4 g protein, 22 g carbohydrates, 4 g fat, 0 mg cholesterol, 480 mg sodium, 7 g dietary fiber
Diet Exchanges: 4 vegetable, 1 fat
Carb Choices: 1

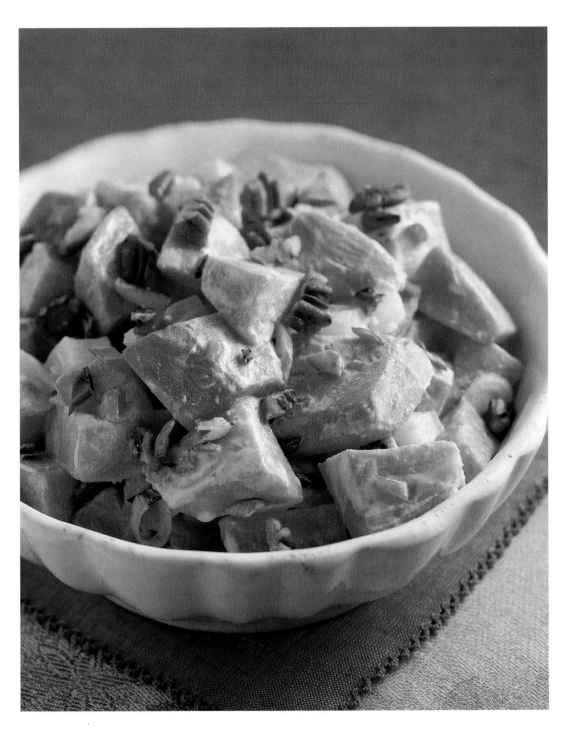

CURRIED SWEET POTATO SALAD

Recipe on page 165

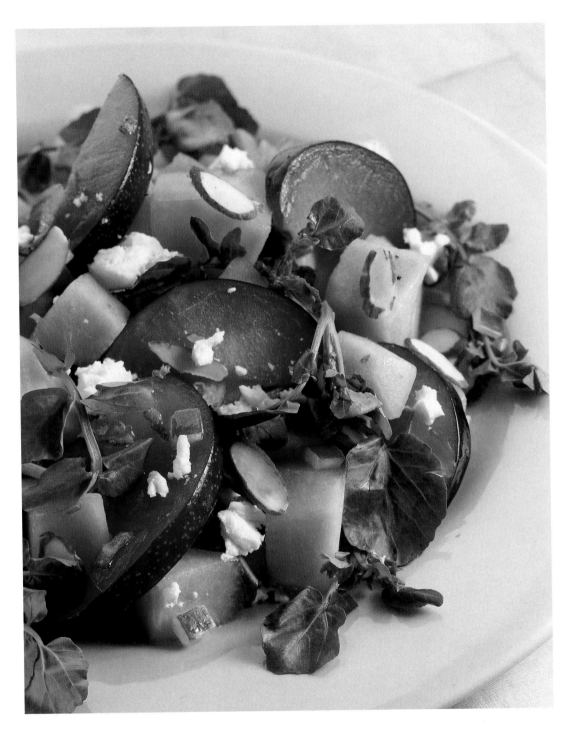

CANTALOUPE AND WATERCRESS SALAD WITH PICKLED ONIONS

Recipe on page 168

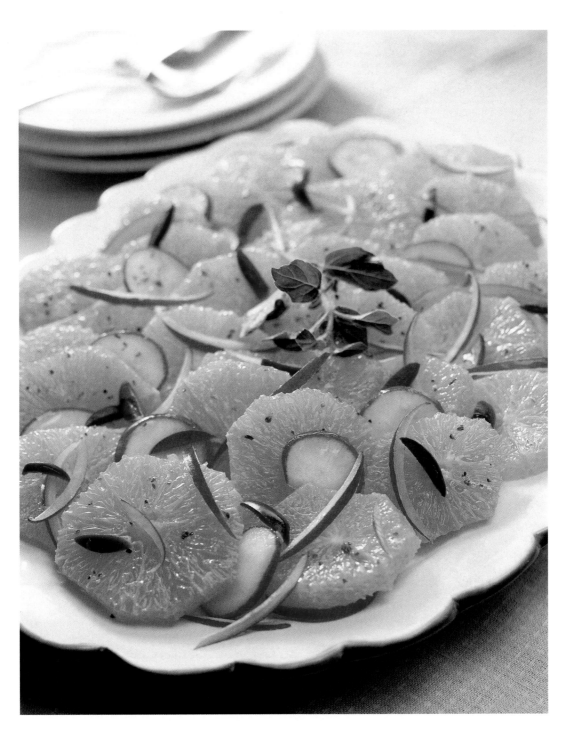

ORANGE AND OLIVE SALAD

Recipe on page 169

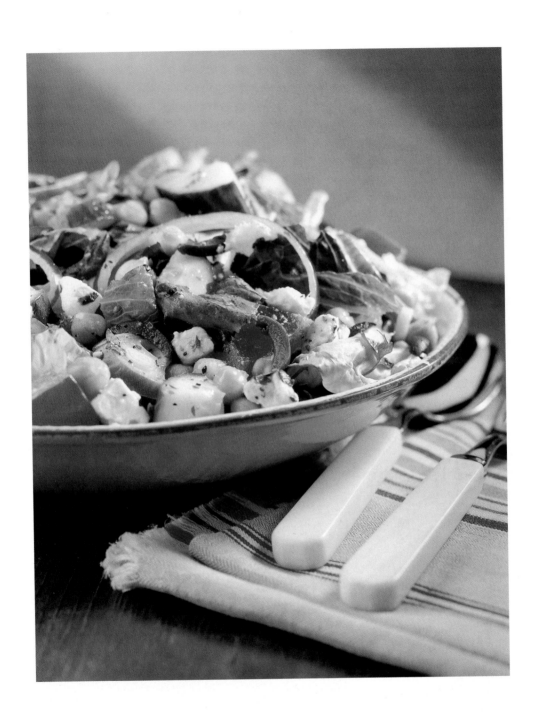

A BIG FAT GREEK SALAD

Recipe on page 173

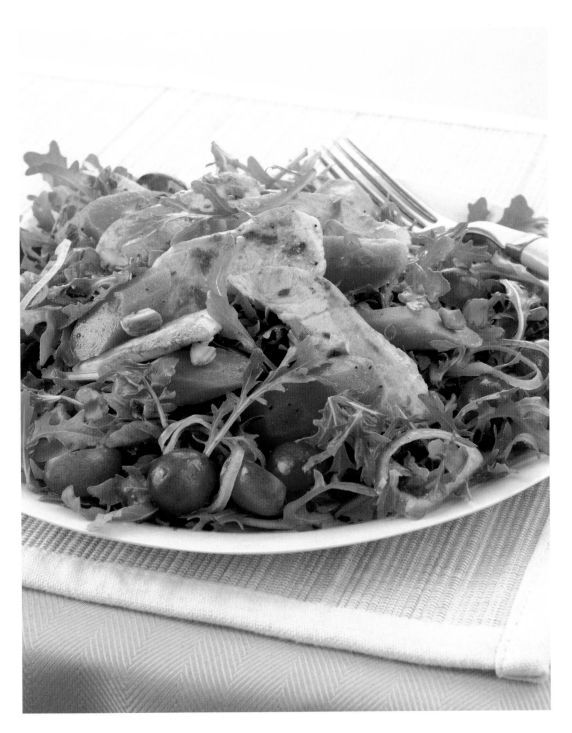

ROASTED CARROT AND CHICKEN SALAD WITH PISTACHIOS

Recipe on page 182

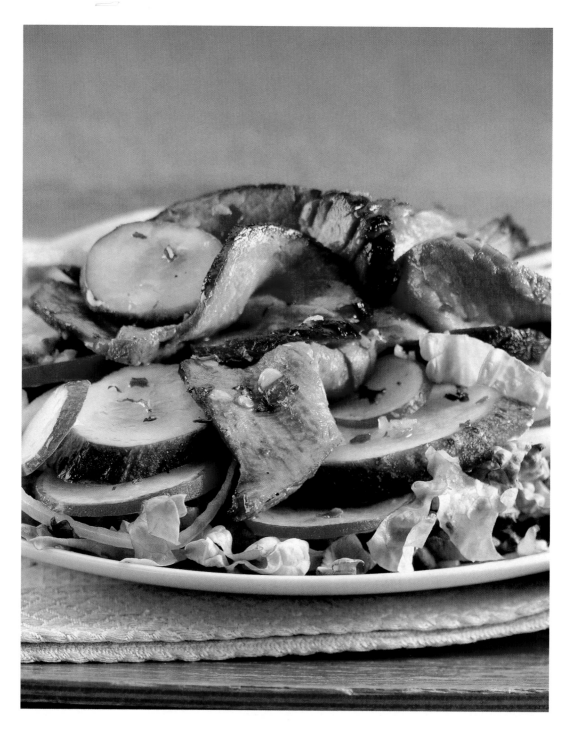

THAI BEEF SALAD

Recipe on page 187

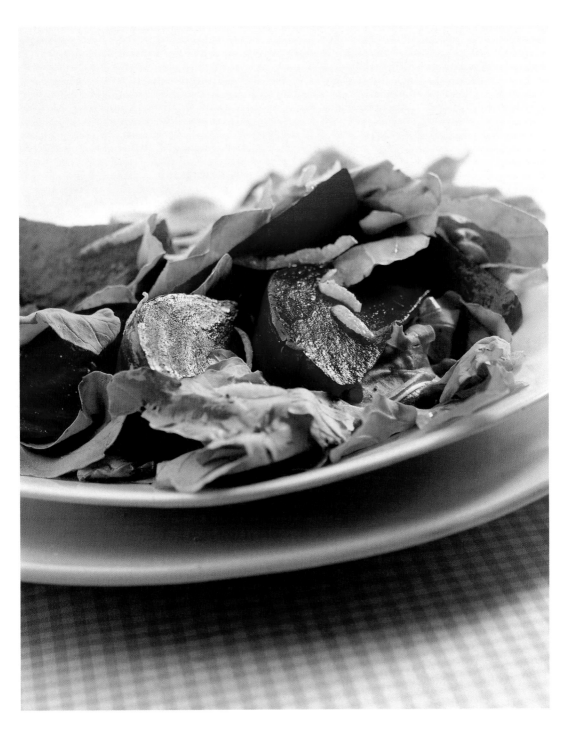

ANISE-SCENTED BALSAMIC BEETS

Recipe on page 197

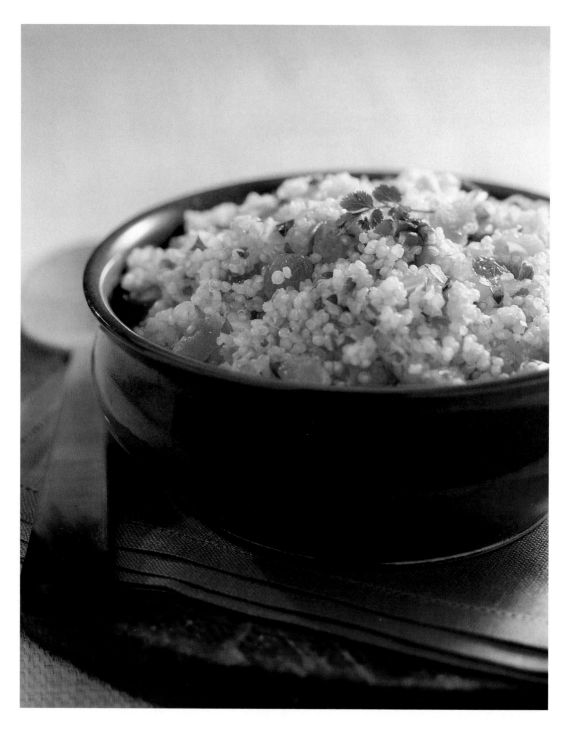

QUINOA WITH RAISINS, APRICOTS, AND PECANS

Recipe on page 226

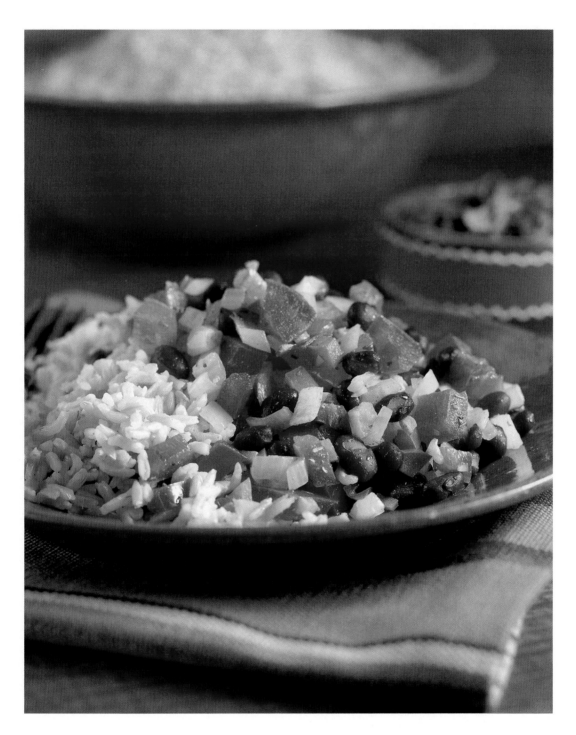

BLACK BEANS AND RICE

Recipe on page 228

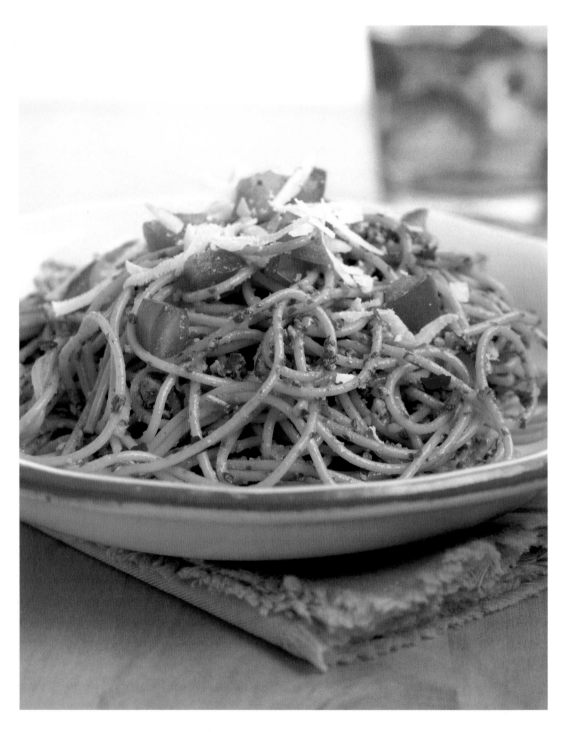

PASTA WITH WALNUT-BASIL PESTO

Recipe on page 233

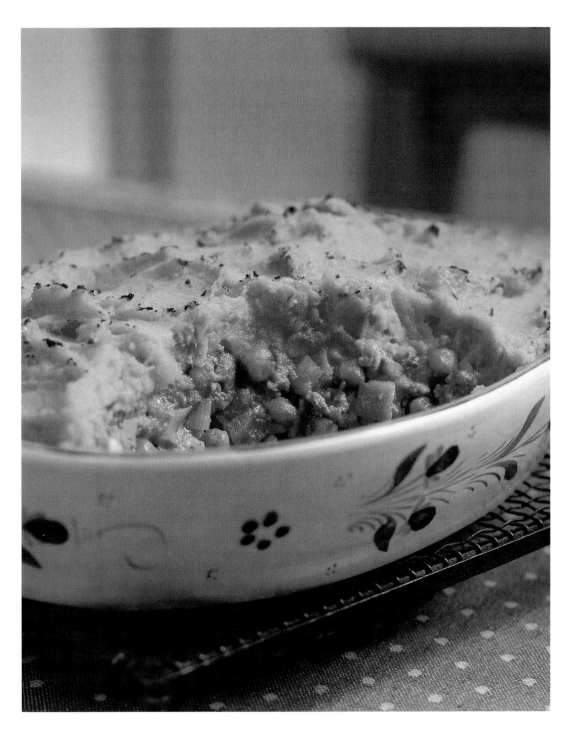

SHEPHERD'S PIE

Recipe on page 243

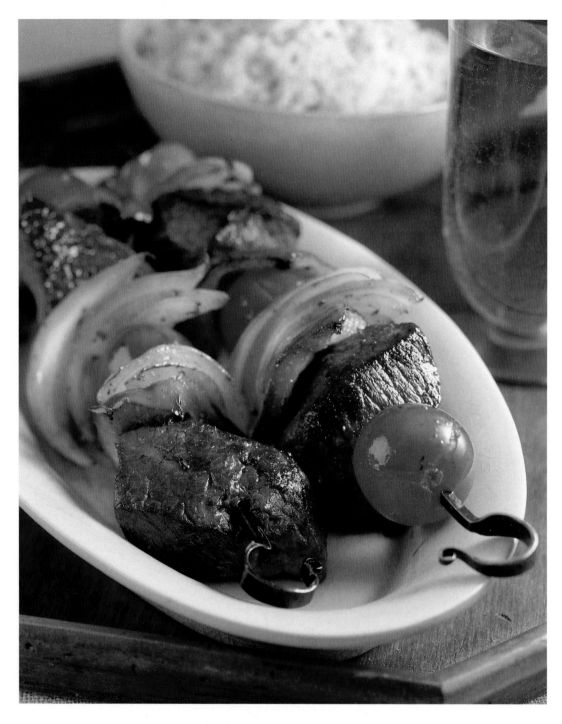

CHINO-LATINO BEEF KEBABS

Recipe on page 244

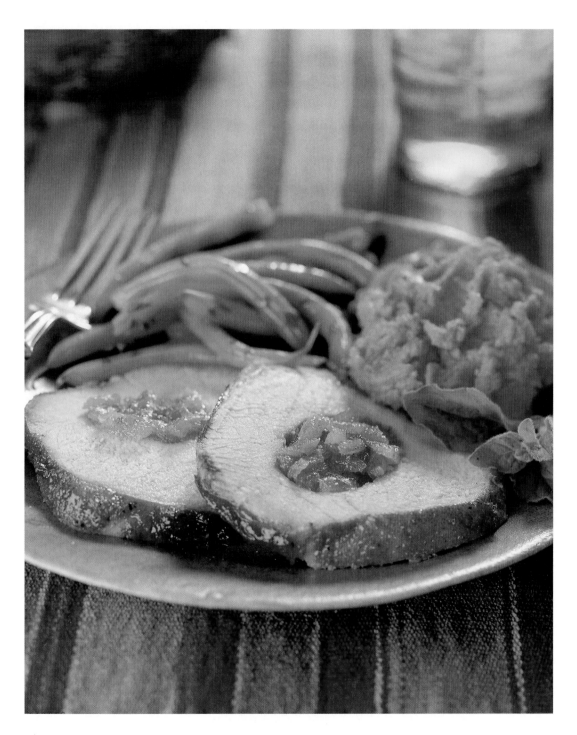

APRICOT-STUFFED PORK LOIN

Recipe on page 249

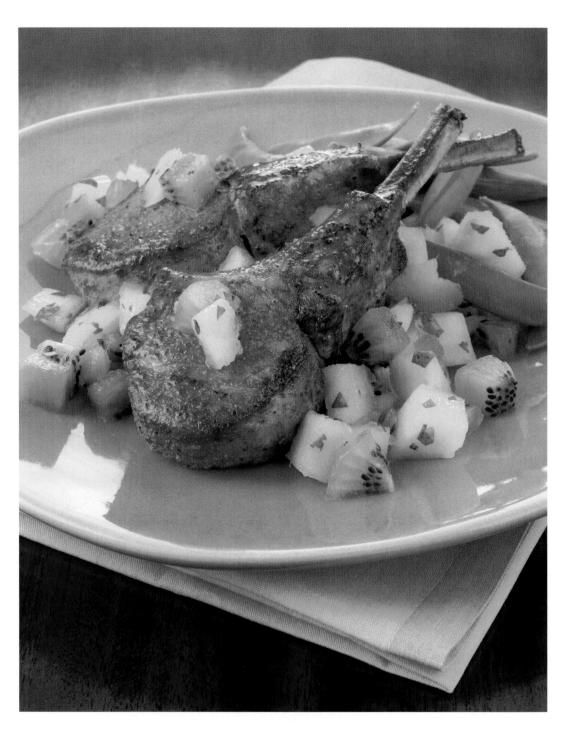

SPICED LAMB CHOPS WITH MANGO-KIWI RELISH

Recipe on page 252

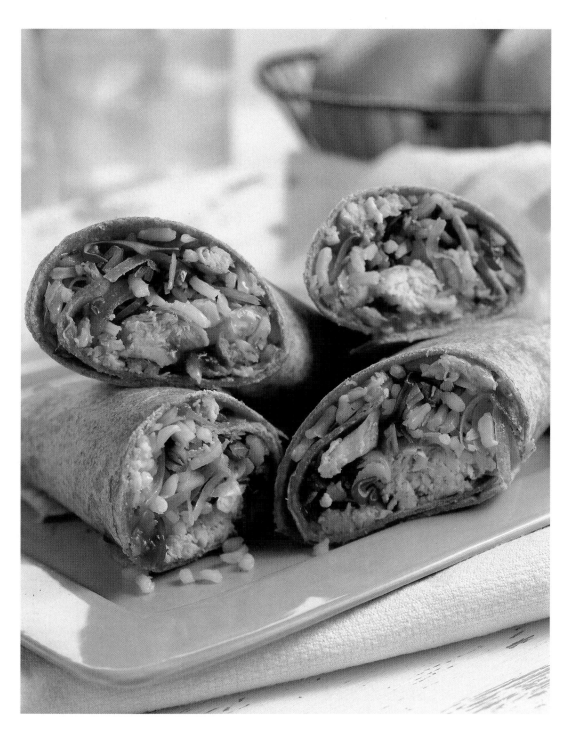

PEKING CHICKEN WRAPS

Recipe on page 259

215

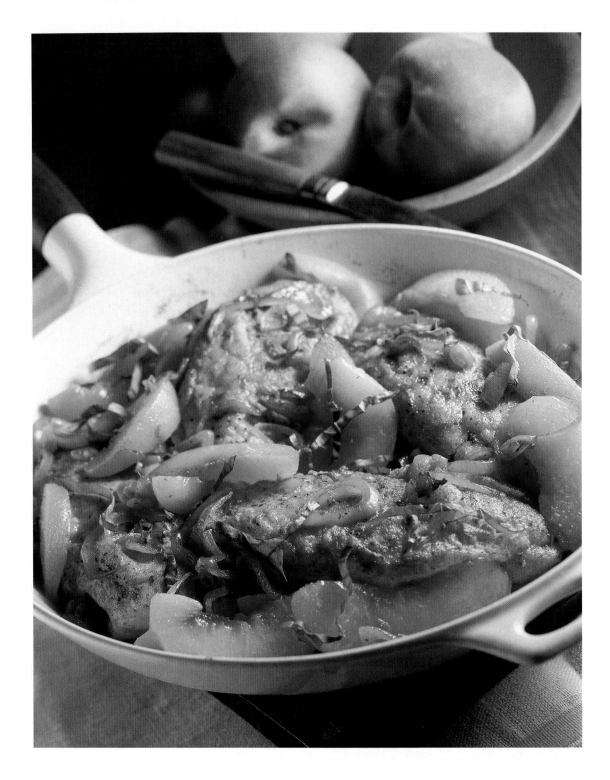

CHICKEN WITH PEACHES AND RED WINE

Recipe on page 260

SAUTÉED STRING BEANS, SWEET ONION, AND GRAPE TOMATOES

This colorful medley is sure to make any entrée look its best. The grape tomatoes are an amazingly sweet addition.

Prep time: 15 minutes • Cook time: 20 minutes

¾ **pound fresh green beans, trimmed and cut in half**

1 **tablespoon olive oil**

1 **small sweet onion, thinly sliced**

1 **red bell pepper, seeded and cut into strips**

2 **cloves garlic, cut into thin slivers**

¼ **teaspoon salt**

⅛ **teaspoon freshly ground black pepper**

1 **pint grape tomatoes, halved**

1 **tablespoon vegetable broth or chicken broth, or water**

2 **teaspoons coarsely chopped fresh marjoram or flat-leaf parsley**

In a large deep skillet, bring ½" water to a boil over high heat. Add the green beans, cover, and cook for 6 to 8 minutes, until tender. Drain.

Dry the skillet. Heat the oil in the same skillet over medium heat. Stir in the onion, bell pepper, garlic, salt, and black pepper. Cook for 6 minutes, stirring often, until tender. Add the tomatoes. Toss well and add the broth or water. Cook for 2 to 3 minutes, stirring often, until the tomatoes start to collapse.

Add the beans and the marjoram or parsley. Toss for 1 minute, until heated through. Serve hot or at room temperature.

Makes 4 servings

Per serving: 90 calories, 2 g protein, 12 g carbohydrates, 3 ½ g fat, 0 mg cholesterol, 90 mg sodium, 5 g dietary fiber
Diet Exchanges: 2 vegetable, 1 fat
Carb Choices: 1

WILD MUSHROOM SAUTÉ

Mushrooms are a favorite diet staple because they are low in calories, high in flavor, and a beautiful complement to any main dish.

Prep time: 15 minutes • Cook time: 14 minutes

1 tablespoon olive oil

½ cup chopped onion

1 package (10 ounces) sliced white mushrooms (see note)

8 ounces shiitake mushrooms, stemmed and halved

6 ounces oyster mushrooms, trimmed and halved

1 teaspoon chopped fresh rosemary

1 tablespoon minced garlic

½ teaspoon salt

⅛ teaspoon freshly ground black pepper

¼ cup Madeira wine or beef broth

Heat the oil in a large nonstick skillet over medium-high heat. Add the onion and cook for 1 minute. Add the mushrooms and rosemary, mounding them in the skillet. Cook for 10 to 12 minutes, stirring occasionally, until the mushrooms give off their liquid and begin to brown. Add the garlic, salt, and pepper and cook for 2 to 3 minutes longer, or until the garlic begins to brown. Pour in the wine or broth and cook for 1 to 2 minutes, or until the liquid evaporates.

Note: Instead of buying separate types of mushrooms, you can use 4 or 5 packages of mixed wild or domestic mushrooms. This dish can be served with beef, chicken, or cooked pasta.

Makes 4 servings

Per serving: 115 calories, 6 g protein, 12 g carbohydrates, 3 g fat, 0 mg cholesterol, 310 mg sodium, 3 g dietary fiber
Diet Exchanges: 2 vegetable, 1 fat
Carb Choices: 1

HONEY-BAKED ACORN SQUASH

Just a spoonful of honey helps the natural sweetness of this fall favorite come through.
A hint of cinnamon is the perfect topper.

Prep time: 5 minutes • Cook time: 1 hour 15 minutes

1 **acorn squash, about 1 ½ pounds**	**Pinch of freshly ground black pepper**
¼ **teaspoon ground cinnamon**	1 **teaspoon olive oil**
¼ **teaspoon salt**	1 **tablespoon honey**

Preheat the oven to 350°F.

Cut the squash in half and scoop out the seeds. Cut each half in half again and place in a 13" × 9" baking dish.

Sprinkle the cinnamon, salt, and pepper over each squash quarter. Drizzle with the oil and then the honey.

Bake for 1 hour 15 minutes to 1 hour 30 minutes, until the squash is lightly golden and tender when pierced with a fork.

Makes 4 servings

Per serving: 80 calories, 1 g protein, 18 g carbohydrates, 1 ½ g fat, 0 mg cholesterol, 75 mg sodium, 2 g dietary fiber
Diet Exchanges: 2 vegetable
Carb Choices: 1

NORTH AFRICAN SPICED SPAGHETTI SQUASH

Spaghetti squash is extraordinary because of what it *doesn't* have:
saturated fat, sodium, or lots of calories.

Prep time: 15 minutes • Cook time: 50 minutes

1 **spaghetti squash (2 ½ pounds), halved and seeded**

⅓ **cup golden raisins**

¼ **cup orange juice**

2 **tablespoons butter**

1 **teaspoon ground cumin**

¾ **teaspoon ground cinnamon**

½ **teaspoon salt**

⅛ **teaspoon cayenne pepper**

1 **teaspoon grated orange zest (optional)**

Preheat the oven to 350°F.

Place the squash halves, cut side down, in a 13" × 9" baking dish. Add enough water to come ½" up the sides of the squash. Bake for 40 to 45 minutes, or until the squash is fork-tender. Remove from the oven and let cool for 10 minutes. Scrape the inside of the squash with a fork to remove spaghetti-like strands. Transfer to a bowl.

Meanwhile, in a small saucepan over medium-high heat, combine the raisins and orange juice. Bring to a boil, then remove from the heat and let stand for 10 minutes.

Melt the butter in a large nonstick skillet over medium heat. Add the cumin, cinnamon, salt, and cayenne pepper and cook for 1 minute, or until the spices are fragrant. Add the squash, raisins, and any remaining juices and cook for 1 minute, or until hot and well combined. Remove from the heat and stir in the orange zest, if using.

Makes 4 servings

Per serving: 185 calories, 3 g protein, 31 g carbohydrates, 8 g fat, 15 mg cholesterol, 400 mg sodium, 5 g dietary fiber
Diet Exchanges: 1 fruit, 3 vegetable, 1 fat
Carb Choices: 2

GLAZED TURNIPS, PEARL ONIONS, AND CARROTS

Flavorful enough for Thanksgiving dinner, easy enough for any night of the week, this attractive trio of vegetables also contains a powerful mix of complex carbohydrates and fiber.

Prep time: 15 minutes • Cook time: 30 minutes

4   peeled turnips ($^3/_4$ pound), cut into 8 wedges each

2   cups frozen small white onions (about 10 ounces), thawed

1   cup baby carrots

1 $^1/_4$ cups chicken broth

2   tablespoons balsamic vinegar

2   tablespoons packed brown sugar

4   teaspoons butter

$^1/_2$ teaspoon ground cumin

$^1/_4$ teaspoon salt

$^1/_8$ teaspoon freshly ground black pepper

2   tablespoons chopped fresh parsley

In a large skillet over medium-high heat, combine the turnips, onions, carrots, broth, vinegar, sugar, butter, cumin, salt, and pepper. Bring to a boil, reduce the heat to medium, and simmer, stirring occasionally, for 20 to 25 minutes, or until the liquid evaporates. Continue cooking, stirring often, for 4 to 6 minutes longer, or until the vegetables are golden and shiny. Remove from the heat and stir in the parsley.

Makes 4 servings

Per serving: 173 calories, 4 g protein, 31 g carbohydrates, 5 g fat, 10 mg cholesterol, 580 mg sodium, 6 g dietary fiber
Diet Exchanges: 4 $^1/_2$ vegetable, 1 fat
Carb Choices: 2

OVEN-ROASTED BRUSSELS SPROUTS

Roasting lends an amazing nuttiness to Brussels sprouts that you might not otherwise notice. And here's even more reason to add them to the menu: A serving of Brussels sprouts has as much or more fiber than 2 slices of whole wheat bread!

Prep time: 10 minutes • Cook time: 18 minutes

1 ½ **pounds Brussels sprouts, quartered**

1 **tablespoon olive oil**

½ **teaspoon salt**

⅛ **teaspoon freshly ground black pepper**

4 **cloves garlic, sliced**

Preheat the oven to 400°F. Coat a baking sheet with cooking spray.

In a large bowl, combine the Brussels sprouts and oil. Spread in a single layer on the baking sheet. Sprinkle with salt and pepper. Roast the Brussels sprouts, shaking the pan occasionally, for 10 minutes. Remove the baking sheet from the oven and stir in the garlic. Return to the oven and roast for 8 to 10 minutes longer, or until the Brussels sprouts are tender and the edges are lightly browned.

Makes 4 servings

Per serving: 108 calories, 6 g protein, 16 g carbohydrates, 4 g fat, 0 mg cholesterol, 330 mg sodium, 7 g dietary fiber
Diet Exchanges: 3 vegetable, 1 fat
Carb Choices: 1

BUTTERMILK-SMASHED RED POTATOES WITH SCALLIONS

FAST
PREP

Sweet, rich buttermilk lends a light tanginess to these mashed potatoes. And the tender skins of red potatoes add extra fiber to the finished dish.

Prep time: 6 minutes • Cook time: 12 minutes

1½ **pounds small red potatoes, scrubbed and halved**

1 **cup fat-free, reduced-sodium chicken or vegetable broth**

½ **cup low-fat buttermilk**

¼ **teaspoon salt**

¼ **teaspoon freshly ground black pepper**

2 **scallions, thinly sliced**

In a heavy large saucepan, place the potatoes, broth, and enough water to barely cover. Bring to a boil over high heat. Reduce the heat to low, partially cover, and simmer for 12 to 15 minutes, until potatoes are very tender.

Reserve ¼ cup of the cooking water. Drain the potatoes and return them to the pot. With a potato masher, mash until fairly smooth.

With a wooden spoon, a bit at a time, beat in the buttermilk and enough of the reserved cooking water to make the potatoes moist but with a chunky texture. Stir in the salt and pepper, and sprinkle with the scallions.

Makes 4 servings

Per serving: 160 calories, 5 g protein, 32 g carbohydrates, 0 g fat, 0 mg cholesterol, 310 mg sodium, 2 g dietary fiber
Diet Exchanges: 2 bread
Carb Choices: 2

CAJUN-SPICED OVEN FRIES

It's hard to believe that fries might actually have some nutritional attributes, but take away the salt and saturated fat and you have a treat that is high in fiber, high in mono-unsaturated fats, and high in flavor. *Photo on page 283.*

Prep time: 10 minutes • Cook time: 35 minutes

4 russet potatoes (about 2 pounds), cut lengthwise into 12 wedges each

1 ½ tablespoons olive oil

1 teaspoon chili powder

1 teaspoon ground cumin

1 teaspoon sweet paprika

1 teaspoon dried oregano

¼ teaspoon dried thyme

1 teaspoon salt

⅛ teaspoon cayenne pepper

Preheat the oven to 450°F. Coat a baking sheet with cooking spray.

In a large bowl, combine the potatoes and oil. Toss well to coat. In a small bowl, combine the chili powder, cumin, paprika, oregano, thyme, salt, and cayenne pepper. Sprinkle the spice mixture over the potatoes, tossing well to coat.

Arrange the potato wedges in a single layer on the baking sheet. Bake for 20 minutes. Turn the potatoes over and bake for 15 to 17 minutes longer, until crisp.

Makes 4 servings

Per serving: 109 calories, 5 g protein, 12 g carbohydrates, 5 g fat, 0 mg cholesterol, 610 mg sodium, 6 g dietary fiber
Diet Exchanges: 1 bread, 1 fat
Carb Choices: 1

CURRIED APPLE COLESLAW

Cabbage is a cook's best friend. It is versatile, easy to prepare, and readily available. It is also a great friend to your health. Members of the cabbage family are packed with nutritious compounds, including fiber and complex carbohydrates that fill you up.

Prep time: 20 minutes • Stand time: 10 minutes

5 cups shredded green cabbage (about ½ medium head)

¾ cup grated carrot (about 1 large)

2 Granny Smith apples, peeled, cored, and grated

2 scallions, chopped

⅓ cup golden raisins

2 tablespoons chopped fresh mint

½ cup light mayonnaise

2 tablespoons apple juice

2 teaspoons madras curry powder

½ teaspoon salt

¼ teaspoon freshly ground black pepper

In a large bowl, combine the cabbage, carrot, apples, scallions, raisins, and mint. In a separate bowl, combine the mayonnaise, apple juice, curry powder, salt, and pepper. Add the mayonnaise mixture to the cabbage mixture and combine well. Let stand for 10 minutes before serving.

Makes 4 servings

Per serving: 206 calories, 3 g protein, 29 g carbohydrates, 10 g fat, 10 mg cholesterol, 560 mg sodium, 5 g dietary fiber
Diet Exchanges: 1 fruit, 2 vegetable, 2 fat
Carb Choices: 2

QUINOA WITH RAISINS, APRICOTS, AND PECANS

Quinoa, once the main staple of the Incas, is one of the best vegetable sources of protein. In this particular dish, it sets the stage for sweet and nutty flavors to mingle perfectly.

Photo on page 208.

Prep time: 15 minutes • Cook time: 20 minutes

3 **tablespoons pecans, chopped**	2 **scallions, finely chopped**
²⁄₃ **cup quinoa**	1 **tablespoon chopped fresh cilantro**
²⁄₃ **cup orange juice**	1 **tablespoon lemon juice**
²⁄₃ **cup water**	1 **tablespoon olive oil**
¹⁄₃ **cup chopped dried apricots**	¹⁄₂ **teaspoon salt**
¹⁄₄ **cup golden raisins**	

Cook the pecans in a small nonstick skillet over medium heat, stirring often, for 3 to 4 minutes, or until lightly toasted. Tip onto a plate and let cool.

Place the quinoa in a fine-mesh strainer and rinse under cold running water for 2 minutes. In a medium saucepan, combine the quinoa, orange juice, and water. Bring to a boil over high heat, reduce the heat to medium-low, cover, and simmer for 12 to 15 minutes, or until the liquid is absorbed. Transfer the quinoa to a large bowl. Add the apricots, raisins, scallions, cilantro, and toasted pecans. Add the lemon juice, oil, and salt, tossing well to distribute.

Makes 4 servings

Per serving: 266 calories, 5 g protein, 42 g carbohydrates, 9 g fat, 0 mg cholesterol, 300 mg sodium, 4 g dietary fiber
Diet Exchanges: 1 ¹⁄₂ fruit, 1 ¹⁄₂ bread, 1 ¹⁄₂ fat
Carb Choices: 3

MACARONI AND CHEESE

Usually America's favorite comfort food has ample supplies of fat, weighing in at 22 grams
for a 1-cup serving. We've scaled back the fat considerably, increased the protein,
and even added a touch of fiber without sacrificing the rich, creamy taste.
Now you can *really* feel comforted!

Prep time: 15 minutes • Cook time: 35 minutes

½ **pound multigrain macaroni**

¼ **cup unbleached flour**

2½ **cups 1% milk**

1 **clove garlic, halved**

½ **teaspoon mustard powder**

¼ **teaspoon salt**

¼ **teaspoon ground red pepper**

1⅓ **cups shredded low-fat extra-sharp
Cheddar cheese**

2 **tablespoons dried bread crumbs**

2 **tablespoons grated Parmesan cheese**

Preheat the oven to 350°F. Coat a medium baking dish with cooking spray.

In a medium saucepan, cook the macaroni according to package directions and drain.

Meanwhile, place the flour in a medium saucepan. Gradually add the milk, whisking constantly,
until smooth. Add the garlic, mustard powder, salt, and red pepper. Place over medium heat. Cook,
whisking constantly, for 7 to 8 minutes, or until thickened. Remove from the heat. Remove the
garlic and discard. Add the Cheddar. Stir until smooth. Add the macaroni. Stir to mix. Pour into the
prepared baking dish.

In a small bowl, combine the bread crumbs and Parmesan. Sprinkle over the casserole. Bake for
15 to 20 minutes, or until bubbling and lightly browned.

Makes 6 servings

Per serving: 300 calories, 19 g protein, 37 g carbohydrates, 9 g fat, 25 mg cholesterol, 350 mg sodium, 3 g dietary fiber
Diet Exchanges: ½ bread, 1 fat, 1 meat, ½ dairy
Carb Choices: 2

BLACK BEANS AND RICE

This hearty side dish not only is high in fiber but also has that magical mix of protein and carbohydrates to keep your energy levels stable. *Photo on page 209.*

Prep time: 15 minutes • Cook time: 40 minutes

½ cup brown basmati rice

1 tablespoon olive oil

2 teaspoons minced garlic

½ cup chopped onion

1 teaspoon dried oregano

1 teaspoon ground cumin

¾ teaspoon ground coriander

½ cup chopped green bell pepper

1 large plum tomato, cored, seeded, and chopped

1 tablespoon red wine vinegar

1 can (15½ ounces) black beans

¼ teaspoon salt

⅛ teaspoon freshly ground black pepper

⅓ cup water

In a medium saucepan, cook the rice according to package directions. Fluff the rice with a fork.

Meanwhile, heat the oil in a medium saucepan over medium heat. Add the garlic, onion, oregano, cumin, and coriander. Cook, stirring occasionally, for 2 minutes, or until the onion begins to soften. Add the bell pepper and cook for 4 minutes longer, or until softened. Stir in the tomato and vinegar and cook for 1 minute. Add the beans, salt, black pepper, and water and simmer, stirring occasionally, for 5 minutes. Serve over the rice.

Makes 4 servings

Per serving: 208 calories, 7 g protein, 40 g carbohydrates, 5 g fat, 0 mg cholesterol, 600 mg sodium, 8 g dietary fiber
Diet Exchanges: 1 vegetable, 2 bread, 1 fat
Carb Choices: 3

BROWN BASMATI FRIED RICE

Basmati rice, long grown at the foot of the Himalaya mountains, is now cultivated in the United States and is widely available.

Prep time: 25 minutes • **Cook time: 57 minutes** • **Stand time: 15 minutes**

²⁄₃ **cup brown basmati rice**

2 **tablespoons sesame oil**

1 **egg, lightly beaten**

2 **teaspoons grated fresh ginger**

1 **teaspoon minced garlic**

2 **scallions, cut into ¼" pieces**

¼ **pound snow peas, trimmed**

½ **cup frozen peas and carrots, thawed**

3 **tablespoons reduced-sodium soy sauce**

In a medium saucepan, cook the rice according to package directions. Fluff the rice with a fork, spread it onto a baking sheet, and allow to cool for at least 15 minutes.

Heat 1 tablespoon of the oil in a large nonstick skillet over medium-high heat. Add the egg and cook, stirring, for 2 minutes, or until firm. Transfer to a bowl and reserve. Heat the remaining 1 tablespoon oil and add the ginger, garlic, scallions, and snow peas to the skillet. Cook, stirring often, for 2 minutes. Add the peas and carrots and the rice and cook for 2 to 3 minutes, or until the vegetables are crisp-tender. Add the soy sauce and cook for 3 to 5 minutes longer, or until the rice is heated through.

Makes 4 servings

Per serving: 228 calories, 6 g protein, 32 g carbohydrates, 9 g fat, 45 mg cholesterol, 530 mg sodium, 4 g dietary fiber
Diet Exchanges: ½ vegetable, 1 ½ bread, 1 ½ fat
Carb Choices: 2

FAST
PREP

TANGY LENTILS VINAIGRETTE

Lentils are a versatile food, high in protein and easy to prepare and add to many dishes. Seventeen grams of fiber never tasted so delicious!

Prep time: 15 minutes ● Cook time: 18 minutes

½ medium onion, root end trimmed but intact

3 cloves garlic

1 bay leaf

4 cups water

1 cup brown lentils, picked over

½ cup finely chopped red onion

½ cup chopped carrots

½ cup chopped celery

½ cup chopped red bell pepper

¼ cup chopped fresh basil

1 tablespoon capers, drained

3 tablespoons balsamic vinegar

2 tablespoons olive oil

½ teaspoon salt

¼ teaspoon freshly ground black pepper

In a large saucepan, combine the onion, garlic, and bay leaf with the water. Bring the water to a boil over medium-high heat. Add the lentils, reduce the heat to medium, and simmer for 18 to 20 minutes, or until tender. Drain the lentils and discard the onion, garlic, and bay leaf.

Transfer the lentils to a large bowl and stir in the red onion, carrots, celery, bell pepper, basil, and capers, tossing well to combine. Add the vinegar, oil, salt, and pepper. Mix well and serve at room temperature or chill to serve cold later.

Makes 4 servings

Per serving: 266 calories, 15 g protein, 37 g carbohydrates, 8 g fat, 0 mg cholesterol, 390 mg sodium, 17 g dietary fiber
Diet Exchanges: 1 vegetable, 2 bread, ½ meat, 1 ½ fat
Carb Choices: 2

MEDITERRANEAN COUSCOUS

Couscous, a North African grain, is now commonly available in the United States. Lucky for us. Now it's easier to reap the benefits of the lean protein and fiber contained in each tiny pearl.

Prep time: 15 minutes • Cook time: 7 minutes • Stand time: 10 minutes

1 ¼ cups water

¾ cup whole wheat couscous

½ teaspoon salt

½ cup canned red kidney beans, rinsed and drained

½ medium cucumber, peeled, seeded, and chopped

½ green bell pepper, chopped

¼ red onion, chopped

½ cup reduced-fat feta cheese

2 tablespoons chopped fresh dill

1 tablespoon capers, drained

2 tablespoons lemon juice

1 tablespoon olive oil

¼ teaspoon freshly ground black pepper

Bring the water to a boil in a medium saucepan over medium-high heat. Stir in the couscous and ¼ teaspoon of the salt. Return to a boil, reduce the heat to low, cover, and simmer for 2 minutes. Remove from the heat and let stand for 5 minutes. Fluff with a fork and cool for 5 minutes longer.

Meanwhile, in a bowl, combine the kidney beans, cucumber, bell pepper, onion, feta, dill, and capers. Add the couscous and toss well. In a small bowl, combine the lemon juice, olive oil, pepper, and the remaining ¼ teaspoon salt. Pour over the couscous and toss well.

Note: This recipe can be made up to 1 day ahead. Store it in an airtight plastic container in your refrigerator.

Makes 4 servings

Per serving: 244 calories, 11 g protein, 41 g carbohydrates, 6 g fat, 5 mg cholesterol, 590 mg sodium, 7 g dietary fiber
Diet Exchanges: ½ vegetable, 2 ½ bread, 1 meat, 1 fat
Carb Choices: 3

COUSCOUS WITH ALMONDS AND DRIED CHERRIES

Perfect warm or at room temperature, alongside roast pork or as a filling for stuffed squash, this versatile side dish will have everyone asking for the recipe.

Prep time: 4 minutes • Cook time: 15 minutes • Stand time: 10 minutes

1 tablespoon olive oil

$\frac{1}{2}$ cup chopped red onion

$\frac{3}{4}$ cup fat-free, reduced-sodium chicken or vegetable broth

$\frac{3}{4}$ cup water

$\frac{1}{4}$ teaspoon ground cinnamon

$\frac{1}{4}$ teaspoon salt

$\frac{1}{8}$ teaspoon freshly ground black pepper

$\frac{3}{4}$ cup whole wheat couscous

$\frac{1}{4}$ cup dried unsweetened cherries

2 tablespoons slivered almonds

2 tablespoons unsalted pepitas (raw pumpkin seeds)

In a medium saucepan, heat the oil over medium heat. Add the red onion and cook for 3 to 4 minutes, stirring often, until tender.

Meanwhile, in a small saucepan, bring the broth and water to a boil.

Stir the cinnamon, salt, and pepper into the onion, then stir in the couscous and dried cherries. Pour in the boiling broth mixture and return to a boil.

Remove the couscous from the heat, cover, and let stand for 10 minutes, or until tender and the water has been absorbed.

Meanwhile, cook the almonds in a small skillet over medium heat for 4 minutes, tossing often, until toasted. Tip onto a plate to stop the cooking.

Fluff the couscous with a fork. Sprinkle with the toasted almonds and pepitas and serve.

Makes 4 servings (4 cups)

Per serving: 160 calories, 5 g protein, 20 g carbohydrates, 7 g fat, 0 mg cholesterol, 230 mg sodium, 4 g dietary fiber
Diet Exchanges: $\frac{1}{2}$ vegetable, 1 bread, 1 $\frac{1}{2}$ fat
Carb Choices: 1

PASTA WITH WALNUT-BASIL PESTO

If you like, coarsely chop and toast 1 tablespoon of the walnuts.
Sprinkle over the top for a little extra crunch. *Photo on page 210.*

Prep time: 9 minutes • Cook time: 10 minutes

1¼ cups packed fresh basil	⅛ teaspoon crushed red-pepper flakes
¼ cup walnuts	8 ounces multigrain angel hair pasta
1 clove garlic, peeled	¼ cup chopped tomato (optional)
1 tablespoon extra-virgin olive oil	¼ cup freshly grated Parmesan cheese
¼ teaspoon salt	

In a food processor, place the basil, walnuts, garlic, oil, salt, and pepper flakes. Process, stopping the machine once or twice to scrape down the sides, until finely pureed. Scrape into a serving bowl.

Meanwhile, bring a medium pot of lightly salted water to a boil. Add the pasta and cook according to package directions. Drain, reserving ½ cup of the cooking water.

Stir 2 or 3 tablespoons of the pasta water into the pesto to warm it and make it creamier. Add the pasta and toss, adding more pasta water if dry. Sprinkle with the tomato, if using, and the cheese.

Makes 4 servings

Per serving: 260 calories, 10 g protein, 34 g carbohydrates, 11 g fat, 5 mg cholesterol, 260 mg sodium, 6 g dietary fiber
Diet Exchanges: 2 bread, 2 fat
Carb Choices: 2

ROMAN PASTA CON PECORINO

Just 1 cup of whole wheat spaghetti contains 5.4 grams of fiber, compared with the white flour variety, which has just 2.2. A sprinkle of Romano cheese adds a punch of protein as well as flavor.

Prep time: 5 minutes • Cook time: 15 minutes

8 ounces whole wheat spaghetti

7 tablespoons grated pecorino Romano cheese

2 tablespoons chopped fresh parsley

1 tablespoon olive oil

¼ teaspoon crushed red-pepper flakes

¼ teaspoon salt

⅛ teaspoon freshly ground black pepper

Bring a large pot of lightly salted water to a boil. Add the pasta and cook according to package directions. Drain the pasta, reserving ½ cup of the cooking water. Transfer pasta to a large bowl. Add 6 tablespoons of the cheese, the parsley, oil, pepper flakes, salt, and pepper. Toss well, adding the pasta water, 1 tablespoon at a time, until the desired consistency is reached. Divide among 4 serving bowls. Sprinkle the dishes with the remaining 1 tablespoon cheese.

Makes 4 servings

Per serving: 272 calories, 12 g protein, 43 g carbohydrates, 7 g fat, 10 mg cholesterol, 280 mg sodium, 7 g dietary fiber
Diet Exchanges: 2½ bread, ½ meat, 1 fat
Carb Choices: 3

SOBA NOODLES WITH PEANUT SAUCE

Americans eat 700 million pounds of peanut butter every year. Maybe that's because the thick and satisfying snack, packed with protein and monounsaturated fat, can actually help you slim down!

Prep time: 10 minutes • **Cook time: 15 minutes**

3 tablespoons peanut butter

2 tablespoons water

1 tablespoon honey

1 tablespoon rice vinegar

1 tablespoon reduced-sodium soy sauce

1 teaspoon grated fresh ginger

1 teaspoon sesame oil

$1/8$ teaspoon crushed red-pepper flakes

4 ounces soba or whole wheat noodles

2 carrots, cut into small matchsticks

2 scallions, chopped

In a small saucepan over medium-high heat, combine the peanut butter, water, honey, vinegar, soy sauce, ginger, oil, and pepper flakes. Bring to a boil and cook, stirring constantly, for 1 minute. Set aside and keep warm.

Bring a pot of water to a boil. Add the noodles and return to a boil. Cook the noodles for 4 minutes, then stir in the carrots. Cook for 2 minutes longer, or until the carrots are crisp-tender. Drain the noodles and transfer to a large bowl. Toss with the scallions and peanut sauce. Serve immediately.

Makes 4 servings

Per serving: 195 calories, 7 g protein, 33 g carbohydrates, 5 g fat, 0 mg cholesterol, 420 mg sodium, 2 g dietary fiber
Diet Exchanges: 1 vegetable, 1 $1/2$ bread, $1/2$ meat, 1 fat
Carb Choices: 2

PARMESAN-PROSCIUTTO CORNMEAL TRIANGLES

This scrumptious side dish completes your meals with a healthy serving
of complex carbohydrates. Make a batch on the weekend and your midweek meal will
come together in no time flat!

Prep time: 15 minutes • Cook time: 13 minutes • Chill time: 4 hours

1 **cup 1% milk**

1 **cup water**

1 **teaspoon minced garlic**

¼ **teaspoon dried thyme**

¼ **teaspoon salt**

⅛ **teaspoon freshly ground black pepper**

1 **cup fine cornmeal**

2 **ounces thinly sliced prosciutto, chopped**

3 **tablespoons chopped fresh parsley**

4 **tablespoons grated Parmesan cheese**

1 **teaspoon olive oil**

Coat an 8" square baking pan with cooking spray.

In a medium saucepan over medium-high heat, combine the milk, water, garlic, thyme, salt, and
pepper. Bring to a boil and gradually whisk in the cornmeal, stirring constantly. Reduce the heat to
low, cover, and cook, stirring occasionally, for 5 minutes, or until thick. Remove from the heat and
stir in the prosciutto, parsley, and 3 tablespoons of the cheese. Spread into the bottom of the prepared pan. Press plastic wrap onto the surface and chill for 4 hours.

Preheat the broiler. Coat a baking sheet with cooking spray.

Remove the cornmeal, or polenta, mixture from the refrigerator and turn out onto a cutting board. Cut into 4 equal triangles. Transfer to the prepared baking sheet and brush with the oil. Sprinkle with the remaining cheese. Broil 4" from the heat for 3 to 4 minutes, or until golden and hot. Serve immediately.

Note: Make ahead by preparing the recipe up to the point of cutting into wedges. Refrigerate for up to 2 days, then follow the recipe as directed.

Makes 4 servings

Per serving: 190 calories, 10 g protein, 27 g carbohydrates, 5 g fat, 10 mg cholesterol, 440 mg sodium, 2 g dietary fiber
Diet Exchanges: ½ milk, 1½ bread, 1 meat, ½ fat
Carb Choices: 2

SATISFYING BEEF AND PORK MAIN DISHES

FAST   SUPER FAST   FAST PREP

GRILLED PEPPERED STEAK WITH MULTIGRAIN TEXAS TOAST

Don't believe the common dieting myth that one must give up beef in order to lose weight. Studies have shown that lean cuts of beef not only are low in fat, but, when combined with complex carbohydrates (such as multigrain bread), can diminish your appetite for sweets.

Prep time: 10 minutes • Cook time: 14 minutes

2 slices multigrain bread

½ teaspoon olive oil

1 clove garlic

½ pound lean boneless sirloin steak, trimmed of all visible fat

¾ teaspoon cracked tricolor peppercorns

2 tablespoons barbecue sauce

2 tablespoons prepared white horseradish sauce

½ tomato, cut into 4 slices

Preheat the oven to 425°F.

Brush 1 side of each slice of bread with the oil. Place oiled side up on a baking sheet and bake for 7 to 8 minutes, or until golden and crisp. Remove from the oven and rub the oiled side lightly with the garlic. Discard the leftover garlic and keep the toast warm.

Place the steak on a plate or work surface and press the peppercorns onto both sides. Coat a grill pan with cooking spray and heat over medium heat. Grill the steak for 3 minutes, then turn and brush with 1 tablespoon of the barbecue sauce. Grill for 3 minutes longer, then turn the steak over and brush with the remaining barbecue sauce. Grill 1 minute longer, or until an instant-read thermometer inserted into the center registers 145°F for medium-rare.

Remove from the grill and slice the steak. Spread 1 tablespoon horseradish sauce on each toasted bread slice and top with half of the sliced steak. Top each steak with 2 tomato slices.

Makes 2 servings

Per serving: 330 calories, 28 g protein, 19 g carbohydrates, 5 g fat, 80 mg cholesterol, 420 mg sodium, 2 g dietary fiber
Diet Exchanges: ½ vegetable, 1 bread, 2½ meat, ½ fat
Carb Choices: 1

BEEF TENDERLOIN STEAKS WITH MUSTARD-HORSERADISH SAUCE

Elegant enough for entertaining but a cinch to prepare, these tender steaks are robed in an unforgettable creamy sauce.

Prep time: 7 minutes • Cook time: 7 minutes

SAUCE

3 tablespoons reduced-fat sour cream

1 small plum tomato, finely chopped

2 tablespoons snipped fresh chives or scallion greens

1 tablespoon prepared white horseradish

1 small shallot, minced

1 teaspoon grainy mustard

STEAKS

4 boneless beef tenderloin steaks (4 ounces each), well-trimmed

$\frac{3}{4}$ teaspoon coarsely ground black pepper

$\frac{1}{4}$ teaspoon salt

1 tablespoon grainy mustard

To make the sauce: In a small bowl, mix the sour cream, plum tomato, chives or scallion greens, horseradish, shallot, and mustard until well blended.

To make the steaks: Preheat the broiler. Coat a broiler-pan rack with olive oil cooking spray.

Sprinkle the steaks on both sides with the pepper and salt. Place on the prepared broiler pan. Broil 2" to 4" from the heat for 4 to 5 minutes, until browned. Turn and spread the tops with the mustard. Cook 3 to 4 minutes longer for medium-rare, or until done the way you like them.

Remove from the heat, transfer to a plate, and let stand for 5 minutes. Serve the steaks with the sauce.

Makes 4 servings

Per serving: 200 calories, 26 g protein, 3 g carbohydrates, 9 g fat, 80 mg cholesterol, 290 mg sodium, 0 g dietary fiber
Diet Exchanges: 3 $\frac{1}{2}$ meat, 1 $\frac{1}{2}$ fat
Carb Choices: 0

ALL-AMERICAN POT ROAST

Researchers in France found that people feel happier after eating a meal with protein, and this savory dish delivers plenty. Now that is something to smile about!

Prep time: 15 minutes • Cook time: 2 hours 25 minutes

4   tablespoons unbleached or all-purpose flour

¾   teaspoon dried oregano

½   teaspoon dried thyme

½   teaspoon salt

¼   teaspoon freshly ground black pepper

1½   pounds boneless eye of round roast, trimmed of all visible fat

1   can (15 ½ ounces) reduced-sodium, fat-free beef broth

½   cup red wine or nonalcoholic wine (optional)

1   teaspoon Worcestershire sauce

2   teaspoons olive oil

1   bay leaf

¾   pound red new potatoes, washed and cut into eighths

¾   pound white turnips, peeled and cut into eighths

1   cup frozen small white onions, thawed

1   cup baby carrots

Preheat the oven to 400°F.

In a large bowl, combine the flour, oregano, thyme, salt, and pepper. Dredge the beef to coat, shaking off the excess, and transfer to a plate. Whisk the broth, wine (if using), and Worcestershire sauce into the remaining flour mixture until smooth.

Heat the oil in an ovenproof pot or Dutch oven. Add the beef and brown for 2 minutes per side. Remove from the heat and stir in the broth mixture and bay leaf. Cover and bake for 1½ hours. Add the potatoes, turnips, onions, and carrots. Cover and return to the oven. Bake for 45 to 55 minutes longer, or until the meat and vegetables are tender. Remove the bay leaf and serve.

Makes 6 servings

Per serving: 254 calories, 29 g protein, 19 g carbohydrates, 7 g fat, 60 mg cholesterol, 330 mg sodium, 5 g dietary fiber
Diet Exchanges: 2 vegetable, ½ bread, 4 meat, 1 fat
Carb Choices: 1

SHEPHERD'S PIE

FAST PREP

Sweet potatoes give this all-American classic a healthy and delicious twist. Their creamy orange interior is loaded with fiber and complex carbohydrates. *Photo on page 211.*

Prep time: 15 minutes • Cook time: 47 minutes

1 ¼ pounds sweet potatoes, peeled and cut into 1" pieces

½ cup fat-free milk

1 tablespoon butter

¾ teaspoon salt

¼ teaspoon freshly ground black pepper

1 pound lean ground sirloin

1 onion, chopped

1 cup frozen peas and carrots

½ teaspoon dried thyme

½ cup reduced-sodium, fat-free beef broth

¼ cup red wine

¼ cup tomato paste

Preheat the oven to 350°F. Coat a 6-cup ovenproof casserole with cooking spray and set aside.

In a small pot, combine the potatoes with enough water to cover by 3". Bring to a boil and cook for 10 to 12 minutes, or until tender. Drain the potatoes, return to the pot, and add the milk, butter, ¼ teaspoon of the salt, and ⅛ teaspoon of the pepper. Mash until smooth and set aside.

Heat a nonstick skillet over medium-high heat. Add the sirloin and cook for 5 to 6 minutes, stirring occasionally, until browned. Drain the fat from the pan and transfer the beef to a bowl. Return the skillet to the heat and add the onion, peas and carrots, and thyme. Cook, stirring occasionally, for 5 to 7 minutes, or until the vegetables are soft.

Return the beef to the skillet and stir in the broth, wine, and tomato paste. Cook for 2 to 3 minutes, or until the liquid is almost evaporated. Stir in the remaining ½ teaspoon salt and ⅛ teaspoon pepper. Transfer the beef mixture to the prepared casserole dish. Spread the reserved sweet potatoes evenly over the top of the beef. Bake for 25 to 30 minutes, or until the potatoes are lightly browned.

Makes 4 servings

Per serving: 377 calories, 28 g protein, 47 g carbohydrates, 8 g fat, 70 mg cholesterol, 610 mg sodium, 7 g dietary fiber
Diet Exchanges: 2 vegetable, 2 bread, 3 meat, 1 fat
Carb Choices: 3

CHINO-LATINO BEEF KEBABS

Each kebab is studded with foods that help balance your blood sugar with a one-two punch. Lean beef provides protein to stop you from overeating, and the onions, green peppers, and tomatoes deliver fiber to block the digestion of excess calories.

Photo on page 212.

Prep time: 20 minutes • Marinating time: 2 hours • Cook time: 8 minutes

1 pound lean boneless sirloin, trimmed of all visible fat

1 tablespoon grated fresh ginger

2 cloves garlic, minced

3 tablespoons reduced-sodium soy sauce

1 teaspoon Worcestershire sauce

1 teaspoon dried oregano

½ teaspoon ground cumin

½ teaspoon sesame oil

1 sweet onion, such as Vidalia, cut into 16 pieces

1 medium green bell pepper, seeded and cut into 16 squares

12 cherry tomatoes

¼ teaspoon salt

With a sharp knife, cut the sirloin into twenty 1" cubes and place in a bowl. In a separate bowl, combine the ginger, garlic, soy sauce, Worcestershire sauce, oregano, cumin, and oil. Add the mixture to the beef and stir well to coat. Cover the bowl and refrigerate for 2 hours or overnight.

Preheat the broiler and coat a broiler-pan rack with cooking spray. Alternately thread 5 beef cubes, 4 onion pieces, 4 bell pepper squares, and 3 cherry tomatoes onto each of four 18" wooden or metal skewers. Place the skewers onto the broiler pan and sprinkle with the salt. Broil 4" from the heat source for 8 to 10 minutes, turning them every 2 minutes, until the vegetables are tender and the beef is cooked through.

Makes 4 servings

Per serving: 188 calories, 23 g protein, 9 g carbohydrates, 7 g fat, 65 mg cholesterol, 360 mg sodium, 2 g dietary fiber
Diet Exchanges: 2 vegetable, 3 meat, 1 fat
Carb Choices: 1

BEEF FAJITAS

For many people, spicy foods are a great way to chase away those salty cravings. This Mexican favorite is guaranteed to heat things up around the dinner table.

Prep time: 15 minutes • Marinating time: 4 hours • Cook time: 18 minutes

1	tablespoon olive oil	1/4	teaspoon salt
4	cloves garlic, minced	2	bell peppers, green or red, seeded and cut into 1/4"-wide strips
2	tablespoons lime juice		
1	teaspoon grated lime zest	1	onion, cut into 1/4"-wide slices
1	teaspoon ground cumin	4	whole wheat tortillas (8" diameter)
1	pound lean round tip sirloin, trimmed of all visible fat	1/2	cup medium-hot salsa
		1/4	cup fat-free sour cream

In a resealable plastic bag, combine the oil, garlic, lime juice, lime zest, and cumin. Add the sirloin and toss well to coat. Refrigerate for 4 hours or overnight.

Preheat the grill or broiler. Remove the sirloin from the marinade, reserving any leftover marinade, and sprinkle with the salt. Grill or broil 4" from the heat for 5 to 6 minutes per side, or until an instant-read thermometer inserted into the center registers 145°F for medium-rare. Transfer to a cutting board and cover loosely with foil.

Heat a nonstick skillet over medium-high heat. Add the bell peppers, onion, and the reserved marinade. Cook, stirring often, for 8 to 9 minutes, or until the vegetables are softened. Warm the tortillas according to package directions.

Thinly slice the sirloin across the grain on a slight angle. To assemble a fajita, place 1 tortilla on a plate and top with one-quarter of the sirloin, one-quarter of the vegetable mixture, 2 tablespoons salsa, and 1 tablespoon sour cream. Repeat with the remaining ingredients.

Makes 4 servings

Per serving: 330 calories, 30 g protein, 33 g carbohydrates, 11 g fat, 50 mg cholesterol, 620 mg sodium, 4 g dietary fiber
Diet Exchanges: 2 vegetable, 1 bread, 3 1/2 meat, 1 1/2 fat
Carb Choices: 2

SUPER-EASY BARBECUE PULLED PORK

Barbecued spareribs contain an astounding 26 grams of fat! Try this hearty high-protein dish instead. It is just as satisfying and will fill you up without weighing you down with lots of saturated fat.

Prep time: 10 minutes • Cook time: 1 hour 45 minutes

1 **tablespoon olive oil**	2 **teaspoons packed brown sugar**
1 ½ **pounds boneless pork loin, trimmed of all visible fat**	2 **teaspoons mustard powder**
	1 ½ **teaspoons garlic powder**
1 **medium onion, chopped (about ½ cup)**	1 **teaspoon Worcestershire sauce**
⅔ **cup ketchup**	¼ **teaspoon freshly ground black pepper**
1 **tablespoon cider vinegar**	1 ½ **cups chicken or vegetable broth**
1 **tablespoon molasses**	

Heat the oil in a medium saucepan over medium-high heat. Add the pork loin and brown, turning occasionally, for 5 minutes. Add the onion, ketchup, vinegar, molasses, sugar, mustard powder, garlic powder, Worcestershire sauce, black pepper, and broth. Stir the mixture well to combine and bring to a boil over medium-high heat. Reduce the heat to low, cover, and simmer, stirring occasionally, for 1 ½ hours. Uncover the saucepan and simmer 10 minutes longer, or until the sauce has thickened slightly and the pork is very tender. Remove from the heat.

Pull the pork into shreds with two forks and serve.

Makes 6 servings

Per serving: 249 calories, 26 g protein, 18 g carbohydrates, 8 g fat, 75 mg cholesterol, 630 mg sodium, 1 g dietary fiber
Diet Exchanges: ½ vegetable, 1 bread, 3 ½ meat, 1 fat
Carb Choices: 1

GRILLED PORK TENDERLOIN WITH GRILLED PEACHES

FAST
PREP

If the peaches in your market aren't ripe, choose ripe nectarines instead. If you don't like spicy, use less cayenne or omit it altogether. But if you do opt for a little heat, you'll find that it's a terrific match for the intensely sweet grilled peaches.

Prep time: 8 minutes • Cook time: 26 minutes

1 whole pork tenderloin (1 pound), trimmed	½ teaspoon freshly ground black pepper
1½ teaspoons sweet paprika	¼ teaspoon cayenne pepper
½ teaspoon mustard powder	2 tablespoons canola oil
½ teaspoon salt	2 large firm-ripe peaches or nectarines

Heat a barbecue grill to medium.

Place the pork tenderloin on a rimmed baking sheet. In a cup, mix the paprika, mustard powder, salt, and peppers. Rub all over the pork. Spoon 1 tablespoon of the oil over the pork and roll it gently in the pan so all sides are coated.

Place the pork on the grill rack. Cover and grill, turning once or twice, for 20 to 25 minutes, or until an instant-read thermometer inserted into the thickest part registers 155°F. Transfer to a platter and cover loosely to keep warm.

Meanwhile, halve and pit the peaches, and brush the insides and outsides with the remaining 1 tablespoon oil.

Place the peach halves on the grill cut side up. Grill, moving them a few times, for 6 to 10 minutes, depending on the ripeness, until the color deepens and the fruit feels soft.

Cut the pork into thin slices and serve with the grilled peaches.

Makes 4 servings

Per serving: 230 calories, 25 g protein, 8 g carbohydrates, 11 g fat, 75 mg cholesterol, 350 mg sodium, 1 g dietary fiber
Diet Exchanges: ½ fruit, 3 ½ meat, 2 fat
Carb Choices: ½

ROASTED PORK LOIN WITH ORANGE AND THYME

Serve this inspired dish with roasted asparagus and mashed sweet potatoes for a fabulous autumn supper. Any leftovers are good cold with an arugula, orange, and red onion salad.

Prep time: 6 minutes • Cook time: 50 minutes

3   cloves garlic, minced

2   teaspoons grated orange zest

3/4   teaspoon dried thyme

1/2   teaspoon salt

1/2   teaspoon freshly ground black pepper

1/4   teaspoon crushed red-pepper flakes

1   center-cut boneless pork-loin roast (1 pound), well-trimmed

Orange wedges or slices

Preheat the oven to 375°F. Line a 9" × 9" baking pan with foil and coat the foil with olive oil cooking spray.

On a cutting board, combine the garlic, orange zest, thyme, salt, black pepper, and red-pepper flakes. Chop together until the garlic is finely minced and the ingredients are well blended. Rub all over the pork.

Place the pork in the prepared pan. Roast for 50 to 60 minutes, or until an instant-read thermometer inserted in the thickest part registers 155°F.

Remove the pork from the oven and let it stand for 10 minutes before carving into thin slices. Serve with orange wedges or slices as a garnish.

Makes 4 servings

Per serving: 170 calories, 25 g protein, 1 g carbohydrates, 7 g fat, 70 mg cholesterol, 370 mg sodium, 0 g dietary fiber
Diet Exchanges: 3 1/2 meat, 1 fat
Carb Choices: 0

APRICOT-STUFFED PORK LOIN

Apricots deliver a healthy dose of fiber at a minimal calorie cost. Each luscious fruit has 1 gram of fiber and only 17 calories. They are also low in fat and contain no cholesterol, so they are ideal for controlling your weight. *Photo on page 213.*

Prep time: 20 minutes • Cook time: 1 hour 10 minutes

1 teaspoon ground cumin	¾ cup dried apricots, finely chopped
1 teaspoon garlic powder	¼ cup chopped fresh parsley
½ teaspoon salt	¼ cup apricot preserves
¼ teaspoon ground allspice	1½ pounds boneless pork loin, trimmed of all visible fat
¼ teaspoon freshly ground black pepper	

Preheat the oven to 375°F. Coat a shallow baking pan with cooking spray and place a wire rack on it. Coat the wire rack with cooking spray as well.

Combine ¾ teaspoon of the cumin, ½ teaspoon of the garlic powder, the salt, ⅛ teaspoon of the allspice, and ⅛ teaspoon of the pepper in a medium bowl. Add the apricots, parsley, and 2 tablespoons of the preserves and mix well.

Using a long, thin knife, cut a 1½"-wide horizontal slit into the end of the pork, cutting through to the other end of the pork to form a deep pocket. Spoon the apricot mixture into the pocket, using the handle from a rubber spatula to pack it in. Combine the remaining ¼ teaspoon cumin, ½ teaspoon garlic powder, ⅛ teaspoon allspice, and ⅛ teaspoon pepper. Rub the spice mixture over the pork.

Place the pork on the wire rack in the prepared pan. Bake for 45 minutes. Brush with the remaining 2 tablespoons preserves. Bake for 25 to 35 minutes longer, or until a meat thermometer inserted in the center registers 160°F and the juices run clear.

Makes 6 servings

Per serving: 222 calories, 24 g protein, 13 g carbohydrates, 7 g fat, 75 mg cholesterol, 250 mg sodium, 1 g dietary fiber
Diet Exchanges: 1 fruit, 3 meat
Carb Choices: 1

LOIN PORK CHOPS BRAISED WITH PORT AND PRUNES

What prunes lack in glamour, they make up for in nutrition. They are an excellent source of fiber, and their bold flavor is the perfect complement to pork.

Prep time: 10 minutes • Cook time: 23 minutes

16 pitted prunes, chopped

¾ cup port wine

4 boneless loin pork chops (4 ounces each)

½ teaspoon salt

1 tablespoon butter

¼ cup finely chopped leeks

¼ cup finely chopped carrots

¼ cup finely chopped celery

1 teaspoon chopped fresh thyme

½ cup reduced-sodium, fat-free beef broth

1 tablespoon red currant jelly or apricot preserves

⅛ teaspoon freshly ground black pepper

In a medium saucepan, combine the prunes and port. Bring to a simmer over medium-low heat and simmer for 7 to 10 minutes, or until the prunes are plump, then remove from the heat.

Sprinkle the pork chops with ¼ teaspoon of the salt. In a large nonstick skillet over medium-high heat, melt ½ tablespoon of the butter and add the pork chops. Cook for 1 minute per side, or until lightly browned. Remove the pork from the pan.

Reduce the heat to medium and add the leeks, carrots, celery, and thyme to the skillet. Cook, stirring occasionally, for 4 to 5 minutes, or until the vegetables are lightly browned. Add the beef broth and the prune mixture to the skillet and bring to a simmer over medium-low heat. Place the pork in the skillet and cook for 4 to 5 minutes, or until the pork is tender and cooked through. Remove the pork chops to a plate and keep warm.

Increase the heat under the skillet to high and bring to a boil. Boil the sauce for 3 to 4 minutes, or until it starts to thicken slightly. Remove from the heat and stir in the jelly or preserves, pepper, and the remaining ½ tablespoon butter and ¼ teaspoon salt. Spoon the sauce and prunes over the pork and serve.

Makes 4 servings

Per serving: 400 calories, 27 g protein, 37 g carbohydrates, 10 g fat, 70 mg cholesterol, 390 mg sodium, 2 g dietary fiber
Diet Exchanges: 2 fruit, ½ vegetable, 3 ½ meat, 2 ½ fat
Carb Choices: 2

HOISIN PORK STIR-FRY

This stir-fry boasts a medley of colorful, high-fiber vegetables and high-quality protein to delight your senses and keep your appetite controlled for hours.

Prep time: 10 minutes • Cook time: 15 minutes

1 **pound pork tenderloin, trimmed of all visible fat**	1 **medium carrot, peeled and sliced on an angle**
2 **tablespoons reduced-sodium soy sauce**	1/4 **teaspoon crushed red-pepper flakes**
1 **tablespoon dry sherry**	1 **tablespoon grated fresh ginger**
1 **tablespoon cornstarch**	2 **cloves garlic, minced**
1 **tablespoon sesame oil**	1/2 **cup orange juice**
3 **cups broccoli florets, from about 1/2 bunch**	3 **tablespoons hoisin sauce**

With a sharp knife, cut the pork into 1 1/2"-long by 1/4"-wide strips and place in a bowl. Add the soy sauce, sherry, and cornstarch, tossing to combine.

Heat the oil in a large nonstick skillet over medium-high heat. Add the broccoli, carrot, and red-pepper flakes. Cook, stirring often, for 3 to 4 minutes. Remove to a plate. Add the ginger and garlic to the pan and cook for 1 minute. Stir in the pork and cook for 4 minutes, or until the pork is no longer pink. Add the broccoli mixture to the pan and toss for 1 minute. Add the orange juice and hoisin sauce and bring the mixture to a boil. Cook for 1 minute longer, stirring to coat, until the mixture thickens slightly.

Makes 4 servings

Per serving: 267 calories, 26 g protein, 16 g carbohydrates, 10 g fat, 75 mg cholesterol, 580 mg sodium, 3 g dietary fiber
Diet Exchanges: 1/2 fruit, 1 vegetable, 1/2 bread, 3 meat, 1 fat
Carb Choices: 1

SPICED LAMB CHOPS WITH MANGO-KIWI RELISH

The "warm" spices—cumin, ginger, cinnamon, and nutmeg—that flavor the lamb chops blend beautifully with the sweet-tart fruit relish. *Photo on page 214.*

Prep time: 12 minutes • Cook time: 10 minutes

- 4 **bone-in rib or loin lamb chops (5 to 6 ounces each), well trimmed**
- ½ **teaspoon ground cumin**
- ½ **teaspoon ground ginger**
- ¼ **teaspoon turmeric**
- ⅛ **teaspoon ground nutmeg**
- ⅛ **teaspoon ground cinnamon**

- ½ **teaspoon salt**
- ½ **teaspoon freshly ground black pepper**
- ¼ **teaspoon sugar**
- 1 **ripe mango, peeled and chopped**
- 2 **ripe kiwifruits, peeled and chopped**
- 2 **tablespoons chopped fresh mint leaves**

If the chops are thick, pound them a little with the flat side of a chef's knife or the flat side of a meat mallet, so that they cook more evenly.

In a cup, mix the cumin, ginger, turmeric, nutmeg, cinnamon, salt, pepper, and sugar. Rub the spice mixture over both sides of the chops. Put the chops on a plate, cover loosely, and let stand while making the mango relish. (This can be done earlier in the day, and the chops refrigerated.)

Preheat the broiler.

In a small bowl, mix the mango, kiwifruits, and mint. Cover and set aside.

Broil the lamb chops 4" from the heat for 5 to 6 minutes per side, turning once, for medium. Serve the chops with the mango-kiwi relish.

Makes 4 servings

Per serving: 250 calories, 31 g protein, 15 g carbohydrates, 7 g fat, 115 mg cholesterol, 360 mg sodium, 3 g dietary fiber
Diet Exchanges: 1 fruit, 4 ½ meat
Carb Choices: 1

HERBED BUTTERFLIED LEG OF LAMB

Begin this dish the night before you plan to serve it and you'll have
the most amazing flavors come together on your grill.

Prep time: 10 minutes • Cook time: 30 minutes • Marinating time: 2 to 3 hours, or overnight

¼ cup dry red wine

1 tablespoon extra-virgin olive oil

2 tablespoons coarsely chopped fresh
rosemary

2 bay leaves

¾ teaspoon dried oregano, crumbled

¾ teaspoon dried mint, crumbled

½ teaspoon coarse-ground black pepper

1 butterflied leg of lamb (2 pounds), well-
trimmed

¾ teaspoon salt

In a shallow glass dish, stir together the wine, oil, rosemary, bay leaves, oregano, mint, and pepper.
Add the lamb and turn to coat with the marinade. Cover and marinate in the refrigerator for 2 to
3 hours or overnight, turning once or twice.

Preheat a barbecue grill to medium. Remove the lamb from the dish, reserving the marinade, and
sprinkle both sides with the salt. Place the lamb on the grill rack and spoon some of the reserved
marinade over. Discard the remaining marinade and bay leaves.

Cover the lamb and grill, turning 2 or 3 times, and moving it away from any hot spots, for 20 to
30 minutes, or until an instant-read thermometer inserted into the thickest part registers 145°F for
medium-rare (the edges will be crispy and more well done).

Place the lamb on a platter to catch the juices and let stand for 10 minutes. Cut into thin slices.

Makes 8 servings

Per serving: 310 calories, 20 g protein, 0 g carbohydrates, 24 g fat, 75 mg cholesterol, 300 mg sodium, 0 g dietary fiber
Diet Exchanges: 3 meat, 3 ½ fat
Carb Choices: 0

HEALTHY POULTRY AND SEAFOOD MAIN DISHES

FAST ◼ SUPER FAST ◼ FAST PREP

GRILLED CHICKEN AND BROCCOLI RABE WITH GARLIC-PARSLEY SAUCE

If you don't feel like firing up the barbie, cook the chicken indoors on a stove-top grill pan. The garlic-parsley sauce makes this dish incredibly satisfying either way.

Prep time: 15 minutes • Cook time: 12 minutes

SAUCE

1 **cup loosely packed flat-leaf parsley sprigs**

3 **tablespoons lemon juice**

2 **tablespoons extra-virgin olive oil**

2 **tablespoons reduced-sodium chicken or vegetable broth, or water**

1 **tablespoon fresh oregano leaves**

1 **clove garlic**

$\frac{1}{4}$ **teaspoon salt**

$\frac{1}{8}$ **teaspoon cayenne pepper (optional)**

$\frac{1}{4}$ **cup finely chopped red bell pepper**

CHICKEN AND BROCCOLI RABE

4 **boneless, skinless chicken breast halves, trimmed**

1 **package (12 ounces) microwaveable cut broccoli rabe**

To make the sauce: In a food processor or blender, combine the parsley, lemon juice, oil, broth or water, oregano, garlic, salt, and cayenne pepper, if using. Process until nearly smooth, stopping the machine once or twice to scrape down the sides. Transfer to a small bowl and stir in the bell pepper.

To make the chicken and broccoli rabe: Place the chicken in a pie plate and spoon 3 tablespoons of the garlic-parsley sauce over. Turn to coat, cover, and let stand while heating a barbecue grill to medium-hot.

Grill the chicken, covered, turning once, for 8 minutes, or until lightly charred and no longer pink in the thickest part. Transfer to a clean plate and cover loosely with foil to keep warm.

Microwave the broccoli rabe according to the package instructions. Divide among 4 plates, and place a chicken breast on top. Spoon the remaining sauce over and serve.

Makes 4 servings ($\frac{1}{2}$ cup sauce)

Per serving: 220 calories, 30 g protein, 6 g carbohydrates, 9 g fat, 65 mg cholesterol, 270 mg sodium, 2 g dietary fiber
Diet Exchanges: 1$\frac{1}{2}$ vegetable, 4 meat, 1$\frac{1}{2}$ fat
Carb Choices: $\frac{1}{2}$

GRILLED CITRUS-HONEY CHICKEN

Balancing the bright flavors of oranges and honey with just the right hint of sweetness makes for a tasty glaze during grilling. Excellent on grilled pork, too.

Prep time: 9 minutes • Cook time: 14 minutes • Marinating time: 1 to 2 hours

1 teaspoon grated orange zest	¼ teaspoon salt
½ cup fresh orange juice	¼ teaspoon ground cinnamon
3 tablespoons lemon juice	4 bone-in chicken breast halves, skinned and trimmed
2 tablespoons honey	Snipped fresh chives (optional)
1 tablespoon olive oil	Orange wedges (optional)
1 clove garlic, minced	
½ teaspoon coarsely ground black pepper	

In a glass measure, with a fork, mix the orange zest, orange juice, lemon juice, honey, oil, garlic, pepper, salt, and cinnamon until well blended. Put the chicken breasts in a large zip-top bag and pour in the juice mixture. Seal the bag and massage gently to coat the chicken with the marinade. Place the bag in a dish or bowl and marinate in the refrigerator for 1 to 2 hours.

Heat a barbecue grill to medium. Drain the chicken marinade into a small saucepan and bring to a boil over medium heat. Boil 2 minutes, until thickened to a glaze.

Place the chicken on the grill and brush with some marinade. Cover and grill, basting two or three times more, and turning once, for about 12 minutes, until golden and cooked through.

If desired, garnish with the chives and serve with the orange wedges.

Makes 4 servings

Per serving: 270 calories, 40 g protein, 14 g carbohydrates, 6 g fat, 100 mg cholesterol, 260 mg sodium, 0 g dietary fiber
Diet Exchanges: ½ fruit, ½ bread, 5 ½ meat, 1 fat
Carb Choices: 1

STIR-FRIED ORANGE CHICKEN AND BROCCOLI

Broccoli is a star member of the cruciferous family. It has a respectable amount of fiber, along with myriad other nutrients that earn it top honors among food researchers.

Prep time: 20 minutes • Cook time: 7 minutes

1 **large bunch broccoli (about 1 ½ pounds)**

½ **cup orange juice**

2 **tablespoons reduced-sodium soy sauce**

2 **teaspoons cornstarch**

2 **tablespoons orange marmalade**

1 **tablespoon canola oil**

1 **pound chicken tenders, trimmed and cut into 1" pieces**

3 **scallions, sliced**

3 **large cloves garlic, minced**

1 **tablespoon minced fresh ginger**

Pinch of red-pepper flakes

⅓ **cup reduced-sodium chicken broth**

1 **red bell pepper, thinly sliced**

Cut the broccoli into small florets. Trim and discard about 2" of the tough broccoli stems. Thinly slice the remaining stems.

In a small bowl, combine the orange juice, soy sauce, cornstarch, and orange marmalade. Stir until blended. Set the sauce aside.

In a wok or large nonstick skillet, heat the oil over high heat. Add the chicken and cook, stirring frequently, for 2 to 3 minutes, or until no longer pink and the juices run clear. Add the scallions, garlic, ginger, and red-pepper flakes and stir to combine. With a slotted spoon, remove the chicken to a plate.

Add the broth and broccoli to the mixture in the wok and reduce the heat to medium. Cover and cook for 2 minutes. Increase the heat to high and add the bell pepper. Cook, stirring frequently, for 2 minutes, or until the broth evaporates and the vegetables are crisp-tender. Stir the sauce and add to the wok along with the chicken. Cook, stirring constantly, for 1 to 2 minutes, or until the sauce thickens and the chicken is hot.

Makes 4 servings

Per serving: 240 calories, 32 g protein, 23 g carbohydrates, 5 g fat, 65 mg cholesterol, 460 mg sodium, 6 g dietary fiber
Diet Exchanges: 2 ½ vegetable, ½ bread, 3 ½ meat, 1 fat
Carb Choices: 2

PEKING CHICKEN WRAPS

Try your hand at this takeout favorite at home. Cabbage is packed with compounds that researchers believe can protect us from heart disease and certain types of cancers. And it is a good source of fiber, as are brown rice, carrots, and whole wheat tortillas.

Photo on page 215.

Prep time: 30 minutes • Cook time: 35 minutes

½ cup brown rice

2 teaspoons dark sesame oil

4 scallions, sliced

¼ pound snow peas, trimmed

1 cup finely shredded red cabbage

1 cup shredded carrot

2 tablespoons unseasoned rice vinegar

2 teaspoons grated fresh ginger

6 whole wheat tortillas (10"–12" diameter)

6 tablespoons hoisin sauce

2 cups shredded cooked chicken breast

Cook the rice according to the package directions. Set aside.

Meanwhile, in a medium nonstick skillet, heat the oil over medium-high heat. Add the scallions and cook, stirring constantly, for 1 minute, or until wilted. Stir into the rice.

Bring a small pot of water to a boil. Add the snow peas and cook for 30 seconds. Drain and rinse with cold water until cool. Pat dry and cut lengthwise into thin strips. In a medium bowl, combine the snow peas, cabbage, carrot, rice vinegar, and ginger.

To assemble the wraps, lay the tortillas on a work surface. Spread each with 1 tablespoon hoisin sauce. Place one-sixth of the chicken in a strip along the bottom of each tortilla, 1" from the edges. Top with the rice and vegetable mixtures. Fold over the bottom edge of each tortilla to cover the filling. Fold the sides in and continue to roll up tightly, burrito style. Cut each in half crosswise with a serrated knife to serve.

Makes 6 servings

Per serving: 290 calories, 23 g protein, 45 g carbohydrates, 4 g fat, 45 mg cholesterol, 490 mg sodium, 5 g dietary fiber
Diet Exchanges: 1 vegetable, 2 ½ bread, 2 ½ meat, ½ fat
Carb Choices: 3

CHICKEN WITH PEACHES AND RED WINE

Skinless chicken breasts provide the high-quality protein you need to feel satisfied for hours. Peaches lend this festive dish a naturally sweet and fruity twist. *Photo on page 216.*

Prep time: 20 minutes • Cook time: 20 minutes

4 boneless, skinless chicken breast halves	3 shallots, thinly sliced
½ teaspoon freshly ground black pepper	½ cup dry red wine or chicken broth
¼ teaspoon salt	2 firm ripe peaches, sliced
3 tablespoons whole grain pastry flour	½ cup loosely packed fresh basil, sliced
1 tablespoon olive oil	

Use your hands to flatten the chicken breasts to an even thickness. Season the chicken with the pepper and the salt. Coat with the flour, patting off the excess.

Heat a large nonstick skillet over medium heat and add 2 teaspoons of the oil. Add the chicken breasts and cook for 12 minutes, turning once, until an instant-read thermometer inserted into the thickest portion registers 160°F and the juices run clear. Remove the chicken to a plate.

Add the remaining oil and the shallots to the skillet. Cook, stirring frequently, for 2 to 3 minutes, or until the shallots soften. Add the wine or broth and stir to scrape up any brown bits. Increase the heat to medium-high and add the peaches. Cook for 2 minutes, stirring frequently, until the wine reduces slightly. Return the chicken and any juices on the plate to the skillet. Cook for 1 to 2 minutes, stirring frequently, or until the chicken is hot. Stir in the basil.

Makes 4 servings

Per serving: 217 calories, 28 g protein, 11 g carbohydrates, 5 g fat, 65 mg cholesterol, 220 mg sodium, 2 g dietary fiber
Diet Exchanges: ½ fruit, ½ vegetable, 4 meat, 1 fat
Carb Choices: 1

COUNTRY CAPTAIN CHICKEN

This hearty dish offers several levels of protection against cravings. A delicious blend of fiber and monosaturated fats keep your appetite in check. *Photo on page 281.*

Prep time: 35 minutes • Cook time: 35 minutes

¼ cup sliced almonds

4 boneless, skinless chicken breast halves

½ teaspoon salt

2 tablespoons whole grain pastry flour

1 tablespoon olive oil

1 medium onion, chopped

2 bell peppers, coarsely chopped

2 cloves garlic, minced

1 tablespoon curry powder

½ teaspoon dried thyme

1 can (16 ounces) diced tomatoes

¼ cup dry red wine or chicken broth

3 tablespoons dried currants

Cook the almonds in a small nonstick skillet over medium heat, stirring often, for 3 to 4 minutes, or until lightly toasted. Tip onto a plate and let cool.

Cut the chicken breasts crosswise in half. Season with ¼ teaspoon of the salt. Lightly coat with the flour, patting off the excess. In a large pot or Dutch oven, heat the oil over medium heat. Add the chicken and cook for 3 minutes on each side, or until lightly browned but not cooked through. Remove the chicken to a plate.

Add the onion and bell peppers to the pot. Cook, stirring frequently, for 5 minutes, or until softened. Stir in the garlic, curry powder, thyme, and remaining ¼ teaspoon salt. Cook for 1 minute, stirring constantly. Add the tomatoes (with juice) and wine or broth and bring to a boil. Reduce the heat and simmer for 5 minutes. Stir in the currants.

Return the chicken to the pot, pushing it down into the sauce. Bring to a boil. Reduce the heat and partially cover the pot. Cook for 10 to 15 minutes, or until an instant-read thermometer inserted into the thickest portion registers 160°F and the juices run clear. Sprinkle with the almonds.

Makes 4 servings

Per serving: 305 calories, 31 g protein, 22 g carbohydrates, 9 g fat, 65 mg cholesterol, 510 mg sodium, 6 g dietary fiber
Diet Exchanges: ½ fruit, 2 vegetable, 4 meat, 1 ½ fat
Carb Choices: 1

OVEN-"FRIED" CHICKEN

Just one serving of traditional fried chicken can have up to 28 grams of fat! Here we offer you a healthier version that's tender and just as delicious.

Chill time: 2 hours • Prep time: 20 minutes • Cook time: 50 minutes

1 cut-up chicken (4 pounds), skin and any visible fat removed

1 cup buttermilk

1 clove garlic, minced

2 tablespoons ground flaxseed

½ cup dry whole wheat bread crumbs

3 tablespoons whole grain pastry flour

3 tablespoons cornmeal

1 teaspoon salt

¾ teaspoon freshly ground black pepper

½ teaspoon ground red pepper

Cut the chicken breasts in half. In a large bowl, combine the buttermilk and garlic. Add the chicken and turn to coat. Cover and refrigerate for 2 hours or overnight.

Preheat the oven to 400°F. Coat a large jelly-roll pan with cooking spray.

In a large food storage bag, shake the ground flaxseed, bread crumbs, flour, cornmeal, salt, and black and red pepper until blended. Drain the chicken in a colander. Pick up the chicken one piece at a time, letting the excess buttermilk drip off. Add to the bag and shake to coat. Place the chicken skinned side up on the prepared pan. Coat the chicken with cooking spray.

Bake for 50 to 55 minutes, or until an instant-read thermometer inserted into the thickest portion registers 170°F and the juices run clear.

Makes 6 servings

Per serving: 258 calories, 35 g protein, 14 g carbohydrates, 6 g fat, 100 mg cholesterol, 560 mg sodium, 2 g dietary fiber
Diet Exchanges: 1 bread, 5 meat, ½ fat
Carb Choices: 1

CHICKEN PESTO PRESTO

This dish couldn't be easier or more delicious. Serve with a big green salad and a quick-cooking grain, like quinoa. Dinner will be ready in a flash.

Prep time: 5 minutes • Cook time: 6 minutes

3–4   plum tomatoes

½   cup shredded part-skim mozzarella cheese

2   tablespoons grated Parmesan cheese

1   pound thinly sliced chicken breast cutlets (8 pieces)

¼   teaspoon salt

¼   teaspoon crushed red-pepper flakes

2   tablespoons prepared pesto sauce

Preheat the broiler. Coat a rimmed baking sheet with olive oil cooking spray.

Thinly slice the tomatoes lengthwise, discarding the core and the outside slices, to get 16 slices. Mix the mozzarella and Parmesan in a small bowl.

Arrange the chicken cutlets on the prepared baking sheet. Sprinkle with the salt and red-pepper flakes, and spread each with equal amounts of pesto.

Broil the chicken 2" to 4" from the heat for 5 minutes, or until no longer pink in the thickest part and the edges are lightly browned.

Remove from the oven. Top each piece of chicken with 2 tomato slices, overlapping if necessary, and sprinkle evenly with the mixed cheeses. Broil for 1 to 2 minutes longer, just until the cheese is melted and the tomatoes are heated. Serve right away.

Makes 4 servings

Per serving: 210 calories, 29 g protein, 3 g carbohydrates, 8 g fat, 75 mg cholesterol, 730 mg sodium, 0 g dietary fiber
Diet Exchanges: 4 ½ meat, 1 fat, ½ vegetable
Carb Choices: 0

OSSO BUCO–STYLE CHICKEN

Osso buco, which means pierced bone in Italian, is typically made with veal shanks. This recipe is a lighter version of the tried-and-true classic.

Prep time: 20 minutes • Cook time: 45 minutes

2   tablespoons olive oil

8   chicken drumsticks (2 pounds), skin removed

½   teaspoon salt

1   medium onion, chopped

2   carrots, chopped

2   ribs celery, chopped

4   cloves garlic, minced

1   can (14 ½ ounces) Italian-style diced tomatoes

1   can (14–19 ounces) chickpeas, rinsed and drained

1   cup chicken or vegetable broth

½   cup white wine or chicken broth

1   bay leaf

¼   cup chopped flat-leaf parsley

1   tablespoon grated lemon peel

In a soup pot or Dutch oven, heat the oil over medium-high heat. Sprinkle the chicken with ¼ teaspoon of the salt. Add the chicken and cook, turning occasionally, for 6 to 8 minutes, or until browned. Remove the chicken to a plate.

Reduce the heat to low and add the onion, carrots, celery, and the remaining ¼ teaspoon salt. Cover and cook for 8 minutes, or until the vegetables soften. Set aside 1 teaspoon garlic. Stir in the remaining garlic and cook for 1 minute. Add the tomatoes (with juice), chickpeas, broth, wine or broth, and bay leaf. Return the chicken to the pot. Bring to a boil. Reduce the heat, cover, and simmer for 30 to 35 minutes, or until the chicken is very tender. Remove and discard the bay leaf.

In a small bowl, combine the parsley, lemon peel, and the reserved 1 teaspoon garlic. Stir until combined. Serve the chicken sprinkled with the parsley mixture.

Makes 8 servings

Per serving: 276 calories, 28 g protein, 18 g carbohydrates, 9 g fat, 80 mg cholesterol, 670 mg sodium, 4 g dietary fiber
Diet Exchanges: 1 ½ vegetable, ½ bread, 3 ½ meat, 1 ½ fat
Carb Choices: 1

ROAST CHICKEN WITH BARLEY STUFFING

Fiber-rich barley is a great alternative to a traditional rice stuffing. Use any combination of your favorite dried fruits to create a signature dish.

Prep time: 35 minutes • Cook time: 1 hour 15 minutes

¾ **cup pearl barley**

1 **large navel orange**

2 **tablespoons olive oil**

1 **medium onion, chopped**

1 **carrot, chopped**

1 **rib celery, chopped**

4 **slices whole wheat bread, toasted and cut into cubes (2½ cups)**

¾ **cup mixed chopped dried fruit**

2 **teaspoons dried thyme**

1 **teaspoon salt**

½ **teaspoon freshly ground black pepper**

1 **cup chicken broth**

3 **cloves garlic, minced**

1 **whole frying chicken (4 pounds)**

Cook the barley according to the package directions. Drain and set aside. Grate the peel from the orange. Peel the orange and chop. Set aside.

In a large skillet, heat 1 tablespoon of the oil over medium-low heat. Add the onion, carrot, and celery. Cook, stirring occasionally, for 10 minutes, or until the onion begins to brown. Remove the skillet from the heat. Add the bread, dried fruit, ¾ teaspoon of the thyme, ¾ teaspoon of the salt, ¼ teaspoon of the pepper, the reserved barley, and the reserved chopped orange. Stir in the chicken broth. Coat a shallow 2-quart baking dish with cooking spray. Turn the stuffing into the dish and cover with foil.

Preheat the oven to 425°F. In a small bowl, combine the garlic, the reserved orange peel, and the remaining 1 tablespoon oil, 1¼ teaspoons thyme, ¼ teaspoon salt, and ¼ teaspoon pepper. Rub the orange mixture under and over the skin and in the cavity. Tie the legs with kitchen string.

Place the chicken on a rack set in a shallow roasting pan. Roast for 30 minutes. Place the stuffing in the oven. Reduce the oven temperature to 350°F and cook the stuffing and chicken for 45 to 55 minutes longer, or until a meat thermometer registers 180°F in the chicken breast and the juices run clear. Remove the foil from the stuffing after 25 minutes, or when hot. Cover the chicken loosely with foil and let rest for 10 minutes. Remove the skin before carving.

Makes 8 servings

Per serving: 320 calories, 27 g protein, 36 g carbohydrates, 8 g fat, 75 mg cholesterol, 610 mg sodium, 6 g dietary fiber
Diet Exchanges: 1 fruit, ½ vegetable, 1 bread, 2½ meat, 2½ fat
Carb Choices: 2

BAKED ZITI WITH TURKEY SAUSAGE

Perfect for a potluck, this lusty casserole is sure to become a family favorite. Even though it's packed with loads of healthy vegetables, the combination of gooey cheese and tender pasta steal the show.

Prep time: 15 minutes • Cook time: 50 minutes

1½ cups (5 ounces) whole wheat ziti, rotelle, or other short pasta

1 teaspoon + 2 tablespoons olive oil

1 pound lean Italian-style turkey sausage (mild or hot), cut into 4" pieces

1 large red bell pepper, chopped

1 small onion, chopped

6 large mushrooms (6 ounces), coarsely chopped

3 cloves garlic, minced

1 teaspoon dried oregano

½ teaspoon dried thyme

1 can (15 ounces) crushed tomatoes

¼ teaspoon salt

¼ teaspoon ground black pepper

1 large ripe tomato, chopped or cut into thin pieces (optional)

¾ cup (3 ounces) shredded mozzarella cheese

Preheat the oven to 375° F. Spray a shallow 3-quart baking dish with cooking spray and set aside.

Cook the pasta according to package directions. Drain and return to the pot. Add 1 teaspoon of the oil and toss to coat.

Heat the remaining 2 tablespoons oil in a large skillet over medium heat. Add the sausage and cook until browned and no longer pink inside, 8 to 10 minutes. Transfer the sausage to a clean plate and allow to cool while preparing the rest of the sauce.

Into the same skillet, add the bell pepper, onion, mushrooms, garlic, oregano, and thyme. Cook until the onion is almost soft, 6 to 7 minutes, stirring occasionally. Stir in the crushed tomatoes and cook for 5 minutes. Season with salt and black pepper.

Cut the sausage into ¼" slices and place in the prepared baking dish along with the sauce and pasta. Toss to combine. Top with fresh tomato (if using), only around the edges if desired, and sprinkle with the cheese. Bake until heated through and the cheese is melted and slightly browned, 20 to 25 minutes.

Makes 4 servings

Per serving: 340 calories, 26 g protein, 27 g carbohydrates, 15 g fat, 60 mg cholesterol, 293 mg sodium, 5 g fiber
Diet Exchanges: 2 vegetable, 1 bread, 3 meat, 2 ½ fat
Carb Choices: 2

SAVORY TURKEY STROGANOFF

Turkey is a superb source of protein, so this meal has the staying power to keep you away from those late-night snacks. *Photo on page 282.*

Prep time: 15 minutes • Cook time: 15 minutes

1 tablespoon olive oil

¾ pound turkey cutlets, cut into thin strips

2 large shallots, thinly sliced

1 box (10 ounces) cremini mushrooms, sliced

1 cup baby carrots, sliced

1 clove garlic, minced

1 teaspoon hot paprika

¼ teaspoon salt

1 cup chicken broth

2 teaspoons tomato paste

2 teaspoons Worcestershire sauce

2 teaspoons cornstarch

⅓ cup reduced-fat sour cream

In a large nonstick skillet, heat 2 teaspoons of the oil over high heat. Add the turkey and cook, stirring frequently, for 3 to 4 minutes, or until no longer pink and just cooked through. Remove to a plate.

Reduce the heat to medium-high and add the remaining 1 teaspoon oil and shallots to the skillet. Cook, stirring, for 1 minute, or until the shallots begin to soften. Add the mushrooms and carrots. Cook, stirring frequently, for 4 minutes, or until the mushrooms soften. Stir in the garlic, paprika, and salt and cook for 1 minute. Remove the skillet from the heat.

In a small bowl, stir the chicken broth, tomato paste, Worcestershire sauce, and cornstarch until blended. Return the skillet to medium heat and add the broth mixture. Cook, stirring frequently, until the sauce comes to a boil and thickens. Simmer for 2 minutes. Stir in the turkey and cook for 1 minute, or until hot. Remove the skillet from the heat and stir in the sour cream.

Makes 4 servings

Per serving: 248 calories, 30 g protein, 11 g carbohydrates, 9 g fat, 70 mg cholesterol, 500 mg sodium, 2 g dietary fiber
Diet Exchanges: 1 ½ vegetable, 4 meat, 1 ½ fat
Carb Choices: 1

TANDOORI TURKEY CUTLETS WITH PEAR-CHERRY CHUTNEY

Tandoori is an Indian term used to describe a method of cooking meats quickly over relatively high heat. While this lively, high-protein dish takes only minutes to prepare, its satisfaction is guaranteed to last.

Prep time: 15 minutes • Cook time: 4 minutes

1 large ripe pear, peeled, cored, and chopped

1 cup pitted fresh or frozen and thawed cherries, quartered

½ small red bell pepper, chopped

¼ cup bottled mango chutney

2 tablespoons finely chopped red onion

2 tablespoons chopped cilantro (optional)

1 tablespoon lime juice

1 teaspoon curry powder

1 teaspoon paprika

1 teaspoon ground cumin

¼ teaspoon salt

4 turkey cutlets (4 ounces each)

In a medium bowl, combine the pear, cherries, bell pepper, chutney, onion, cilantro (if using), and lime juice. Set aside.

In a small bowl, combine the curry powder, paprika, cumin, and salt. Sprinkle both sides of the turkey cutlets with the spice mixture, patting to coat.

Heat a grill pan over medium heat. Coat the pan with cooking spray. Cook the cutlets for 2 minutes on each side, or until no longer pink. Serve with the chutney.

Makes 4 servings (2 cups chutney)

Per serving: 223 calories, 27 g protein, 21 g carbohydrates, 4 g fat, 60 mg cholesterol, 200 mg sodium, 3 g dietary fiber
Diet Exchanges: 1 fruit, 1 vegetable, 4 meat
Carb Choices: 1

TURKEY AND BEAN CHILI

Thanks to an abundance of fiber, high-quality protein, and a zesty mix of seasonings, you can say *adiós* to cravings with our tasty version of this popular Mexican dish.

Prep time: 20 minutes • Cook time: 1 hour 10 minutes

1 pound ground turkey breast

1 large onion, chopped

2 red or yellow bell peppers, chopped

4 large cloves garlic, minced

3 tablespoons tomato paste

2 tablespoons chili powder

1 tablespoon ground cumin

1 teaspoon dried oregano

1 teaspoon salt

1 large sweet potato, peeled and cut into ½" cubes

1 can (28 ounces) diced tomatoes

1 can (14 ounces) chicken broth

1 chipotle chile pepper in adobo sauce, minced (optional)

2 cans (15–16 ounces each) mixed beans for chili, rinsed and drained

1 zucchini, chopped

In a large soup pot or Dutch oven, over medium-high heat, cook the turkey, onion, and bell peppers, stirring frequently, for 8 minutes, or until the turkey is cooked through. Add the garlic, tomato paste, chili powder, cumin, oregano, and salt. Cook, stirring constantly, for 1 minute.

Add the sweet potato, diced tomatoes (with juice), chicken broth, and chipotle chile, if using. Bring to a boil. Reduce the heat to low and simmer, covered, stirring occasionally, for 30 minutes.

Stir in the beans and zucchini. Return to a simmer. Cover and simmer for 30 minutes longer, stirring occasionally, or until the flavors are well-blended and the vegetables are tender.

Makes 8 servings

Per serving: 227 calories, 17 g protein, 29 g carbohydrates, 5 g fat, 45 mg cholesterol, 680 mg sodium, 10 g dietary fiber
Diet Exchanges: 2 vegetable, 1 bread, 2 meat
Carb Choices: 2

TURKEY SAUSAGE–STUFFED PEPPERS

Some research indicates that chile peppers may make you burn calories faster and increase metabolism. They are a perfect complement to this deliciously robust meal.

Prep time: 30 minutes • Cook time: 1 hour 5 minutes

¼ cup brown rice

1 large red bell pepper, cut in half lengthwise

1 large yellow bell pepper, cut in half lengthwise

¼ pound turkey sausage, casing removed

½ medium onion, chopped

1 clove garlic, minced

3 cups shredded spinach

2 ounces (½ can) chopped green chiles, rinsed and drained

¼ teaspoon ground cumin

⅛ teaspoon salt

1 tomato, chopped

½ cup shredded hot Pepper Jack cheese

Cook the rice according to the package directions. Set aside.

Preheat the oven to 350°F. Bring a large pot of water to a boil. Add the red and yellow peppers to the boiling water, cook for 3 minutes, and drain.

In a large nonstick skillet, over medium heat, cook the sausage, stirring frequently to break up, for 6 minutes, or until no longer pink. Remove with a slotted spoon to a large bowl. Add the onion to the skillet and cook, stirring frequently, for 6 to 8 minutes, or until golden brown. Stir in the garlic and cook for 1 minute. Add the spinach, chiles, cumin, and salt. Cook, stirring occasionally, for 5 minutes, or until the spinach wilts. Add to the sausage. Stir in the rice, half of the tomato, and ¼ cup of the cheese.

Fill the pepper halves with the rice mixture. Place in a shallow baking dish. Spoon the remaining tomato over the filling. Cover the dish loosely with foil. Bake for 30 minutes. Uncover and sprinkle with the remaining ¼ cup cheese. Bake for 10 minutes longer, or until the cheese melts and the filling is hot.

Makes 4 servings

Per serving: 186 calories, 11 g protein, 15 g carbohydrates, 9 g fat, 60 mg cholesterol, 390 mg sodium, 3 g dietary fiber
Diet Exchanges: 2 vegetable, ½ bread, 1 ½ meat, 1 fat
Carb Choices: 1

SKILLET TURKEY TETRAZZINI

Nothing is more comforting than a creamy stove-top casserole, and this updated
classic fits the bill perfectly. Just a quick pass under the broiler guarantees
a wonderful, crunchy-topped finish.

Prep time: 20 minutes • Cook time: 30 minutes

½ **pound whole wheat pasta, such as penne**

1 **bag (10 ounces) fresh spinach, large leaves
torn in half**

1 **tablespoon olive oil**

1 **pound turkey cutlets, cut into ¾" pieces**

1 **box (8 ounces) sliced mushrooms**

1 **small onion, finely chopped**

¾ **cup chicken broth**

¾ **cup 1% milk**

2 **tablespoons cornstarch**

½ **cup frozen peas**

¾ **cup freshly grated Parmesan cheese**

2 **tablespoons ground flaxseed**

Prepare the pasta according to package directions. Before draining, add the spinach and stir until
wilted. Drain the pasta.

In a large ovenproof skillet, heat the oil over medium-high heat. Add the turkey and cook, stirring
frequently, for 3 to 4 minutes, or until no longer pink. Remove to a plate.

Reduce the heat to medium-low and add the mushrooms and onion to the skillet. Cook, stirring
frequently, for 5 minutes, or until softened. Add the chicken broth and bring to a boil.

Preheat the broiler. In a small bowl, combine the milk and cornstarch. Stir until the cornstarch dis-
solves. Stir into the broth mixture. Add the peas and bring to a boil, stirring frequently. Reduce the
heat and simmer for 3 minutes, stirring frequently. Stir ½ cup of the cheese, turkey, and pasta into
the sauce. Sprinkle with the flaxseed and remaining ¼ cup cheese. Broil for 2 to 3 minutes, or until
the cheese melts.

Makes 6 servings

Per serving: 383 calories, 28 g protein, 39 g carbohydrates, 14 g fat, 70 mg cholesterol, 480 mg sodium, 8 g dietary fiber
Diet Exchanges: 1 vegetable, 2 bread, 3 ½ meat, 1 fat
Carb Choices: 3

SANTA FE TURKEY PIZZAS

Fill up fast with this high-fiber, high-protein meal. Of course, all you'll taste is a lively blend of turkey and vegetables with a south-of-the-border twist!

Prep time: 15 minutes • Cook time: 16 minutes

4   whole wheat tortillas (8" diameter)

6   ounces ground turkey breast

1   small red bell pepper, chopped

1   small zucchini, thinly sliced

¼   cup chopped red onion

1   cup fresh or frozen and thawed corn

1   cup canned salt-free black beans, rinsed and drained

1   tablespoon chili powder

1 ½   cups mild chunky salsa

2   tablespoons chopped cilantro

⅓   cup reduced-fat shredded Mexican cheese blend (see note)

2   tablespoons chopped pickled jalapeño chile pepper (optional)

2   cups loosely packed shredded escarole

¼   cup reduced-fat sour cream (optional)

Preheat the oven to 450°F. Arrange the oven racks to divide the oven into thirds. Place the tortillas on 2 baking sheets.

In a large nonstick skillet over medium-high heat, cook the turkey, bell pepper, zucchini, and onion, stirring frequently to break up the turkey, for 5 minutes, or until the turkey is no longer pink. Stir in the corn, beans, chili powder, and ¾ cup of the salsa. Cook for 2 minutes, stirring, until heated through. Stir in the cilantro.

Top the tortillas with the turkey mixture, spreading up to ½" from the edges. Bake for 8 minutes, rotating the cookie sheets halfway through, or until the tortillas are crisp and browned at the edges. Sprinkle with the cheese and bake for 1 to 2 minutes, or until melted. Sprinkle with the jalapeño (if using) and the escarole. Serve with the sour cream, if you wish, and the remaining ¾ cup salsa on the side.

Note: If Mexican cheese blend is not available, use reduced-fat Cheddar cheese.

Makes 4 servings

Per serving: 350 calories, 23 g protein, 51 g carbohydrates, 6 g fat, 35 mg cholesterol, 620 mg sodium, 5 g dietary fiber

Diet Exchanges: 2 vegetable, 2 bread, 3 meat, 1 fat

Carb Choices: 3

CHILI-SPICED TURKEY-BEAN BURGERS WITH GUACAMOLE

These spirited burgers, loaded with spices and topped with a spoonful of guacamole, are love at first bite. *Photo on page 283.*

Prep time: 20 minutes • Cook time: 20 minutes

GUACAMOLE

1 ripe avocado

2 tablespoons chopped sweet white onion

1 tablespoon salsa

1 tablespoon fresh lime juice

Salt

BURGERS

$^2\!/_3$ cup canned black beans, rinsed and drained

1 large egg

1 tablespoon + 2 teaspoons chili powder

$^1\!/_2$ teaspoon ground cumin

$^1\!/_2$ teaspoon salt

1 pound lean ground turkey breast

4 small whole grain hamburger buns, split

4 slices tomato

To make the guacamole: In a small bowl, mash the avocado with a fork until fairly smooth. Mix in the onion, salsa, lime juice, and salt. Cover tightly and set aside.

To make the burgers: Preheat the broiler. Coat the broiler pan rack with olive oil cooking spray.

In a medium bowl, mash the beans to a chunky texture. Stir in the egg, chili powder, cumin, and salt until well blended. Add the ground turkey and mix first with a spoon, then gently with your hands, until well blended (mix lightly so burgers don't get tough). With moistened hands, shape mixture into 4 equal-sized patties. Place on the prepared broiler-pan rack.

Broil the patties 4" to 6" from the heat for 6 to 7 minutes per side, until lightly browned, firm, and cooked through. Transfer to a plate. Place the buns on the broiler pan and toast.

Place toasted buns on 4 plates. On the bun bottom, place a tomato slice and a burger. Spoon 2 tablespoons guacamole over each, cover with the bun top, and serve.

Makes 4 servings

Per serving: 350 calories, 37 g protein, 34 g carbohydrates, 9 g fat, 125 mg cholesterol, 820 mg sodium, 8 g dietary fiber
Diet Exchanges: 2 bread, 1 fat, 4 meat
Carb Choices: 2

GRILLED ROSEMARY-LEMON TURKEY

This summery dish is wonderful served alongside fresh sliced tomatoes
and cucumbers or a bulgur and parsley salad.

Prep time: 12 minutes • Marinating time: 1 to 2 hours • Cook time: 8 minutes

2　**tablespoons chopped fresh rosemary
　leaves**

1 ½　**teaspoons grated lemon zest**

2　**tablespoons lemon juice**

1　**tablespoon extra-virgin olive oil**

½　**teaspoon freshly ground black pepper**

¼　**teaspoon salt**

2　**cloves garlic, peeled and smashed**

1　**pound turkey cutlets (4 ounces each)**

　Lemon wedges

In a pie plate, mix 1 ½ tablespoons rosemary, lemon zest, lemon juice, oil, pepper, and salt. Add the garlic and turkey cutlets and turn to coat with the marinade. Cover and marinate in the refrigerator for 1 to 2 hours.

Heat a barbecue grill to medium-hot. Turn the turkey once more in the marinade and place on the grill. Cover and grill, turning once, for 2 to 4 minutes per side, until just cooked through.

Sprinkle the turkey cutlets with the remaining ½ tablespoon chopped rosemary and serve with lemon wedges.

Makes 4 servings

Per serving: 160 calories, 28 g protein, 1 g carbohydrates, 4 g fat, 45 mg cholesterol, 250 mg sodium, 0 g dietary fiber
Diet Exchanges: 3 ½ meat, 1 fat
Carb Choices: 0

TURKEY KEBABS WITH MANGO-PINEAPPLE SALSA

Fresh, fruity salsa gives this protein-rich meal a deliciously exotic touch.

Prep time: 35 minutes • Marinating time: 1 hour • Cook time: 12 minutes

TURKEY AND MARINADE

1½ pounds turkey tenderloin, trimmed and cut into eighteen 1" pieces

1 teaspoon grated orange peel

½ cup orange juice

2 tablespoons soy sauce

1 tablespoon honey

2 cloves garlic, minced

½ teaspoon freshly ground black pepper

SALSA

1 large ripe mango, peeled and chopped

1½ cups chopped fresh or canned unsweetened pineapple

2 tablespoons chopped red onion

1 chipotle chile pepper in adobo sauce, minced

1 tablespoon seasoned rice vinegar

2 tablespoons chopped fresh mint

½ teaspoon salt

2 large red onions, cut into 6 wedges each

1 large red bell pepper, cut into twelve 1" pieces

1 medium zucchini, cut into 12 slices

To make the turkey and marinade: Place the turkey in a food storage bag. In a small bowl, combine the orange peel, orange juice, soy sauce, honey, garlic, and pepper. Whisk until blended. Pour over the turkey. Seal the bag and turn to coat. Marinate for 1 hour.

To make the salsa: In a medium bowl, combine the mango, pineapple, onion, chile, vinegar, mint, and ¼ teaspoon salt. Stir to mix. Set aside at room temperature.

Coat a grill rack with cooking spray. Preheat the grill. Remove the turkey from the marinade and set the marinade aside. Thread the turkey, onion, bell pepper, and zucchini evenly onto skewers.

Grill the kebabs, turning frequently and brushing with the marinade, for 12 to 15 minutes, or until the juices run clear. Sprinkle with the remaining ¼ teaspoon salt. Serve with the salsa.

Makes 6 servings

Per serving: 223 calories, 29 g protein, 25 g carbohydrates, 2 g fat, 55 mg cholesterol, 590 mg sodium, 3 g dietary fiber
Diet Exchanges: 1 fruit, 1 vegetable, ½ bread, 3 ½ meat
Carb Choices: 2

CITRUS-DRIZZLED WHOLE STRIPED BASS

The striped bass is sometimes called a striper on the Atlantic Coast and a rockfish in the Chesapeake Bay area. If you want outstanding flavor, buy only fresh bass. It should have bright eyes and a firm silver body that will not hold fingerprints when it's handled.

Prep time: 15 minutes • Cook time: 35 minutes

1 whole striped bass (3–3 ½ pounds), cleaned (head and tail on)

1 tablespoon olive oil

6 sprigs fresh thyme

20 fresh basil leaves

2 scallions, chopped

2 tablespoons lime juice

2 tablespoons lemon juice

2 tablespoons orange juice

2 teaspoons grated lime zest

2 teaspoons grated orange zest

½ teaspoon salt

¼ teaspoon freshly ground black pepper

2 navel oranges, peeled and cut into segments

Preheat the oven to 500°F. Coat a baking pan with cooking spray.

With a sharp knife, make 4 deep crosswise cuts, down to the bone, on each side of the fish. Rub the oil over both sides of the fish.

Arrange 3 sprigs of the thyme, 10 basil leaves, and half of the chopped scallions in a row down the center of the baking pan. Place the fish on top. Drizzle with the lime juice, lemon juice, and orange juice, then rub both sides with the lime and orange zest. Season the fish with the salt and pepper. Top with the remaining thyme, basil, and scallions. Loosely cover the fish with aluminum foil and pour ½ cup water into the baking pan. Bake for 30 minutes.

Remove the fish from the oven and top with the orange segments. Re-cover the fish with the aluminum foil and bake for 5 to 10 minutes longer, or until the fish flakes easily with a fork.

Makes 4 servings

Per serving: 243 calories, 31 g protein, 14 g carbohydrates, 7 g fat, 135 mg cholesterol, 410 mg sodium, 4 g dietary fiber
Diet Exchanges: 1 fruit, 4 ½ meat, 1 fat
Carb Choices: 1

STOVETOP-SMOKED TROUT WITH APPLE-HORSERADISH SAUCE

Fresh trout has a delicate taste and firm texture. It is a great source of protein, so it will help keep your appetite in check for hours.

Prep time: 45 minutes • Chill time: 2 hours • Cook time: 25 minutes

SAUCE

¼ cup light mayonnaise

3 tablespoons reduced-fat sour cream

½ small Granny Smith apple, peeled and finely chopped

4 teaspoons prepared horseradish, drained

½ teaspoon Dijon mustard

TROUT

1 quart water

½ teaspoon salt

2 cloves garlic, minced

2 tablespoons packed brown sugar

2 tablespoons honey

4 trout fillets (4–6 ounces each), such as rainbow, brook, or farm raised

1 cup mesquite wood chips, soaked in water for 30 minutes (see note)

¾ cup granulated sugar

¾ cup uncooked rice

To make the sauce: Combine the mayonnaise, sour cream, apple, horseradish, and mustard in a bowl. Refrigerate until ready to use.

To make the trout: In a large bowl, combine the water, salt, garlic, brown sugar, and honey. Add the trout and refrigerate for 2 hours.

In a small bowl, combine the wood chips, granulated sugar, and rice. Line a heavy Dutch oven or large cast-iron skillet with a double layer of heavy-duty aluminum foil. Spread the sugar mixture evenly over the bottom of the Dutch oven. Set a wire rack 1 $\frac{1}{2}$" to 2" above the sugar mixture in the Dutch oven. Remove the trout from the salt solution and rinse with cold water.

Place the trout on the wire rack. Cover the Dutch oven and set over high heat. When the pan begins to smoke, reduce the heat to low and cook for 15 to 20 minutes. Remove from the heat and let stand for 4 minutes.

Note: Make sure you have a well-ventilated kitchen or a good exhaust fan before making this dish.

Makes 4 servings ($\frac{3}{4}$ cup sauce)

Per serving: 280 calories, 24 g protein, 13 g carbohydrates, 14 g fat, 75 mg cholesterol, 510 mg sodium, 1 g dietary fiber
Diet Exchanges: 1 bread, 3 meat, 2 fat
Carb Choices: 1

MACKEREL IN A SAFFRON-TOMATO BROTH

Mackerel is one of the healthiest finfish you can buy. It is loaded with omega-3 fatty acids, which protect your heart. For best results, cook shortly after purchase.

Prep time: 15 minutes • Cook time: 54 minutes

2   cups clam broth

½   cup white wine or nonalcoholic wine

3   tablespoons tomato paste

1   cup finely chopped onion

3   cloves garlic, minced

3   sprigs fresh thyme

1   teaspoon saffron, lightly crushed

1   teaspoon fennel seed

¼   teaspoon salt

¼   teaspoon black pepper

2   tablespoons thinly sliced fresh basil

1   russet potato, about 8 ounces, peeled and cut into ¼" cubes

2   medium carrots, peeled and cut into ¼" cubes

4   mackerel fillets (4 ounces each), skin on, pinbones removed

In a medium saucepan over medium heat, heat the broth, wine, and tomato paste. Add the onion, garlic, thyme, saffron, and fennel seed. Bring to a boil, reduce the heat to medium-low, and simmer, covered, for 25 minutes. Uncover and cook for 20 minutes longer. Season with the salt and ⅛ teaspoon of the pepper. Strain the broth and return it to the saucepan. Stir in the basil and keep warm.

In a medium saucepan over high heat, combine the potato with enough water to cover by 4". Bring to a boil and cook for 4 minutes. Stir in the carrots and cook for 1 minute longer. Remove from the heat and let stand for 1 minute. Drain the vegetables and keep warm.

Heat a large nonstick skillet over medium-high heat. Coat the skillet with cooking spray. Season the mackerel with the remaining ⅛ teaspoon pepper. Add to the skillet skin side up and cook for 2 minutes. Turn and cook for 2 to 3 minutes longer, or until the fish flakes easily with a fork.

Divide the saffron-tomato broth among 4 shallow bowls. Place the potatoes and carrots in the center of each bowl. Top the vegetables with a mackerel fillet.

Makes 4 servings

Per serving: 370 calories, 25 g protein, 26 g carbohydrates, 16 g fat, 80 mg cholesterol, 600 mg sodium, 4 g dietary fiber
Diet Exchanges: 2 vegetable, ½ bread, 3 meat, 2 ½ fat
Carb Choices: 1

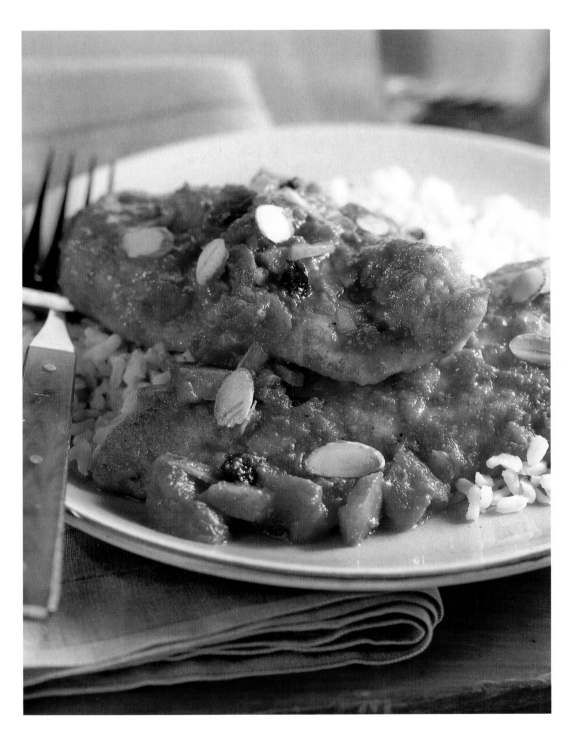

COUNTRY CAPTAIN CHICKEN

Recipe on page 261

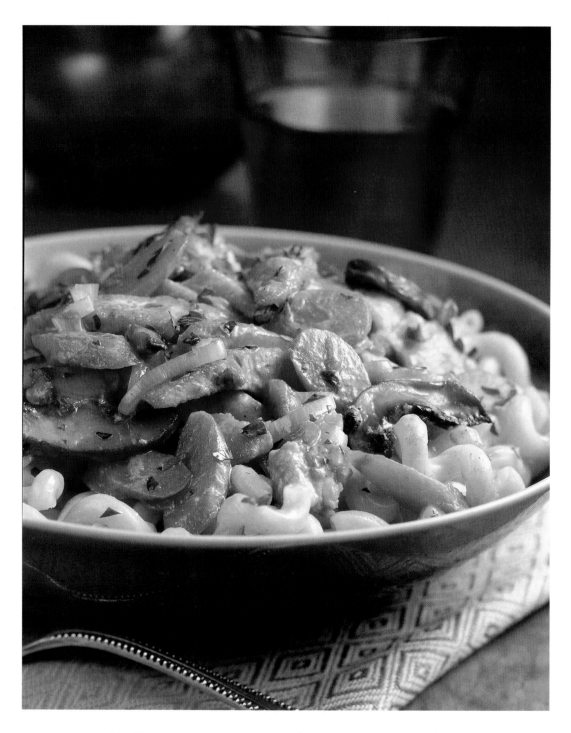

SAVORY TURKEY STROGANOFF (OVER MULTIGRAIN PASTA)

Recipe on page 268

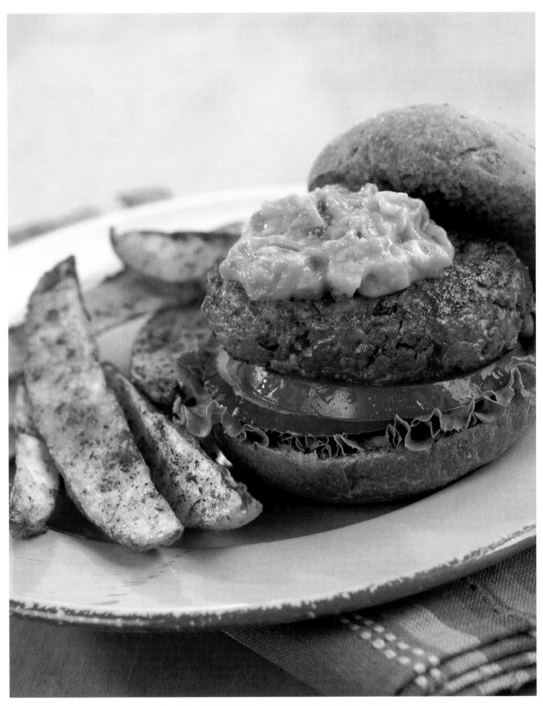

CAJUN-SPICED OVEN FRIES *(LEFT) AND*
CHILI-SPICED TURKEY-BEAN BURGERS WITH GUACAMOLE *(RIGHT)*

Recipes on pages 224 and 274

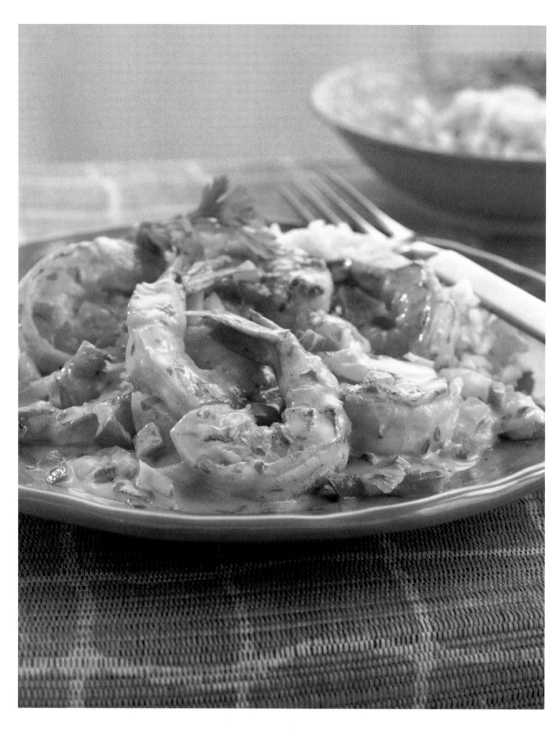

SHRIMP-COCONUT CURRY

Recipe on page 302

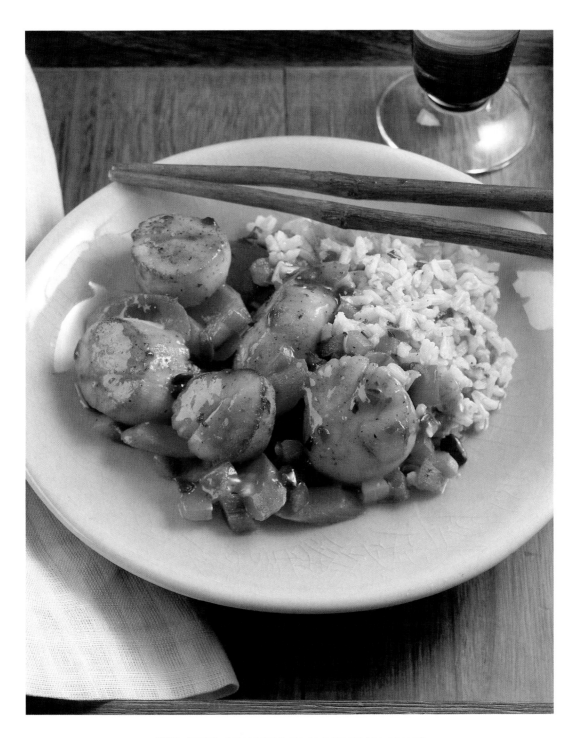

STIR-FRIED SCALLOPS IN BLACK BEAN SAUCE

Recipe on page 305

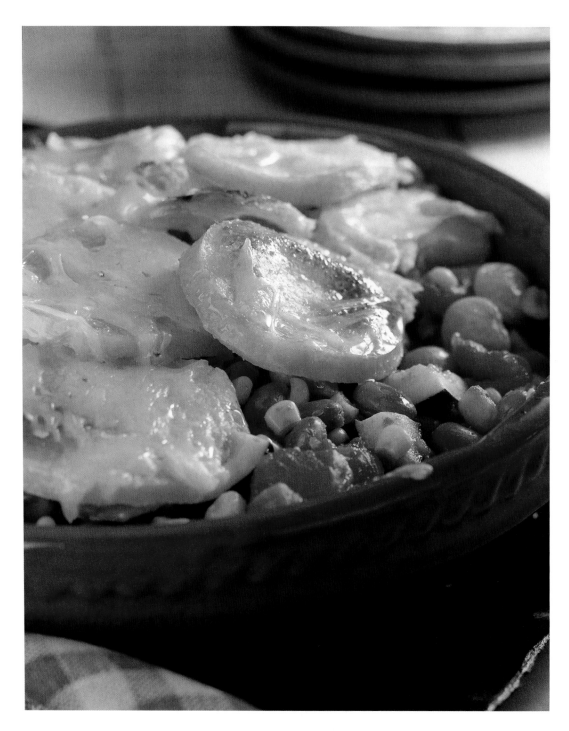

SPEEDY TAMALE PIE

Recipe on page 310

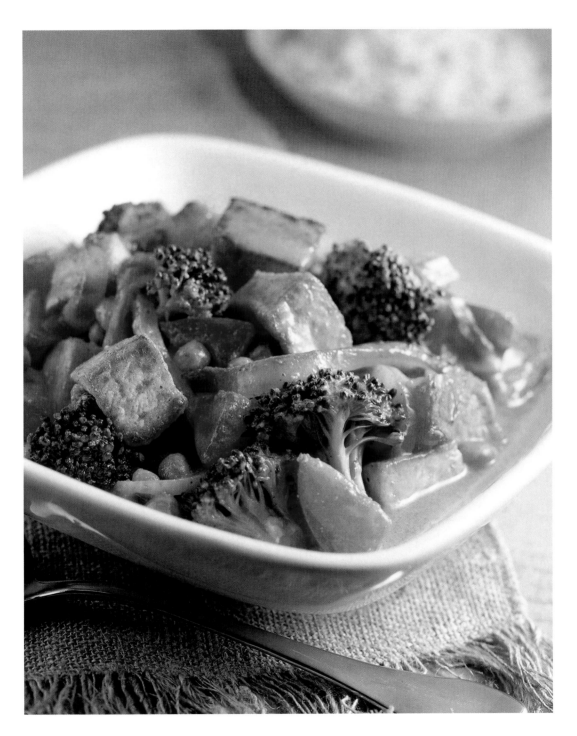

CURRIED TOFU

Recipe on page 311

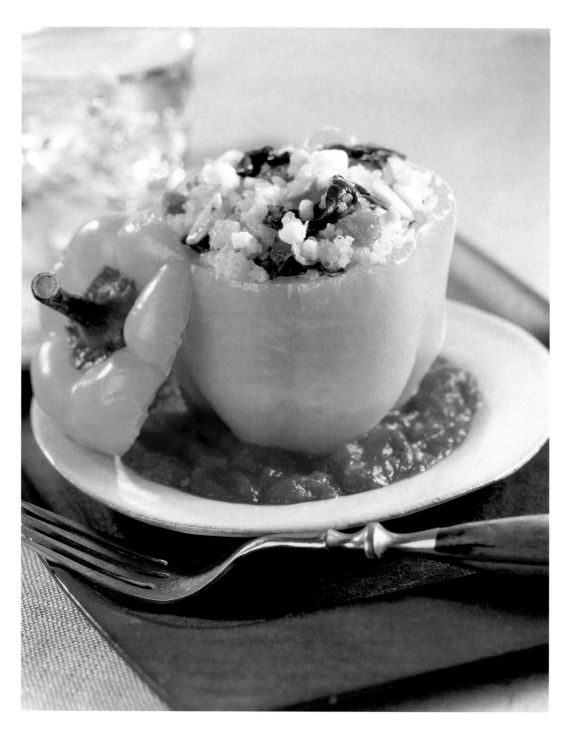

QUINOA-STUFFED PEPPERS

Recipe on page 314

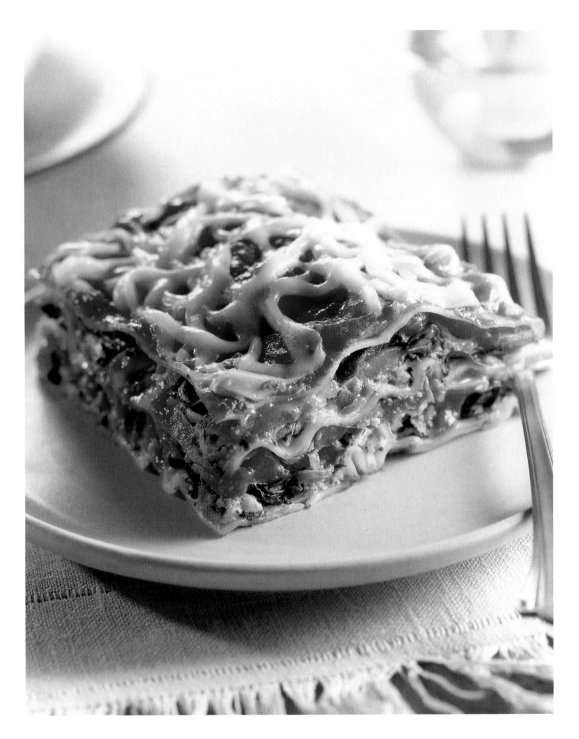

ROASTED VEGETABLE LASAGNE

Recipe on page 324

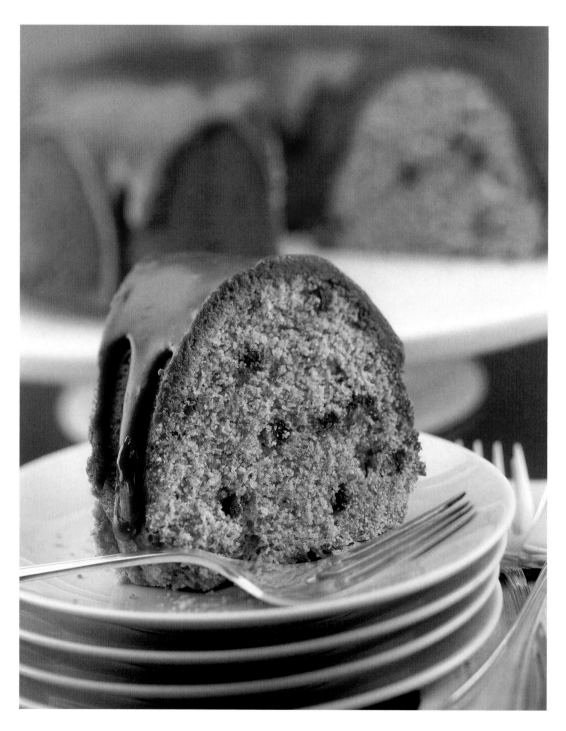

PEANUT BUTTER BUNDT CAKE

Recipe on page 340

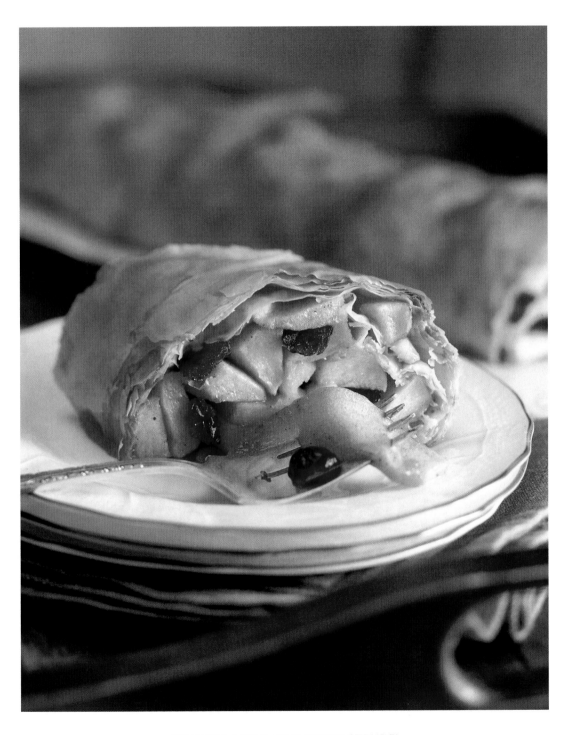

ROASTED APPLE-CRANBERRY STRUDEL

Recipe on page 346

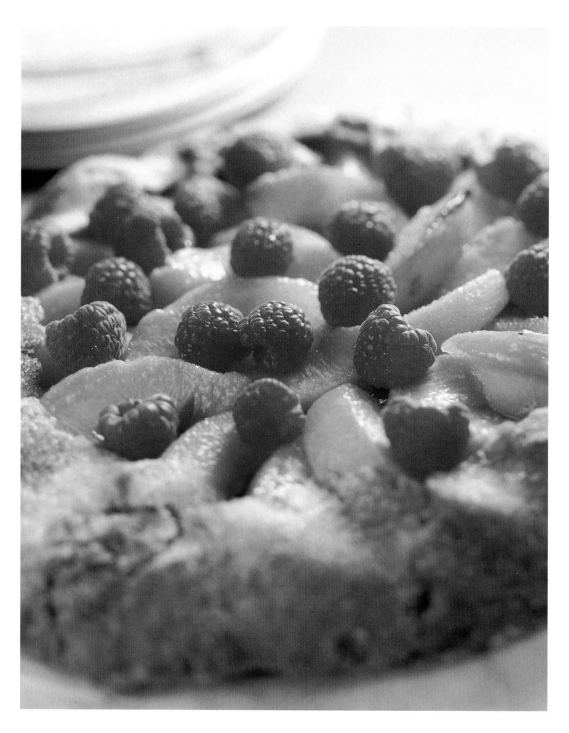

PEACH AND RASPBERRY CROSTATA

Recipe on page 350

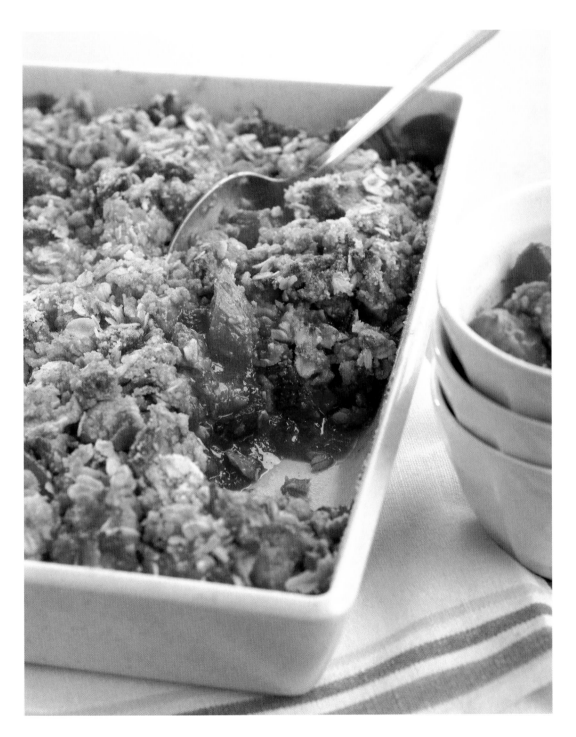

STRAWBERRY-RHUBARB CRISP

Recipe on page 352

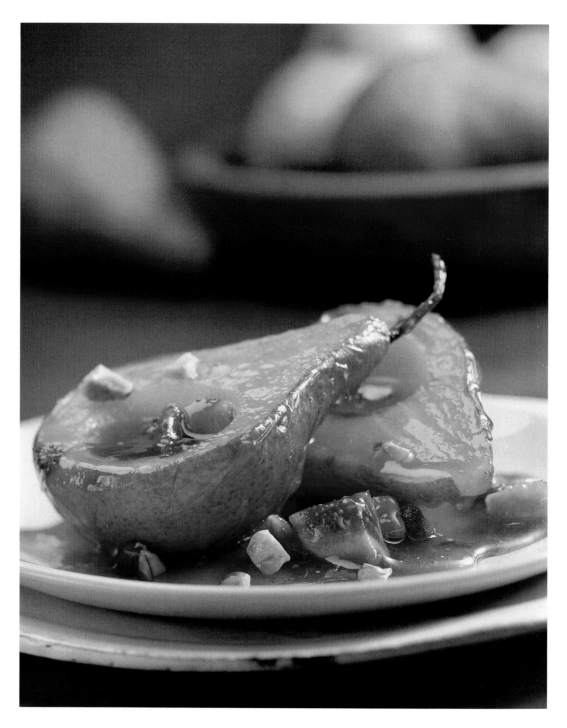

ROASTED PEARS WITH ORANGE-CARAMEL SAUCE

Recipe on page 353

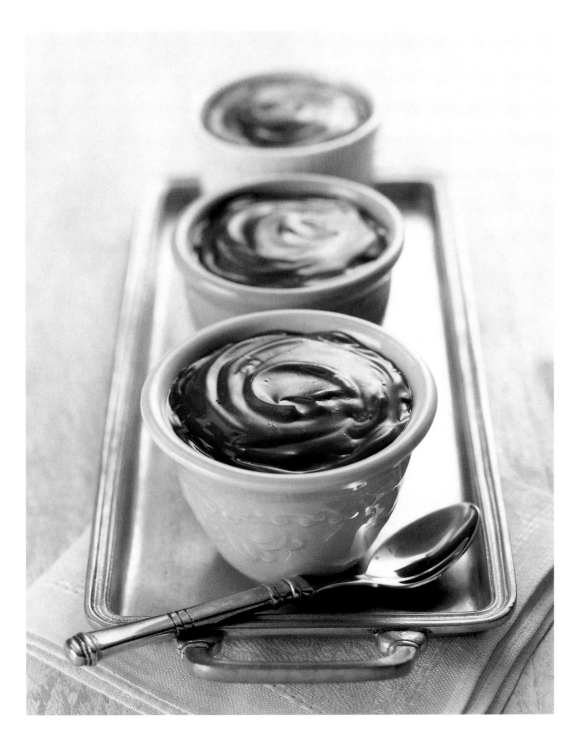

DARK CHOCOLATE PUDDING

Recipe on page 355

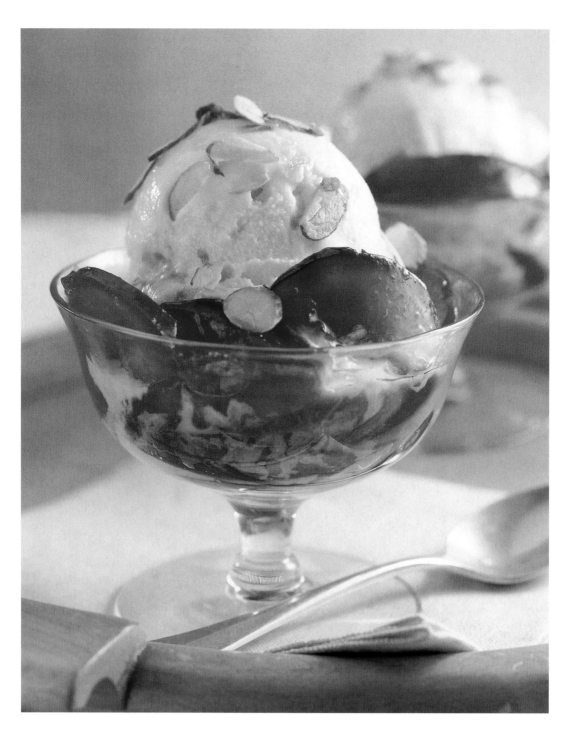

GINGER FROZEN YOGURT WITH SWEET PLUM SAUCE

Recipe on page 358

ROSEMARY-SCENTED SWORDFISH KEBABS

Swordfish's tough exterior makes it ideal for kebabs. It is an excellent source of protein so you are less likely to fall victim to those late-night munchies.

Prep time: 10 minutes • Marinating time: 1 ½ hours • Cook time: 8 minutes

2 cloves garlic, minced

1 medium shallot, minced

2 tablespoons Dijon mustard

2 tablespoons orange juice

1 tablespoon chopped fresh rosemary

2 teaspoons olive oil

2 teaspoons grated orange zest

4 swordfish steaks (6 ounces each), about ¾" thick

½ teaspoon salt

¼ teaspoon freshly ground black pepper

In a medium bowl, combine the garlic, shallot, mustard, orange juice, rosemary, oil, and orange zest. Add the swordfish to the bowl and coat with the mustard mixture. Refrigerate for 1 ½ hours.

Preheat the grill to medium hot. Remove the swordfish from the marinade and wipe off the excess. Sprinkle the swordfish with the salt and pepper and grill for 4 to 5 minutes per side, or until the fish is cooked through.

Makes 4 servings

Per serving: 233 calories, 32 g protein, 3 g carbohydrates, 9 g fat, 60 mg cholesterol, 620 mg sodium, 0 g dietary fiber
Diet Exchanges: 4 ½ meat, 1 fat
Carb Choices: 0

DILLED SALMON EN PAPILLOTE

Fresh salmon is a terrific source of omega-3 fatty acids. The deeper the color, the more omega-3s it provides. Even better, your tastebuds will appreciate its flavor!

Prep time: 20 minutes • Cook time: 15 minutes

1 **small onion, chopped**

1 **clove garlic, minced**

1 **package frozen spinach (10 ounces), thawed and excess liquid squeezed out**

1 **tablespoon + 2 teaspoons lemon juice**

2 **tablespoons chopped fresh dill**

4 **teaspoons Dijon mustard**

4 **salmon fillets (4 ounces each), skin and pinbones removed**

½ **teaspoon salt**

⅛ **teaspoon freshly ground black pepper**

4 **teaspoons drained capers**

4 **teaspoons light butter**

Preheat the oven to 400°F. Coat 4 sheets of aluminum foil 12" × 20" with cooking spray. Fold the aluminum foil sheets in half crosswise.

Coat a medium skillet with cooking spray and heat over medium-high heat. Add the onion and garlic and cook for 1 minute. Add the spinach and cook for 2 minutes, or until hot. Add 1 tablespoon of the lemon juice and cook for 30 seconds, stirring. Remove from the heat and stir in 1 tablespoon of the dill. Cool for 10 minutes.

In a small bowl, combine the mustard and the remaining 1 tablespoon dill and 2 teaspoons lemon juice.

Sprinkle the salmon with the salt and the pepper. Unfold the foil sheets and place one-quarter of the spinach mixture on half of each sheet. Top each mound of spinach with 1 salmon fillet. Spread the mustard mixture over the tops and sides of each fillet. Sprinkle 1 teaspoon of the capers over each fillet. Top each fillet with 1 teaspoon of the butter. Fold the foil over the salmon and, starting at one end, crimp the edges of the foil together to make a tight seal.

Transfer the foil packets to a large baking sheet. Bake for 12 to 15 minutes, or until the packets are puffed (they may not all puff). Arrange on dinner plates and cut open at the table.

Makes 4 servings

Per serving: 207 calories, 19 g protein, 7 g carbohydrates, 12 g fat, 55 mg cholesterol, 650 mg sodium, 2 g dietary fiber
Diet Exchanges: 1 vegetable, 2 ½ meat, 1 fat
Carb Choices: 1

TUSCAN TUNA CAKES

Beyond being delicious, fresh tuna is one of the most healthful fishes you can buy.
It's loaded with niacin and vitamins A and B$_{12}$.

Prep time: 20 minutes • Cook time: 12 minutes

1 **pound yellowfin tuna, chopped coarsely**	2 **teaspoons grated lemon zest**
1 **large egg**	1 **teaspoon chopped fresh oregano**
1 **large egg white**	1½ **cups fresh bread crumbs**
¼ **cup finely chopped fennel**	½ **teaspoon salt**
1 **small onion, finely chopped**	½ **teaspoon freshly ground black pepper**
1 **tablespoon drained capers**	2 **tablespoons olive oil**
1 **tablespoon lemon juice**	4 **fresh lemon wedges**

Place the tuna into a large bowl. Add the egg, egg white, fennel, onion, capers, lemon juice, lemon zest, and oregano. Mix the tuna until well combined. Gently fold in 1 cup of the bread crumbs, salt, and pepper until just combined.

Spread the remaining ½ cup bread crumbs on a plate. Divide the tuna mixture into 8 equal portions. Roll each portion in the bread crumbs, then shape each into a disk approximately 3½" in diameter and ½" thick. Heat 1 tablespoon of the oil in a large nonstick skillet over medium heat. Add 4 tuna cakes and cook for 3 to 4 minutes per side, or until the cakes are golden and cooked through. Repeat with the remaining 1 tablespoon oil and 4 tuna cakes. Serve with fresh lemon wedges.

Makes 4 servings

Per serving: 297 calories, 38 g protein, 11 g carbohydrates, 10 g fat, 120 mg cholesterol, 530 mg sodium, 1 g dietary fiber
Diet Exchanges: ½ vegetable, ½ bread, 5 meat, 1½ fat
Carb Choices: 1

TERIYAKI-GLAZED TUNA STEAKS WITH ASIAN SLAW

Perfect for a summer evening, the sweet and salty glaze that coats this fish is the perfect complement to the tangy bite of the crunchy Asian vegetables.

Prep time: 15 minutes • Cook time: 10 minutes

SLAW

½ small head napa cabbage

1 cup snow peas, trimmed

1 carrot, peeled and grated

1 scallion, chopped

2 tablespoons rice vinegar

1 tablespoon reduced-sodium soy sauce

2 teaspoons honey

¼ teaspoon sesame oil

TUNA STEAKS

2 teaspoons cornstarch

¼ cup orange juice

3 tablespoons reduced-sodium soy sauce

5 teaspoons honey

⅛ teaspoon crushed red-pepper flakes

2 teaspoons sesame oil

4 yellowfin tuna steaks (6 ounces each), about ¾" thick

To make the slaw: Using a sharp knife, thinly shred the cabbage (yielding about 4 cups) and transfer to a large bowl. Cut the snow peas into thin strips and add to the cabbage along with the carrot and scallion. Add the vinegar, soy sauce, honey, and oil and toss well.

To make the tuna steaks: Dissolve the cornstarch in 1 tablespoon water. In a small saucepan over medium-high heat, combine the orange juice, soy sauce, honey, and red-pepper flakes. Bring the mixture to a boil and cook for 1 minute. Stir in the dissolved cornstarch. Return the mixture to a boil and cook for 1 minute, or until thickened.

In a large nonstick skillet, heat the oil over medium-high heat. Add the tuna steaks and cook for 4 minutes. Turn the tuna and brush with the thickened soy sauce mixture. Cook for 3 to 5 minutes longer, or until the tuna is pink in the center and cooked through. Transfer to a serving platter or dinner plates and brush with any remaining glaze. Serve with the slaw.

Makes 4 servings

Per serving: 300 calories, 43 g protein, 21 g carbohydrates, 5 g fat, 75 mg cholesterol, 660 mg sodium, 2 g dietary fiber
Diet Exchanges: 1 vegetable, 1 bread, 5 meat, $\frac{1}{2}$ fat
Carb Choices: 1

SHRIMP-COCONUT CURRY

Shrimp is preferred by more Americans than any other shellfish. This protein-rich crus-tacean is short of stature but stands tall when it comes to satisfying your appetite. When buying fresh shrimp, make sure they smell of the sea with no hint of ammonia.

Photo on page 284.

Prep time: 15 minutes • Cook time: 30 minutes

1 **cup brown basmati rice**	1 **cup chopped onion**
1 **tablespoon olive oil**	1 **teaspoon Thai green curry paste**
1 ½ **pounds large shrimp, peeled and deveined**	1 **can (13 ½ ounces) light coconut milk**
1 **teaspoon grated fresh ginger**	3 **teaspoons fish sauce**
1 **clove garlic, minced**	1 **tablespoon packed brown sugar**
1 **cup finely chopped red bell pepper**	2 **tablespoons chopped fresh cilantro**

Cook the rice according to package directions. Fluff the rice with a fork.

Meanwhile, heat 2 teaspoons of the oil in a large nonstick skillet over medium-high heat. Add the shrimp and cook for 2 to 3 minutes per side, or until lightly browned and opaque. Transfer the shrimp to a bowl and reserve. Heat the remaining 1 teaspoon oil in the skillet, add the ginger and garlic, and cook for 30 seconds, or until fragrant. Add the bell pepper and onion and cook for 3 minutes. Stir in the curry paste and cook, stirring often, for 1 minute.

Reduce the heat to medium and add the coconut milk, fish sauce, and sugar. Cook for 3 minutes, stirring occasionally, until heated through. Add the shrimp and cook for 1 minute longer, or until hot. Remove from the heat and stir in the cilantro. Serve over rice.

Makes 4 servings

Per serving: 450 calories, 37 g protein, 45 g carbohydrates, 13 g fat, 235 mg cholesterol, 620 mg sodium, 3 g dietary fiber
Diet Exchanges: 1 vegetable, 2 ½ bread, 5 meat, 3 fat
Carb Choices: 3

AEGEAN SEAS SHRIMP

A few boiled small potatoes or steamed rice will complete this meal beautifully.

Prep time: 20 minutes • Cook time: 12 minutes

1 **pound large shrimp, thawed if frozen, peeled and deveined, rinsed and patted dry**

3 **large cloves garlic, minced**

2 **tablespoons extra-virgin olive oil**

2 **tablespoons lemon juice**

2 **tablespoons chopped fresh oregano or marjoram, or ½ teaspoon dried**

½ **teaspoon sweet paprika**

¼ **teaspoon salt + a pinch**

¼ **teaspoon freshly ground black pepper**

1 **bag (9 ounces) baby spinach**

¼ **cup crumbled feta cheese**

Lemon wedges (optional)

On a rimmed baking sheet, place the shrimp in a mound. Drizzle with 2 minced garlic cloves, 1 tablespoon of the oil, the lemon juice, oregano or marjoram, paprika, the ¼ teaspoon salt, and the pepper. Toss to mix.

Preheat the broiler.

Stir the remaining 1 tablespoon oil and 1 minced garlic clove in a large nonstick skillet over medium heat. Cook, stirring, for 2 minutes, or until the garlic is fragrant. Add the spinach, in batches if necessary, tossing until wilted. Sprinkle with the pinch of salt. Remove from the heat and cover to keep warm.

Broil the shrimp 4" from the heat, turning once, for 3 minutes, or until pink and just firm. Sprinkle with the feta and broil 1 to 2 minutes longer, just until the cheese softens a little (it won't really melt).

Transfer the spinach to a large platter and spoon the shrimp and the pan juices on top. If desired, serve with lemon wedges.

Makes 4 servings

Per serving: 220 calories, 24 g protein, 9 g carbohydrates, 10 g fat, 200 mg cholesterol, 570 mg sodium, 3 g dietary fiber
Diet Exchanges: 1 vegetable, 3 meat, 2 fat
Carb Choices: ½

LINGUINE WITH RED CLAM SAUCE

Clams are little purses of nutrition! Also, 1 serving (about 20 small clams) contains an astounding 44-day supply of vitamin B_{12} and a 2-day supply of iron. When buying hard-shelled clams, be sure they are tightly closed. Discard any that don't open during cooking.

Prep time: 10 minutes • Cook time: 20 minutes

8 **ounces multigrain linguine or spaghetti**	2 **cloves garlic, minced**
½ **cup clam juice**	¼ **teaspoon crushed red-pepper flakes**
½ **cup white wine or nonalcoholic wine**	1 **can (15 ounces) crushed tomatoes**
1 **tablespoon chopped fresh oregano**	½ **teaspoon salt**
24 **littleneck clams, scrubbed**	⅛ **teaspoon freshly ground black pepper**
1 **tablespoon olive oil**	1 **tablespoon butter**

Bring a large pot of lightly salted water to a boil. Add the linguine or spaghetti and cook according to package directions. Drain and keep warm.

Meanwhile, in a separate pot, combine the clam juice, wine, and 2 teaspoons of the oregano over high heat. Bring the mixture to a boil and add the clams. Cover the pot and cook for 6 to 8 minutes, or until the clams open. Remove the pot from the heat and transfer the clams to a bowl. Strain and reserve 1 cup of the broth from the pot.

Wipe out the pot and return to the stove over medium-high heat. Add the oil, garlic, and red-pepper flakes. Cook for 1 minute, or until the garlic is fragrant. Add the tomatoes and the remaining 1 teaspoon oregano. Cook, stirring occasionally, for 4 minutes, or until slightly thickened. Add the salt, pepper, and reserved clam broth and cook for 4 minutes longer. Stir in the butter and cook for 1 minute. Add the clams and stir until combined.

Divide the pasta among 4 plates and top each with one-quarter of the clams and one-quarter of the sauce.

Makes 4 servings

Per serving: 360 calories, 19 g protein, 49 g carbohydrates, 8 g fat, 25 mg cholesterol, 570 mg sodium, 6 g dietary fiber
Diet Exchanges: 1 ½ vegetable, 2 ½ bread, 1 ½ meat, 1 ½ fat
Carb Choices: 3

STIR-FRIED SCALLOPS IN BLACK BEAN SAUCE

Scallops are reasonably low in calories—3 ounces contain only 75 calories—so they are ideal for dieters. They also contain high-quality protein to keep your appetite reined in. When buying fresh scallops, be sure their color ranges from pale beige to creamy pink. Scallops that look pure white have been soaked in water, which leaches out some of the flavor.

Photo on page 285.

Prep time: 10 minutes • Cook time: 30 minutes

1 cup brown basmati rice

1 tablespoon olive oil

1 tablespoon grated fresh ginger

2 cloves garlic, minced

1 pound sea scallops, drained

2 scallions, chopped

1 large carrot, sliced

1 green bell pepper, seeded and chopped

2 teaspoons fermented black beans, or
   2 tablespoons black bean sauce

3 tablespoons sake

1 tablespoon reduced-sodium soy sauce

1 teaspoon honey

Cook the rice according to package directions. Fluff the rice with a fork.

Meanwhile, heat 2 teaspoons of the oil in a large nonstick skillet over medium-high heat. Add the ginger and garlic and cook for 30 seconds, or until fragrant. Stir in the scallops and cook for 3 to 4 minutes, or until opaque. Transfer the scallops to a bowl and reserve.

Heat the remaining 1 teaspoon oil and add the scallions, carrot, and bell pepper. Cook, stirring often, for 2 to 3 minutes, or until the vegetables are crisp-tender. Add the black beans or black bean sauce, sake, soy sauce, and honey and cook for 45 seconds. Drain any liquid from the scallops, then add to the skillet, tossing, and cook for 1 minute, or until hot. Serve over the rice.

Makes 4 servings

Per serving: 410 calories, 35 g protein, 47 g carbohydrates, 7 g fat, 75 mg cholesterol, 550 mg sodium, 3 g dietary fiber
Diet Exchanges: 1 vegetable, 2 ½ bread, 4 ½ meat, 1 fat
Carb Choices: 3

IT-CAN'T-BE-VEGETARIAN MAIN DISHES

■ FAST   ■ SUPER FAST   ■ FAST PREP

BEAN AND VEGGIE BURGERS

Topped with zippy yogurt sauce, these hearty burgers contain a boatload of flavorful vegetables, beans, and grains.

Prep time: 25 minutes • Cook time: 35 minutes

BURGERS

¼ cup bulgur

1 small onion, finely chopped

¾ cup shredded zucchini

½ cup shredded carrot

½ cup chopped red bell pepper

1 tablespoon minced garlic

2 cups chopped spinach

1½ teaspoons ground cumin

½ teaspoon salt

4 ounces firm tofu

1 can (15–16 ounces) chickpeas, rinsed and drained

¼ cup ground flaxseed

6 whole wheat buns, split

SAUCE

⅓ cup low-fat plain yogurt

3 tablespoons chopped cilantro

1 scallion, finely chopped

1 jalapeño chile pepper, seeded and minced (wear plastic gloves when handling)

⅛ teaspoon salt

Green leaf lettuce and sliced tomatoes

To make the burgers: Preheat the oven to 400°F. Coat a baking sheet with cooking spray. Prepare the bulgur according to package directions and set aside.

In a large nonstick skillet, over medium heat, combine the onion, zucchini, carrot, bell pepper, and garlic. Cook, stirring frequently, for 8 minutes, or until the vegetables are crisp-tender. Increase the heat to medium-high. Stir in the spinach, cumin, and salt. Cook for 2 minutes, or until the spinach wilts. Cool for 10 minutes.

Pat the tofu dry with paper towels. Crumble the tofu into a large bowl and add the chickpeas. With a potato masher, mash until smooth. Add the vegetable mixture to the bulgur. Stir until well blended. Shape into 6 burgers, 3" in diameter. Coat with the flaxseed. Place on the prepared baking sheet. Bake for 10 minutes. Coat the burgers with cooking spray, and turn over. Bake 15 minutes longer, or until browned.

To make the sauce: In a small bowl, combine the yogurt, cilantro, scallion, chile pepper, and salt. Stir until blended.

Serve each burger on a bun with lettuce, tomato, and yogurt sauce.

Makes 6 servings

Per serving: 260 calories, 13 g protein, 41 g carbohydrates, 7 g fat, 0 mg cholesterol, 620 mg sodium, 9 g dietary fiber
Diet Exchanges: 1 vegetable, 3 bread, ½ meat, ½ fat
Carb Choices: 3

SPEEDY TAMALE PIE

Fiber and high-quality protein are a dieter's strongest weapon. This spicy mix of beans and tomatoes comes together quickly, making this dish perfect for weeknight meals.

Photo on page 286.

Prep time: 15 minutes • Cook time: 40 minutes

2 **cans (15 ounces each) salt-free pinto beans, rinsed and drained**

2 **medium zucchini, cut into ¾" chunks**

1 **can (14 ½ ounces) Mexican-style stewed tomatoes**

1 **cup fresh or frozen corn kernels**

1 **cup frozen lima beans**

1 **cup medium-spicy chunky salsa**

2 **teaspoons chili powder**

1 **tube (16–18 ounces) prepared polenta, cut into ½"-thick slices**

1 **cup shredded reduced-fat Cheddar or Monterey Jack cheese**

Preheat the oven to 400°F. Coat a shallow 2 ½-quart baking dish with cooking spray.

In a large soup pot or Dutch oven, combine the beans, zucchini, stewed tomatoes, corn, lima beans, salsa, and chili powder. Bring to a boil. Reduce the heat and simmer, covered, for 10 minutes. Turn into the prepared baking dish. Arrange the polenta on top, overlapping the slices slightly if necessary. Bake for 25 minutes, or until bubbly at the edges. Sprinkle with the cheese and bake for 3 minutes, or until melted. Let stand for 10 minutes before serving.

Makes 6 servings

Per serving: 408 calories, 19 g protein, 77 g carbohydrates, 4 g fat, 5 mg cholesterol, 475 mg sodium, 13 g dietary fiber
Diet Exchanges: 1 ½ vegetable, 4 ½ bread, 2 meat
Carb Choices: 5

CURRIED TOFU

FAST
PREP

Tofu is an excellent source of vegetable protein. Firm tofu has 34 percent more protein and slightly more vitamins and minerals than regular tofu does. *Photo on page 287.*

Prep time: 15 minutes • Cook time: 50 minutes • Stand time: 10 minutes

1 **cup brown basmati rice**

1 **package (14 ounces) firm tofu, drained and cut into ¾" cubes**

1 **tablespoon canola oil**

½ **teaspoon salt**

1 **large onion, halved and thinly sliced**

1–2 **tablespoons red curry paste (see note)**

½ **teaspoon curry powder**

4 **cups broccoli florets**

1 **cup light coconut milk**

¾ **cup vegetable broth**

1 **cup frozen green peas**

1 **large tomato, cut into ¾" pieces**

2 **tablespoons lime juice**

Cook the rice according to package directions. Place the tofu between layers of paper towels and let stand for 10 minutes.

Heat the oil in a large nonstick skillet over medium-high heat. Add the tofu and cook, turning once, for 6 to 8 minutes, or until golden brown. Sprinkle with ¼ teaspoon of the salt. With a slotted spoon, remove to a plate.

Add the onion to the skillet and cook, stirring frequently, for 3 to 4 minutes, or until browned. Stir in the curry paste, curry powder, and the remaining ¼ teaspoon salt. Add the broccoli, coconut milk, broth, and peas. Bring to a boil. Reduce the heat to low. Cover and simmer for 3 to 4 minutes, or until the broccoli is crisp-tender. Stir in the tomato, lime juice, and the reserved tofu. Simmer, stirring occasionally, for 2 to 3 minutes, or until the tofu is hot. Serve over the rice.

Note: The heat level of red curry pastes can vary, so start out with 1 tablespoon and then taste.

Makes 6 servings

Per serving: 265 calories, 11 g protein, 37 g carbohydrates, 11 g fat, 0 mg cholesterol, 390 mg sodium, 5 g dietary fiber
Diet Exchanges: 1 ½ vegetable, 2 bread, 1 meat, 1 ½ fat
Carb Choices: 2

BROWN RICE WITH SQUASH AND CHICKPEAS

Chickpeas get high marks for fiber. One-half cup of these buff-colored legumes has 7 grams of fiber. This delicious recipe combines chickpeas with brown rice and lentils, which means you get a triple dose of blood sugar balancing benefits!

Prep time: 15 minutes • Cook time: 1 hour 10 minutes

4 teaspoons olive oil	¾ teaspoon salt
1 medium onion, halved and thinly sliced	1 can (15–19 ounces) chickpeas, rinsed and drained
3 large cloves garlic, minced	
1 tablespoon grated fresh ginger	2 cups frozen cubed butternut squash
2½ cups water	2 bunches broccoli rabe, trimmed and cut into 2" pieces
1 cup brown rice	
½ cup lentils	¼–½ teaspoon red-pepper flakes

Heat 2 teaspoons of the oil in a large deep skillet over medium heat. Add the onion. Cook, stirring frequently, for 8 minutes, or until the onion is lightly browned. Add half of the garlic and the ginger. Cook for 1 minute, stirring constantly. Add the water, rice, lentils, and ½ teaspoon of the salt. Bring to a boil. Cover, reduce the heat, and simmer for 30 minutes. Stir in the chickpeas and squash. Cover and cook for 15 to 20 minutes longer, or until the rice is tender.

Meanwhile, bring a large pot of water to a boil. Stir in the broccoli rabe and cook for 2 minutes. Drain, reserving ¼ cup of the cooking water.

In the same pot, heat the remaining 2 teaspoons oil over low heat. Add the red-pepper flakes and the remaining garlic. Cook, stirring constantly, for 1 minute, or until the garlic is sizzling but not brown. Add the broccoli rabe and the remaining ¼ teaspoon salt. Cook, stirring occasionally, for 10 to 12 minutes, or until the broccoli rabe is tender, adding the reserved cooking water if necessary. Serve the rice topped with the broccoli rabe.

Makes 6 servings

Per serving: 312 calories, 13 g protein, 57 g carbohydrates, 5 g fat, 0 mg cholesterol, 490 mg sodium, 11 g dietary fiber
Diet Exchanges: 2 vegetable, 3 bread, 1 meat, ½ fat
Carb Choices: 4

CAJUN RICE WITH RED BEANS AND CORN

Kick up your heels with this spicy dish from the Big Easy. In this meatless version, corn adds just a hint of sweetness to mellow the heat.

Prep time: 15 minutes • Cook time: 1 hour 25 minutes

2 teaspoons canola oil	1 box (10 ounces) frozen corn
1 large onion, chopped	1 green bell pepper, chopped
1 tablespoon minced garlic	1 rib celery, chopped
1 tablespoon Cajun or Creole seasoning	1 can (14 $\frac{1}{2}$ ounces) diced tomatoes
2$\frac{1}{4}$ cups water	1 scallion, thinly sliced (optional)
1 can (15–19 ounces) red or kidney beans, rinsed and drained	Salt
	Hot-pepper sauce
1 cup brown rice	

Heat the oil in a large, deep skillet over medium heat. Add the onion and cook for 5 minutes, or until softened. Stir in the garlic and cook for 1 minute. Stir in the Cajun or Creole seasoning. Remove $\frac{1}{2}$ cup of the onion mixture and set aside. Add the water, beans, and rice. Stir to combine and bring to a boil. Cover, reduce the heat to low, and simmer for 30 minutes. Stir in the corn and cook for 15 to 20 minutes longer, or until the rice is tender.

Meanwhile, in a large saucepan, combine the bell pepper, celery, and the reserved $\frac{1}{2}$ cup onion mixture. Cook over low heat for 10 minutes, or until the vegetables soften. Stir in the tomatoes (with juice) and bring to a boil. Cover, reduce the heat, and simmer for 20 minutes, or until the sauce thickens slightly.

Spoon the rice mixture onto plates and top with the sauce. Sprinkle with the scallion, if using. Add the salt to taste. Serve with the hot-pepper sauce on the side.

Makes 6 servings

Per serving: 250 calories, 8 g protein, 50 g carbohydrates, 3 g fat, 0 mg cholesterol, 210 mg sodium, 8 g dietary fiber
Diet Exchanges: 1 vegetable, 3 bread, $\frac{1}{2}$ fat
Carb Choices: 3

QUINOA-STUFFED PEPPERS

When you pick a peck of peppers, you are choosing one of the most nutrient-dense vegetables you can buy, especially when it comes to vitamin C and beta-carotene (the redder the pepper, the more beta-carotene it contains). Their bell shape make them ideal for holding this delicious mix of protein, fiber, and monounsaturated fats. *Photo on page 288.*

Prep time: 25 minutes • Cook time: 1 hour 45 minutes

⅓ cup slivered almonds

1½ cups water

¼ teaspoon salt

¾ cup quinoa

4 large red, green, or yellow bell peppers

1 teaspoon olive oil

1 medium onion, chopped

2 large cloves garlic, minced

1 package (10 ounces) fresh spinach, tough stems removed, torn into large pieces

½ cup crumbled feta cheese

¼ cup dried currants or raisins

1 can (14½ ounces) diced tomatoes

2 tablespoons tomato paste

¼ teaspoon dried Italian seasoning

Preheat the oven to 375°F.

Cook the slivered almonds in a small nonstick skillet over medium heat, stirring often, for 3 to 4 minutes, or until lightly toasted. Tip onto a plate and let cool.

In a saucepan, bring the water and salt to a boil. Place the quinoa in a fine-mesh strainer and rinse under cold running water for 2 minutes. Stir into the boiling water. Reduce the heat, cover, and simmer for 20 minutes, or until the water is absorbed and the quinoa is tender. Uncover and set aside.

Bring a large pot of water to a boil. Cut off and reserve the tops of the peppers. Remove the seeds and ribs. Add the peppers and tops to the boiling water and cook for 5 minutes. Drain.

In the same pot, heat the oil over medium heat. Add the onion and cook, stirring occasionally, for 6 minutes, or until golden brown. Stir in the garlic. Remove 2 tablespoons of the onion mixture and set aside.

Add the spinach to the pot and cook, stirring frequently, for 5 minutes, or until wilted and any water evaporates. Remove the pot from the heat. Add the feta, currants or raisins, almonds, and quinoa to the spinach mixture. Stir to combine. Arrange the peppers in a shallow baking dish. Spoon in the stuffing, mounding to fill, and replace the tops. Add $\frac{1}{2}$" water to the baking dish. Cover loosely with foil and bake for 40 to 45 minutes, or until the peppers are tender.

Meanwhile, in a saucepan, combine the tomatoes (with juice), tomato paste, Italian seasoning, and the reserved 2 tablespoons onion mixture. Bring to a boil. Reduce the heat, cover, and simmer for 30 minutes, or until thickened. Spoon the sauce onto plates and top with the peppers.

Makes 4 servings

Per serving: 330 calories, 14 g protein, 50 g carbohydrates, 11 g fat, 10 mg cholesterol, 700 mg sodium, 9 g dietary fiber
Diet Exchanges: $\frac{1}{2}$ fruit, 4 vegetable, 1 $\frac{1}{2}$ bread, 1 meat, 2 fat
Carb Choices: 4

STUFFED PORTOBELLOS

Although nearly half the calories of hummus come from fat, virtually none of it is saturated. Add olive oil and walnuts and you have a delectable dose of monounsaturated fats, too.

Prep time: 20 minutes • Cook time: 35 minutes

1 cup brown rice

2 teaspoons olive oil

1 small onion, chopped

4 cups sliced escarole or Swiss chard

2 large cloves garlic, minced

½ cup rinsed and chopped roasted red peppers

4 large portobello mushrooms (4 ½"–5" diameter), stems discarded (see note)

½ cup prepared hummus, preferably basil flavored

3 plum tomatoes, sliced

¼ cup walnuts, chopped

¼ cup grated Parmesan cheese

Preheat the oven to 400°F.

Cook the rice according to package directions.

Meanwhile, heat the oil in a medium skillet over medium-low heat. Add the onion and cook, stirring occasionally, for 5 minutes, or until softened. Add the escarole or Swiss chard and the garlic. Cook, stirring occasionally, for 5 minutes, or until wilted. Remove from the heat and stir in the rice and peppers.

Place the mushrooms gill side up on a baking sheet with sides. Spread the hummus on the mushrooms and spoon on the rice mixture, spreading it to the edges. Arrange the tomato slices on top and sprinkle with the walnuts and cheese. Bake for 25 to 30 minutes, or until the mushrooms are tender. Let stand for 10 minutes before serving.

Note: To prevent the mushrooms from being waterlogged, remove any sand or dirt with a brush and wipe with damp paper towels instead of rinsing with water.

Makes 4 servings

Per serving: 260 calories, 10 g protein, 30 g carbohydrates, 12 g fat, 5 mg cholesterol, 250 mg sodium, 7 g dietary fiber
Diet Exchanges: 3 vegetable, 1 bread, 1 meat, 2 fat
Carb Choices: 2

ITALIAN VEGETABLE STIR-FRY OVER POLENTA

FAST PREP

Polenta is a common accompaniment to northern Italian dishes. This colorful, high-fiber dish is especially satisfying when combined with cheese.

Prep time: 20 minutes • Cook time: 35 minutes

POLENTA

4 cups water

¼ teaspoon salt

1 cup yellow cornmeal

½ cup grated Parmesan cheese

STIR-FRY

1 tablespoon olive oil

1 small red onion, thinly sliced

1 red bell pepper, thinly sliced

1 small fennel bulb, trimmed, quartered, cored, and thinly sliced

1 large zucchini, halved lengthwise and thinly sliced

1 can (15–19 ounces) chickpeas, rinsed and drained

1 tablespoon minced garlic

¼ teaspoon red-pepper flakes

¼ teaspoon salt

2 large tomatoes, coarsely chopped

¼ cup chopped fresh basil

To make the polenta: In a large saucepan, bring the water and salt to a boil. Slowly whisk in the cornmeal. Reduce the heat to low. Cover and simmer, stirring frequently, for 30 to 35 minutes, or until the polenta thickens. Stir in the cheese. Cover and keep warm.

To make the stir-fry: Heat the oil in a large nonstick skillet over medium-high heat. Add the onion, bell pepper, and fennel. Cook, stirring frequently, for 2 to 3 minutes, or until the vegetables begin to soften. Add the zucchini, chickpeas, garlic, red-pepper flakes, and salt. Cook, stirring constantly, for 2 to 3 minutes, or until the vegetables are crisp-tender. Add the tomatoes. Cook, stirring frequently, for 1 minute, or until the tomatoes soften. Stir in the basil. Serve over the polenta.

Makes 6 servings

Per serving: 246 calories, 10 g protein, 38 g carbohydrates, 7 g fat, 5 mg cholesterol, 580 mg sodium, 7 g dietary fiber
Diet Exchanges: 1 ½ vegetable, 2 bread, ½ meat, 1 fat
Carb Choices: 3

CHUNKY VEGETABLE SHEPHERD'S PIE

Shepherd's pie was originally conceived as a resourceful way to make use of leftovers from a Sunday meal. There is nothing *leftover* about this dish! It is thick with hearty ingredients.

Prep time: 30 minutes • Cook time: 1 hour 10 minutes

3 pounds sweet potatoes, peeled and cut into large chunks	1 teaspoon seasoning blend, such as Mrs. Dash original
1 tablespoon olive oil	1 can (15–19 ounces) cannellini beans, rinsed and drained
1 large onion, coarsely chopped	
3 medium carrots, sliced	1 box (9 ounces) frozen Italian green beans
1 large rib celery, sliced	1 can (14 ounces) vegetable broth
½ pound cremini mushrooms, halved	3 tablespoons whole grain pastry flour
1 tablespoon minced garlic	4 plum tomatoes, cut into ¾" pieces

In a soup pot or Dutch oven, cover the potatoes with cold water. Bring to a boil. Cover, reduce the heat, and simmer for 15 to 20 minutes, or until tender. Drain in a colander and set aside.

Preheat the oven to 375°F.

In the same pot, heat the oil over medium heat. Add the onion, carrots, and celery. Cook, stirring occasionally, for 5 minutes, or until the onion softens. Stir in the mushrooms, garlic, and seasoning blend. Cook, stirring frequently, for 5 minutes, or until the mushrooms soften. Add the cannellini, green beans, and broth. Bring to a boil. In a small bowl, whisk ½ cup cold water and the flour until smooth. Stir into the vegetables. Reduce the heat and simmer for 3 minutes. Stir in the tomatoes. Pour the vegetable mixture into a 13" × 9" baking dish.

In the same pot, mash the sweet potatoes. Spoon the potatoes around the edge of the baking dish. Bake for 35 minutes, or until bubbly in the center. Let stand for 5 minutes before serving.

Makes 8 servings

Per serving: 299 calories, 10 g protein, 63 g carbohydrates, 2 g fat, 0 mg cholesterol, 460 mg sodium, 11 g dietary fiber
Diet Exchanges: 2 vegetable, 3 ½ bread
Carb Choices: 4

SQUASH AND GREENS GRATIN

Butternut squash deserves a spot on every plate! The sweet interior is high in fiber and deliciously sweet, which makes it perfect for any occasion.

Prep time: 35 minutes • Cook time: 1 hour 10 minutes

1 tablespoon olive oil

3 leeks (1 ½ pounds), white and pale green parts only, halved lengthwise, sliced, and rinsed

1 red bell pepper, thinly sliced

½ teaspoon salt

¼ teaspoon freshly ground black pepper

3 large carrots, thinly sliced

1 large butternut squash (3 pounds), peeled, seeded, and cut lengthwise into ½"-thick slices

1 box (10 ounces) frozen chopped kale, thawed and squeezed dry

1 cup shredded Gruyère or Swiss cheese

½ cup grated Parmesan cheese

1 cup vegetable broth

Preheat the oven to 375°F. Coat a shallow 3-quart baking dish with cooking spray.

Heat the oil in a large skillet over medium heat. Add the leeks and bell pepper. Add ¼ teaspoon of the salt and ⅛ teaspoon of the pepper. Cook, stirring frequently, for about 5 minutes, or until softened. Stir in the carrots and cook for 5 minutes.

Arrange one-third of the squash in the prepared baking dish. Season with some of the remaining salt and pepper. Top with half of the kale, ½ cup of the Gruyère or Swiss, half of the carrot mixture, and 3 tablespoons of the Parmesan. Repeat the layering. Top with the remaining squash. Pour the vegetable broth over and sprinkle with the remaining salt and pepper. Cover the dish with foil and bake for 45 minutes.

Remove the foil and sprinkle with the remaining Parmesan. Bake for 15 minutes longer, or until the vegetables are tender. Let stand for 15 minutes before serving.

Makes 8 servings

Per serving: 246 calories, 11 g protein, 37 g carbohydrates, 8 g fat, 20 mg cholesterol, 480 mg sodium, 8 g dietary fiber
Diet Exchanges: 6 vegetable, 1 meat, 1 fat
Carb Choices: 2

TOMATO AND SPINACH CRUSTLESS QUICHE

Perfect for a weekend brunch or light supper, this tasty quiche is so satisfying
·you won't miss the crust at all.

Prep time: 20 minutes • Cook time: 45 minutes

2   teaspoons olive oil

4   plum tomatoes, halved lengthwise

½   cup chopped red onion

1   clove garlic, minced

1   package (10 ounces) spinach, rinsed and
drained, tough stems removed

¾   cup shredded reduced-fat Cheddar cheese

3   large eggs

1   cup 1% milk

2   tablespoons grated Parmesan cheese

1½   teaspoons Dijon mustard

⅛   teaspoon freshly ground black pepper

Preheat the oven to 350°F. Coat a 9" pie plate with cooking spray.

Heat the oil in a large nonstick skillet over medium-high heat. Add the tomatoes cut side down.
Cook for 5 minutes, or until browned. Turn the tomatoes over and add the onion and garlic. Cook,
stirring occasionally, for 2 minutes, or until the onion softens. Arrange the tomatoes cut side up in
the pie plate. Spoon the onion and garlic around the tomatoes.

Add half of the spinach to the skillet and reduce the heat to medium. Cook for 4 minutes, or until
wilted, and drain in a colander. Repeat with the remaining spinach. When cool enough to handle,
squeeze the spinach until dry. Coarsely chop. Sprinkle the spinach in between the tomatoes. Top
with the Cheddar.

Whisk the eggs in a medium bowl. Add the milk, Parmesan, mustard, and pepper. Whisk until well
blended. Pour into the pie plate. Bake for 30 to 35 minutes, or until golden brown and puffed.
Remove to a wire rack to cool. Serve warm or at room temperature, cut into wedges.

Makes 6 servings

Per serving: 127 calories, 11 g protein, 7 g carbohydrates, 6 g fat, 115 mg cholesterol, 260 mg sodium, 2 g dietary fiber
Diet Exchanges: ½ milk, 1 vegetable, 1 meat, 1 fat
Carb Choices: 0

MOO SHU VEGETABLE ROLL-UPS

A traditional moo shu roll-up is a thin pancake stuffed with shredded pork, egg, and various seasonings. This vegetarian version has the same tantalizing taste plus an impressive 18 grams of protein and 7 grams of fiber that will have you saying *sayonara* to hunger pangs.

Prep time: 15 minutes • Cook time: 7 minutes

4 **whole wheat tortillas (10" diameter)**

2 **teaspoons canola oil**

4 **large eggs, beaten**

¼ **pound shiitake mushrooms, stems discarded, thinly sliced**

4 **cups shredded coleslaw mix**

1 **cup shredded carrots**

3 **scallions, thinly sliced**

2 **tablespoons light teriyaki sauce**

¼ **cup chopped unsalted peanuts**

¼ **cup hoisin sauce**

Preheat the oven to 350°F. Wrap the tortillas in foil and place in the oven to heat through, for 5 minutes.

Meanwhile, heat 1 teaspoon of the oil in a large nonstick skillet over medium heat. Add the eggs and cook, stirring frequently, for 1 to 2 minutes, or until the eggs are scrambled, but still moist. Turn the eggs out onto a plate and set aside.

Add the remaining 1 teaspoon oil to the skillet and increase the heat to medium-high. When hot, add the mushrooms. Cook, stirring frequently, for about 2 minutes, or until softened. Add the coleslaw mix and carrots. Cook, stirring constantly, for 3 to 4 minutes, or until crisp-tender. Stir in the scallions and teriyaki sauce and cook for 1 minute. Remove the skillet from the heat. Gently stir in the peanuts and the reserved eggs.

To serve, spread some of the hoisin sauce on the center of the tortillas. Top with the vegetable mixture and roll up.

Makes 4 servings

Per serving: 370 calories, 16 g protein, 42 g carbohydrates, 16 g fat, 210 mg cholesterol, 700 mg sodium, 6 g dietary fiber
Diet Exchanges: 2 vegetable, 2 bread, 1 ½ meat, 2 ½ fat
Carb Choices: 3

GREEK PITA PIZZAS

Studies show that people in Greece have the lowest heart disease rates in the world, and researchers believe that their diet may be one of the reasons. Many of their traditional foods are made with olives and olive oil, rich sources of monounsaturated fats that have the added benefit of protecting your heart!

Prep time: 15 minutes • Cook time: 17 minutes

1   **box (9 ounces) frozen artichoke hearts, thawed and chopped**

1   **medium zucchini, coarsely shredded (2 cups)**

1   **teaspoon minced garlic**

¾   **teaspoon dried oregano**

6   **pitted kalamata olives, chopped**

4   **whole wheat pitas (6 ½" diameter)**

⅓   **cup crumbled reduced-fat basil-tomato feta cheese**

1   **cup grape tomatoes, halved lengthwise**

½   **cup reduced-fat shredded mozzarella cheese**

1   **scallion, thinly sliced**

Preheat the oven to 425°F. Pat the artichokes dry with paper towels. In a large nonstick skillet, over medium-high heat, cook the artichokes, zucchini, garlic, and oregano for 4 to 5 minutes, or until the zucchini is tender. Stir in the olives.

Place the pitas on a baking sheet and spread with the zucchini mixture. Sprinkle with the feta. Top with the tomatoes. Bake for 10 minutes, or until the pitas are crisp. Sprinkle with the mozzarella and bake for 3 to 4 minutes longer, or until the cheese is melted. Sprinkle with the scallion and let stand for a few minutes before serving.

Makes 4 servings

Per serving: 290 calories, 15 g protein, 47 g carbohydrates, 7 g fat, 10 mg cholesterol, 700 mg sodium, 9 g dietary fiber
Diet Exchanges: 2 vegetable, 2 ½ bread, 1 meat, 1 fat
Carb Choices: 3

SKINNY PASTA PRIMAVERA

Pasta is a staple in kitchens all over the world. It feels "heavier" in your stomach than high-fat foods do but doesn't have the high calories. Whole grain pasta is best because it's higher in fiber than pasta made with heavily processed semolina flour.

Prep time: 25 minutes • Cook time: 15 minutes

⅔ cup reduced-fat ricotta cheese

1 cup vegetable broth

1 tablespoon olive oil

1 shallot, finely chopped

¼ pound white button mushrooms, sliced

½ pound plum tomatoes, chopped

2 large cloves garlic, minced

¼ teaspoon salt

¼ teaspoon freshly ground black pepper

½ pound multigrain spaghetti

3 cups small broccoli florets

1 medium carrot, julienned

¼ pound asparagus, cut into 1" diagonal pieces

¾ cup frozen shelled green soybeans (edamame), thawed

½ cup fresh basil, thinly sliced

⅓ cup grated Parmesan cheese

In a food processor, combine the ricotta and broth. Process until smooth. Set aside. Bring a large pot of water to a boil.

Heat the oil in a large nonstick skillet over medium-high heat. Add the shallot and mushrooms. Cook, stirring frequently, for 3 minutes, or until the mushrooms begin to brown. Reduce the heat to medium. Stir in the tomatoes, garlic, salt, and pepper. Cook for 2 minutes, or until the tomatoes begin to soften. Reduce the heat to very low and cover to keep warm.

Cook the pasta according to package directions. Two minutes before the pasta is finished cooking, add the broccoli, carrot, asparagus, and soybeans. Drain.

Return the hot pasta and vegetables to the pot. Add the basil, the reserved mushroom mixture, and the reserved ricotta. Toss to combine. Serve sprinkled with the Parmesan.

Makes 4 servings

Per serving: 390 calories, 13 g protein, 55 g carbohydrates, 10 g fat, 15 mg cholesterol, 440 mg sodium, 9 g dietary fiber
Diet Exchanges: 4 vegetable, 2 ½ bread, 1 meat, 2 fat
Carb Choices: 4

ROASTED VEGETABLE LASAGNA

Ricotta cheese is an excellent source of protein. Combine it with a medley of fiber-rich vegetables and you have a perfect Italian meal! *Photo on page 289.*

Prep time: 35 minutes • Cook time: 1 hour 10 minutes

3 medium zucchini, cut into ¼"-thick lengthwise slices

2 large red bell peppers, cut into 1"-wide strips

1 tablespoon olive oil

1 box (8 ounces) sliced mushrooms

4 medium carrots, coarsely shredded

1 package (10 ounces) frozen chopped spinach, thawed and squeezed dry

1 container (15 ounces) reduced-fat ricotta cheese

⅓ cup grated Parmesan cheese

1 large egg

1 jar (26 ounces) spaghetti sauce

9 no-boil lasagna noodles

1½ cups shredded reduced-fat mozzarella cheese

Preheat the oven to 450°F. Coat bottoms and sides of 2 baking sheets with cooking spray. Arrange the zucchini and peppers on the baking sheets. Coat with cooking spray. Roast for 15 to 20 minutes, or until tender, moving the sheets to the opposite oven racks once. Remove sheets and reduce the oven temperature to 350°F.

Heat the oil in a large nonstick skillet over medium-high heat. Add the mushrooms and cook, stirring frequently, for 4 minutes, or until lightly browned. Stir in the carrots and cook for 1 minute longer. Set aside.

In a medium bowl, stir the spinach, ricotta, Parmesan, and egg until blended.

Spread $\frac{1}{2}$ cup of the spaghetti sauce over the bottom of a 13" × 9" × 2" baking dish. Top with 3 of the noodles, overlapping if necessary. Spoon on one-half of the ricotta mixture, spreading to cover the noodles. Top with one-half of the roasted vegetables and one-half of the mushroom mixture. Spoon $\frac{1}{2}$ cup of the sauce over the vegetables and sprinkle with $\frac{1}{2}$ cup of the mozzarella. Repeat the layering. Top with the remaining 3 noodles. Spread the remaining sauce over the noodles. Cover the dish with foil. Bake for 30 minutes. Uncover and sprinkle with the remaining $\frac{1}{2}$ cup mozzarella. Bake for 20 to 25 minutes longer, or until hot and bubbly. Let stand for 15 minutes before serving.

Note: This can be served with additional pasta sauce to spoon over the top, if desired.

Makes 8 servings

Per serving: 320 calories, 19 g protein, 35 g carbohydrates, 12 g fat, 75 mg cholesterol, 670 mg sodium, 6 g dietary fiber
Diet Exchanges: 3 vegetable, 1 $\frac{1}{2}$ bread, 2 $\frac{1}{2}$ meat, 2 fat
Carb Choices: 3

TO-DIE-FOR

DESSERTS

■ FAST ■ SUPER FAST ■ FAST PREP

CHOCOLATE ALMOND MERINGUE COOKIES

Light as a cloud, these crunchy, nutty treats are guaranteed to please a crowd.
Why wait for a special occasion? Whip up a batch tonight!

Prep time: 20 minutes • Cook time: 2 hours

½ **cup blanched almonds**

5 **tablespoons sugar**

3 **large egg whites, at room temperature**

¼ **teaspoon cream of tartar**

2 **tablespoons unsweetened cocoa powder**

¼ **cup raspberry or strawberry all-fruit preserves**

Preheat the oven to 250°F. Line a baking sheet with parchment paper or foil.

Place the almonds and 2 tablespoons of the sugar in a food processor. Process until finely ground.

Place the egg whites and cream of tartar in a large bowl. Using an electric mixer on high speed, beat until frothy. Gradually add the remaining 3 tablespoons sugar and beat until stiff, glossy peaks form. Gently fold in the cocoa and ground almonds.

Spoon the meringue into 1½" mounds on the prepared baking sheet. Using the back of a spoon, depress the centers and build up the sides of each meringue to form a shallow cup.

Bake for 1 hour. Turn off the oven and allow the meringues to stand with the oven door closed for 1 hour. Remove from the sheet and place onto a rack to cool completely.

Store in an airtight container. To serve, fill each meringue with ¼ teaspoon of the preserves.

Makes 16

Per cookie: 61 calories, 2 g protein, 9 g carbohydrates, 2 g fat, 0 mg cholesterol, 10 mg sodium, 1 g dietary fiber
Diet Exchanges: ½ bread, ½ fat
Carb Choice: 1

MEXICAN WEDDING COOKIES

Pecans contain a good amount of fiber, and most of their fat is monounsaturated. That means these tasty nuts will help balance your blood sugar long after you've eaten the last tasty crumb.

Prep time: 20 minutes • Cook time: 12 minutes

¾ **cup whole pecans**

1½ **cups whole grain pastry flour**

¼ **cup cornstarch**

¼ **teaspoon salt**

1 ¼ **cups confectioners' sugar**

5 **tablespoons butter, sliced into chunks**

2 **tablespoons safflower or light olive oil**

2 **tablespoons reduced-fat sour cream**

2 **teaspoons vanilla extract**

Preheat the oven to 350°F. Place the pecans on paper towels. Microwave on high power for 1½ to 2 minutes, or until heated and fragrant. Place in a food processor while still warm and process with pulses just until finely chopped. (Some small pieces may remain.) Add the flour, cornstarch, and salt and process with pulses until combined. Scrape out onto a sheet of waxed paper. Do not wipe out the processor bowl.

Add ¾ cup of the sugar and the butter to the processor. Process until the butter is in small pieces. Add the oil, sour cream, and vanilla and process for 1 minute, or until creamy. Add the flour mixture and pulse just until combined, scraping down the sides of the processor bowl as needed.

Using a rounded measuring teaspoonful, roll the dough into ¾" balls and place on a baking sheet, 1" apart. Bake for 10 to 12 minutes, or until golden on the bottom. Remove from the pans to a sheet of waxed paper. While the cookies are still warm, spoon the remaining ½ cup sugar into a sieve and sprinkle evenly over the tops of the cookies. Let cool and store airtight for up to 1 week, or freeze for up to 1 month.

Makes about 36

Per cookie: 63 calories, 1 g protein, 6 g carbohydrates, 4 g fat, 5 mg cholesterol, 0 mg sodium, 6 g dietary fiber
Diet Exchanges: ½ bread, 1 fat
Carb Choices: ½

OATMEAL COOKIES WITH CHERRIES

When you'd kill for a cookie, turn to one of these healthy indulgences. Cherries contain a moderate amount of calories and very little fat, so they lend natural sweetness to these tasty delights.

Prep time: 15 minutes • Cook time: 10 minutes

1 cup whole grain pastry flour	¼ cup unsweetened applesauce
1 teaspoon baking powder	2 tablespoons canola oil
½ teaspoon ground cinnamon	1 large egg
½ teaspoon baking soda	1 teaspoon vanilla extract
½ teaspoon salt	1½ cups old-fashioned rolled oats
½ cup packed brown sugar	¾ cup dried cherries
⅓ cup granulated sugar	

Preheat the oven to 375°F. Coat 2 large baking sheets with cooking spray.

In a small bowl, combine the flour, baking powder, cinnamon, baking soda, and salt.

In a large bowl, combine the brown sugar and granulated sugar, applesauce, oil, egg, and vanilla. Stir until well blended. Add the flour mixture and stir until combined. Stir in the oats and cherries.

Drop the batter by rounded teaspoonfuls, 2" apart, onto the prepared baking sheets. Bake for 10 to 12 minutes, or until golden brown. Let stand on the baking sheets for 2 minutes before removing to a rack to cool completely.

Makes 30

Per cookie: 43 calories, 1 g protein, 7 g carbohydrates, 1 g fat, 5 mg cholesterol, 80 mg sodium, 1 g dietary fiber
Diet Exchanges: ½ bread
Carb Choices: ½

BISCOTTI WITH FIGS, ALMONDS, AND CHOCOLATE

After dinner, this intensely crunchy treat is loaded with ingredients to indulge your sweet tooth. The monounsaturated fats in almonds, the wholesome morsels of figs, and the bittersweet chocolate will also help you withstand those late-night munchies.

Prep time: 40 minutes • Cook time: 1 hour • Stand time: 30 minutes

½ cup almonds

½ cup sugar

2 large eggs

2 teaspoons vanilla extract

1 ⅔ cups whole grain pastry flour

¾ teaspoon baking soda

¾ teaspoon salt

½ cup dried figs, stemmed and finely chopped

4 ounces bittersweet chocolate, cut into ¼" chunks

Preheat the oven to 300°F. Coat a baking sheet with cooking spray.

Spread the almonds on a separate, ungreased baking sheet. Bake for 10 minutes, or until lightly toasted. Let cool, then coarsely chop the almonds.

In a large bowl, combine the sugar, eggs, and vanilla. With an electric mixer on medium speed, beat for 1 minute. Add the flour, baking soda, and salt. With the mixer on low speed, beat until blended. Stir in the figs, chocolate, and almonds.

Lightly flour a work surface. Divide the dough in half. Roll each piece of dough on the floured surface to a 12" log. Transfer the logs to the prepared baking sheet, allowing space in between. Bake for 30 minutes, or until firm to the touch. Let cool on the baking sheet for 30 minutes.

Loosen the logs with a spatula and slide them one at a time onto a cutting board. With a serrated knife, on the diagonal, cut the log into ½"-thick slices. Place the slices upright on the baking sheet, 1" apart. Bake for 20 minutes, or until the cut sides of the biscotti feel dry to the touch. Let stand on the baking sheets for 2 minutes before removing to a rack to cool completely. Store in an airtight container.

Makes 36

Per cookie: 60 calories, 1 g protein, 10 g carbohydrates, 2 g fat, 10 mg cholesterol, 80 mg sodium, 1 g dietary fiber
Diet Exchanges: ½ bread, ½ fat
Carb Choices: 1

CRUNCHY PEANUT SQUARES

These delicious squares dress up a common healthy and satisfying treat. Air-popped popcorn is usually lower in fat and calories than the kinds that are cooked in oil. For the healthiest popcorn, use a hot-air popper and omit the butter and salt.

Prep time: 5 minutes • Cook time: 3 minutes

1 tablespoon butter	3 cups plain air-popped popcorn
⅓ cup honey	2 cups crisp rice cereal
¼ cup packed brown sugar	2 cups oat circle cereal
⅓ cup natural peanut butter	⅓ cup unsalted peanuts, chopped
1 teaspoon vanilla extract	⅓ cup chocolate chips (optional)

Line a 13" × 9" × 2" baking pan with foil, extending the foil at the ends. Coat the foil with cooking spray.

In a large nonstick saucepan, melt the butter, honey, and brown sugar over low heat, stirring frequently. Remove the saucepan from the heat. Add the peanut butter and vanilla. Return the saucepan to the heat and cook, stirring constantly, for 2 minutes, until the mixture is well blended and melts.

Remove the pan from the heat and add the popcorn, rice and oat cereals, and peanuts. Stir until evenly coated with the peanut butter mixture. Turn into the prepared pan. Spray hands with cooking spray and press the mixture firmly into the pan. Sprinkle with chocolate chips, if using. Cool completely on a rack.

Remove from the pan using the foil. Discard the foil. Cut into squares to serve.

Makes 24

Per square: 82 calories, 2 g protein, 12 g carbohydrates, 3 g fat, 0 mg cholesterol, 65 mg sodium, 1 g dietary fiber
Diet Exchanges: ½ bread, ½ fat
Carb Choices: 1

PUMPKIN-CARROT SNACK BARS

You can do more with pumpkins than carve Halloween jack-o'-lanterns. They have a delicate flavor and are loaded with fiber. Topped with a sprinkling of nuts, they're the perfect treat.

Prep time: 15 minutes • Cook time: 22 minutes

1 **cup canned solid-pack pumpkin**

1 **cup shredded carrot**

½ **cup sugar**

⅓ **cup dried cranberries or raisins, chopped**

¼ **cup canola oil**

2 **large eggs**

1 **cup whole grain pastry flour**

1 **teaspoon baking powder**

1 **teaspoon ground cinnamon**

½ **teaspoon baking soda**

¼ **teaspoon salt**

¼ **cup shelled pumpkin seeds or chopped walnuts (optional)**

Preheat the oven to 350°F. Coat a 13" × 9" × 2" baking pan with cooking spray.

In a large bowl, combine the pumpkin, carrot, sugar, cranberries or raisins, oil, and eggs. Stir until well blended. Add the flour, baking powder, cinnamon, baking soda, and salt. Mix until blended.

Pour the batter into the prepared pan and spread evenly. Sprinkle with the pumpkin seeds or walnuts, if using. Bake for 22 to 25 minutes, or until the top springs back when pressed lightly. Cool completely in the pan on a rack.

Makes 16

Per bar: 99 calories, 2 g protein, 14 g carbohydrates, 4 g fat, 25 mg cholesterol, 150 mg sodium, 1 g dietary fiber
Diet Exchanges: ½ bread, 1 fat
Carb Choices: 1

OATMEAL-DATE BARS

Dates have a history that spans over 5,000 years. It's been said that the name comes from the Greek word for *finger*, after the shape of this fruit. They have an intensely sweet flavor and are loaded with fiber, an ideal combination for fans of sugary snacks.

Prep time: 30 minutes • Cook time: 35 minutes

FILLING

1 cup cinnamon applesauce, sweetened with apple juice concentrate

1 cup chopped dates

1/2 teaspoon pumpkin pie spice

1 teaspoon vanilla extract

CRUST

1 cup whole grain pastry flour

1 cup old-fashioned rolled oats

1/2 teaspoon baking powder

1/2 teaspoon baking soda

1/2 teaspoon salt

2/3 cup packed brown sugar

3 tablespoons butter, at room temperature

3 tablespoons reduced-fat sour cream

Preheat the oven to 375°F. Line a 10 1/2" × 7" baking dish with foil and coat with cooking spray.

To make the filling: In a small nonstick saucepan, combine the applesauce, dates, and pumpkin pie spice. Bring to a bare simmer and cook 10 minutes, or until thickened, stirring and mashing occasionally with a heatproof spatula. Stir the vanilla into the filling until blended and set the filling aside to cool while preparing the crust.

To make the crust: In a medium bowl, whisk together the flour, oats, baking powder, baking soda, and salt. Place the mixture on a sheet of waxed paper. In the same bowl, beat the sugar, butter, and sour cream with an electric mixer on high speed for 1 minute. Stir in the oat mixture with a wooden spoon until combined.

Set a sheet of plastic wrap on a small baking sheet. Remove 1 cup of the dough and crumble it onto the plastic wrap. Cover loosely with the plastic and freeze while assembling the bars. Drop the remaining dough by spoonfuls into the prepared baking dish. Cover with a sheet of plastic wrap coated with cooking spray and press the dough into an even layer. Remove the wrap.

Drop the filling by spoonfuls over the dough and spread in an even layer. Crumble the chilled dough evenly over the filling.

Bake for 25 minutes, or until golden brown. Cool completely in the pan on a rack. Remove from the pan and gently remove the foil. Cut into 18 squares, cutting in thirds lengthwise and sixths crosswise. Store airtight for up to 1 week, or freeze for up to 2 months.

Makes 18

Per bar: 96 calories, 2 g protein, 18 g carbohydrates, 3 g fat, 5 mg cholesterol, 135 mg sodium, 2 g dietary fiber
Diet Exchanges: 1 fruit, ½ bread, ½ fat
Carb Choices: 1

DOUBLE CHERRY–CORNMEAL TEA BREAD

Made from dried corn kernels, cornmeal is low in fat and sodium and high in fiber. Its coarse texture mixed with the sweetness of cherries will give your tastebuds a delightful surprise.

Prep time: 20 minutes ● Cook time: 55 minutes ● Stand time: 10 minutes

3 **tablespoons dried cherries**	⅓ **cup plain low-fat yogurt**
1 ⅓ **cups whole grain pastry flour**	¼ **cup unsweetened applesauce**
⅔ **cup yellow cornmeal**	2 **tablespoons butter, melted**
1 **teaspoon baking powder**	1 **egg**
½ **teaspoon baking soda**	1 **tablespoon grated orange or lemon peel**
¼ **teaspoon salt**	1 **cup fresh cherries, pitted and quartered**
⅔ **cup sugar**	

Preheat the oven to 350°F. Coat an 8 ½" × 4 ½" loaf pan with cooking spray. In a small dish, combine the dried cherries with enough hot water to cover. Let stand for 10 minutes, or until softened.

Meanwhile, in a medium bowl, whisk together the flour, cornmeal, baking powder, baking soda, and salt until blended. In a medium bowl, whisk together the sugar, yogurt, applesauce, butter, egg, and orange or lemon peel until well blended. Drain the dried cherries well and coarsely chop. Stir the fresh and dried cherries into the yogurt mixture. Add the flour mixture in 2 additions, stirring just until combined. Scrape the batter into the prepared pan.

Bake for 55 minutes, or until a wooden pick inserted into the center comes out clean. Cool in the pan on a rack for 10 minutes. Turn out onto the rack and cool completely.

Makes 12 servings

Per serving: 141 calories, 3 g protein, 25 g carbohydrates, 3 g fat, 25 mg cholesterol, 180 mg sodium, 2 g dietary fiber
Diet Exchanges: 1 ½ bread, ½ fat
Carb Choices: 2

HARVEST APPLE CAKE

Apples are bursting with pectin, a fiber that slows the digestion of nutrients. Getting more pectin in your diet is an excellent strategy for helping to control your blood sugar.

Prep time: 35 minutes • Cook time: 35 minutes • Stand time: 30 minutes

2 Granny Smith apples, peeled, cored, and cut into ½" cubes

¾ cup packed brown sugar

1 ½ cups whole grain pastry flour

1 teaspoon baking soda

1 teaspoon ground cinnamon

1 teaspoon ground ginger

½ teaspoon ground nutmeg

½ teaspoon salt

⅓ cup canola oil

⅓ cup low-fat buttermilk

1 large egg

1 teaspoon vanilla extract

½ cup chopped walnuts

½ cup raisins

Preheat the oven to 350°F. Coat a 9" × 9" square baking pan with cooking spray.

In a large bowl, combine the apples and brown sugar, stirring to coat the apples well. Let stand for 30 minutes, stirring occasionally.

In a medium bowl, combine the flour, baking soda, cinnamon, ginger, nutmeg, and salt.

In a small bowl, stir the oil, buttermilk, egg, and vanilla until blended. Add to the apple mixture along with the walnuts and raisins. Stir until combined. Add the flour mixture and stir until blended. Pour the batter into the prepared pan and spread evenly. Bake for 35 to 40 minutes, or until a wooden pick inserted into the center comes out clean.

Cool in the pan on a rack. Serve warm or at room temperature.

Makes 9 servings

Per serving: 290 calories, 4 g protein, 41 g carbohydrates, 14 g fat, 25 mg cholesterol, 300 mg sodium, 3 g dietary fiber
Diet Exchanges: 1 fruit, 2 bread, 2 ½ fat
Carb Choices: 3

LEMON PUDDING CAKE

With zesty flavor and intensely moist texture, a slice of this wholesome and healthy cake is a lively endnote to any meal.

Prep time: 25 minutes • Cook time: 40 minutes

½ **cup sugar**

3 **tablespoons whole grain pastry flour**

⅛ **teaspoon ground nutmeg**

1 **cup 1% milk or unsweetened light soymilk**

¼ **cup lemon juice**

2 **tablespoons butter, melted**

1 **egg yolk**

1 ½ **teaspoons grated lemon peel**

2 **large egg whites**

⅛ **teaspoon salt**

Preheat the oven to 350°F. Set a 1-quart soufflé or baking dish in a small roasting pan.

In a medium bowl, combine the sugar, flour, and nutmeg. Make a well in the center. Add the milk or soymilk, lemon juice, butter, egg yolk, and lemon peel. Mix by hand until blended.

With an electric mixer on medium-high speed, beat the egg whites and salt in a medium bowl until soft peaks form. Spoon the whites into the batter and fold together until smooth. (The batter will be thin.) Pour into the soufflé or baking dish. Add boiling water to the roasting pan to come halfway up the side of the dish.

Bake for 40 minutes, or until the top is golden and a pudding has formed underneath. (Cut a small slit in the center to ensure that the cake layer is done.) Remove the baking dish to a rack and cool for 15 minutes. Serve warm or at room temperature.

Makes 4 servings

Per serving: 214 calories, 5 g protein, 33 g carbohydrates, 8 g fat, 70 mg cholesterol, 210 mg sodium, 1 g dietary fiber
Diet Exchanges: 2 bread, 1 ½ fat
Carb Choices: 2

LEMON-BLUEBERRY COBBLER

A traditional cobbler is topped with a thick biscuit crust. You won't miss the saturated fat in our version, made with cornmeal and whole wheat pastry flour. Eat it warm and you'll enjoy one of the healthiest comfort foods imaginable.

Prep time: 20 minutes • Cook time: 45 minutes

5 **cups fresh or frozen and thawed blueberries**

2 **teaspoons grated lemon peel**

$1/2$ **cup sugar**

2 **tablespoons + 1 cup whole grain pastry flour**

1 **cup 1% milk or unsweetened light soymilk**

1 **egg**

3 **tablespoons butter, melted**

1 **tablespoon lemon juice**

$1/2$ **cup cornmeal**

1 $1/2$ **teaspoons baking powder**

$1/4$ **teaspoon baking soda**

$1/4$ **teaspoon salt**

Light vanilla frozen yogurt

Preheat the oven to 375°F. Coat the inner sides of a 2-quart baking dish (8" × 11 $1/2$") with cooking spray. Add the blueberries, lemon peel, $1/4$ cup of the sugar, and the 2 tablespoons flour. Toss together until combined. Using the back of a spoon, spread the fruit mixture level.

In a medium bowl, whisk together the milk or soymilk, egg, butter, lemon juice, cornmeal, and the remaining $1/4$ cup sugar until blended. Add the baking powder, baking soda, salt, and the 1 cup flour. Whisk together just until combined. Pour the batter evenly over the fruit mixture.

Bake for 45 to 50 minutes, or until the fruit is bubbly and a knife inserted into the center of the topping comes out clean. Serve warm with frozen yogurt.

Makes 6 servings

Per serving: 270 calories, 5 g protein, 49 g carbohydrates, 7 g fat, 50 mg cholesterol, 330 mg sodium, 4 g dietary fiber
Diet Exchanges: 1 $1/2$ fruit, 2 $1/2$ bread, 1 $1/2$ fat
Carb Choices: 4

PEANUT BUTTER BUNDT CAKE

It's difficult to believe that peanut butter could be a diet food, but its creamy rich texture helps make this cake taste like a real indulgence—and it reduces the amount of butter typically called for in similar recipes. *Photo on page 290.*

Prep time: 25 minutes • Cook time: 55 minutes

CAKE

1½ cups whole grain pastry flour	½ cup butter, at room temperature
1 cup cake flour	1 cup sugar
2 teaspoons baking powder	2 egg whites
½ teaspoon baking soda	1 tablespoon vanilla extract
½ teaspoon salt	⅓ cup mini chocolate chips
½ cup reduced-fat peanut butter	1½ cups low-fat buttermilk

GLAZE

1 tablespoon unsweetened cocoa powder	½ teaspoon vanilla extract
2 tablespoons peanut butter	½ cup confectioners' sugar
1½–2 tablespoons water	Pinch of salt

To make the cake: Preheat the oven to 350°F. Coat a 10" Bundt pan with cooking spray.

In a medium bowl, whisk together the whole grain and cake flours, baking powder, baking soda, and salt. In another medium bowl with an electric mixer at medium speed, beat together the peanut butter and butter for 1 minute, or until creamy. Add the sugar, egg whites, and vanilla and beat for 2 minutes, or until light and fluffy. Beat in the chocolate chips on low speed, just until combined.

With the mixer set on the lowest speed, alternately add the flour mixture and the buttermilk in 3 additions, beginning and ending with the flour mixture. Scrape the batter into the prepared pan and spread level.

Bake for 55 to 60 minutes, or until a wooden pick inserted into the center comes out clean and the cake begins to pull away from the sides of the pan. Cool in the pan on a rack for 10 minutes. Loosen the sides with a spatula and invert onto a serving plate. Slip strips of waxed paper under the edges of the cake, for glazing.

To make the glaze: Meanwhile, in a small bowl, stir together the cocoa, peanut butter, water, and vanilla until blended. Stir in the confectioners' sugar and salt until smooth. Drizzle the glaze over the cake using a spoon. Set aside until the glaze is firm. Remove the waxed paper strips.

Makes 16 servings

Per serving: 270 calories, 6 g protein, 37 g carbohydrates, 12 g fat, 15 mg cholesterol, 290 mg sodium, 2 g dietary fiber
Diet Exchanges: 2 ½ bread, ½ meat, 3 fat
Carb Choices: 3

ORANGE–OLIVE OIL CAKE WITH FRESH BERRIES

Olive oil makes this dessert luxuriously rich and adds a healthy dash of monounsaturated fats. If fresh berries aren't available, substitute frozen.

Prep time: 25 minutes • Cook time: 20 minutes

CAKE

- ¾ cup whole grain pastry flour
- ¼ cup cornmeal
- 1 teaspoon baking powder
- ¼ teaspoon baking soda
- ¼ teaspoon salt
- ⅓ cup + 1 tablespoon sugar

- 3 tablespoons olive oil
- ½ cup fat-free plain yogurt
- 2 large eggs
- 1 tablespoon grated orange peel
- 2 tablespoons orange juice
- ¼ teaspoon ground cinnamon

BERRIES

- 1 cup fresh blackberries
- 1 tablespoon sugar
- 1 tablespoon orange juice

- 1 cup fresh blueberries
- 1 cup fresh raspberries

To make the cake: Preheat the oven to 350°F. Coat a 9" springform pan with cooking spray.

In a small bowl, combine the flour, cornmeal, baking powder, baking soda, and salt.

In a large bowl, combine the ⅓ cup sugar and the oil. With an electric mixer on high speed, beat for 2 minutes. Add the yogurt, eggs, orange peel, and orange juice. Beat for 1 minute. Add the flour mixture and beat until blended. Pour the batter into the prepared pan.

In a small bowl, combine the cinnamon and the 1 tablespoon sugar. Sprinkle over the batter. Bake for 20 to 25 minutes, or until a wooden pick inserted into the center comes out clean. Cool completely in the pan on a rack.

To make the berries: In a food processor or blender, puree $3/4$ cup of the blackberries, the sugar, and the orange juice until smooth. Strain the puree through a sieve into a small bowl and discard the seeds. Cut the cake into wedges and serve with the berry sauce spooned over it and the blueberries, raspberries, and remaining blackberries on top.

Note: This cake is best served the day it is made. When you use an electric mixer to beat citrus peel into a batter, a lot of the peel can cling to the beaters, so be sure to scrape any peel from the beaters back into the batter.

Makes 8 servings

Per serving: 189 calories, 4 g protein, 30 g carbohydrates, 7 g fat, 55 mg cholesterol, 200 mg sodium, 3 g dietary fiber
Diet Exchanges: 1 fruit, 1 bread, 1 fat
Carb Choices: 2

PEAR-TOPPED TRIPLE GINGERBREAD

With over 5,000 varieties of pears to choose from, you could eat a different one every day and never have the same taste twice. Pears are best when they are picked unripe and then ripened at room temperature. They are ready to eat when their flesh gives slightly and they have a sweet, fruity fragrance.

Prep time: 15 minutes • Cook time: 40 minutes

1 large pear, peeled, halved, and cored	½ cup dark molasses
1 tablespoon lemon juice	⅓ cup packed brown sugar
1¾ cups whole grain pastry flour	3 egg whites
1¼ teaspoons baking soda	3 tablespoons canola oil
1 teaspoon ground cinnamon	3 tablespoons finely chopped candied ginger (optional)
¾ teaspoon ground ginger	1½ teaspoons grated fresh ginger
½ teaspoon pumpkin pie spice or nutmeg	
¼ teaspoon salt	

Preheat the oven to 350°F. Coat a 9" × 1" round (or square) cake pan with cooking spray. Slice the pear into thin wedges. Gently toss the slices with the lemon juice.

In a medium bowl, whisk together the flour, baking soda, cinnamon, ginger, pie spice or nutmeg, and salt until combined. In a large bowl, whisk together the molasses, sugar, egg whites, oil, candied ginger (if using), and fresh ginger until blended. Add the flour mixture and stir just until blended. Scrape the batter into the prepared pan and arrange the pear slices on top, in a spoke fashion.

Bake for 40 to 45 minutes, or until a wooden pick inserted in the center comes out clean. Place the pan onto a rack to cool for at least 15 minutes. Cut into wedges and serve warm.

Makes 10 servings

Per serving: 153 calories, 3 g protein, 27 g carbohydrates, 5 g fat, 0 mg cholesterol, 245 mg sodium, 2 g dietary fiber
Diet Exchanges: ½ fruit, 1½ bread, 1 fat
Carb Choices: 2

CHOCOLATE-RASPBERRY CAKE

This dazzling cake is a showstopper! Layers of chocolate, whipped topping, and fruit make this dessert worthy of any special occasion.

Prep time: 15 minutes • Cook time: 35 minutes

1 cup whole grain pastry flour	2 large egg yolks, at room temperature
½ cup sugar	1 teaspoon vanilla extract
3 tablespoons unsweetened cocoa powder	2 large egg whites, at room temperature
1 teaspoon baking powder	1¼ cups reduced-fat whipped topping
¼ teaspoon salt	1½ cups raspberries
1 container (8 ounces) low-fat vanilla yogurt	½ cup raspberry all-fruit preserves, melted
2 tablespoons canola oil	Mint sprigs (optional)

Preheat the oven to 350° F. Coat an 8" round baking pan with cooking spray.

In a medium bowl, mix the flour, sugar, cocoa, baking powder, and salt. In a large bowl, mix the yogurt, oil, egg yolks, and vanilla. Place the egg whites in a medium bowl. Using an electric mixer on high speed, beat until stiff peaks form.

Stir the flour mixture into the yogurt mixture just until blended. Fold in the egg whites until no streaks of white remain. Pour into the prepared pan. Bake for 35 minutes, or until a wooden pick inserted into the center comes out clean. Cool on a rack for 5 minutes. Remove from the pan and place on the rack to cool completely.

To serve, split the cake horizontally into 2 layers. Spread 1 cup of whipped topping over 1 layer. Top with 1 cup of the raspberries and drizzle with the preserves. Top with the remaining cake layer and spoon 12 dollops of the remaining whipped topping around the cake. Top each with a few of the remaining raspberries and garnish with the mint, if using.

Makes 12 servings

Per serving: 161 calories, 4 g protein, 27 carbohydrates, 5 g fat, 35 mg cholesterol, 115 mg sodium, 3 g dietary fiber
Diet Exchanges: 1 bread, 1 fat
Carb Choices: 2

ROASTED APPLE-CRANBERRY STRUDEL

High-fiber foods don't have to be boring! Granny Smith apples and cranberries give this strudel a tangy kick. *Photo on page 291.*

Prep time: 35 minutes • Cook time: 32 minutes • Stand time: 10 minutes

4 large Granny Smith apples (2 ¼ pounds), peeled, cored, and thinly sliced

⅓ cup dried cranberries

1 tablespoon brandy or water

½ teaspoon pumpkin pie spice or ground nutmeg

⅓ cup + 1 ½ tablespoons packed brown sugar

¾ teaspoon ground cinnamon

5 sheets phyllo dough (17" × 12")

3 tablespoons butter, melted

Preheat the oven to 400°F. Line 2 large baking sheets with foil and coat with cooking spray.

Spread the apple slices in an even layer on one of the baking sheets. Bake for 12 minutes, or until tender, turning them over with a fork or spatula halfway through the cooking (for microwave directions, see note). Meanwhile, in a small microwaveable bowl, combine the cranberries and brandy or water. Cover loosely with plastic wrap and microwave on high for 40 seconds, or until the liquid just begins to simmer. Let stand for at least 10 minutes.

Spoon the apples into a medium bowl (you should have about 2 ½ cups). Stir in the pie spice or nutmeg, the ⅓ cup sugar, ½ teaspoon of the cinnamon, and the cranberries. Set aside to cool.

In a small dish, stir together the 1 ½ tablespoons sugar and the remaining ¼ teaspoon cinnamon. Lay 1 sheet of phyllo on a sheet of waxed paper and lightly brush with the butter. Sprinkle evenly with about one-quarter of the cinnamon sugar. Repeat with the remaining phyllo, butter, and cinnamon sugar, coating the last phyllo with butter only, layering the phyllo sheets on top of each other.

Mound the apple mixture down the long side of the phyllo stack, leaving a 2" border on the long side and the ends. Loosely roll up the strudel, using the waxed paper as a guide. Tuck in the ends and transfer to the prepared baking sheet. Brush the top of the strudel with the remaining butter. Using a serrated knife, divide the strudel into 8 equal portions by cutting lightly through the top of the strudel (just to the filling), on the diagonal. Do not cut all the way through.

Bake for 20 to 25 minutes, or just until golden brown. Cool in the pan on a rack for at least 10 minutes. Slide the strudel onto a board and cut along the scored marks. Serve warm.

Note: To "bake" apples in the microwave, place them in a microwaveable glass bowl and microwave on high power for 2 to 3 minutes, stirring once. Apples should be tender enough to pierce with fork.

Makes 8 servings

Per serving: 188 calories, 1 g protein, 35 g carbohydrates, 5 g fat, 10 mg cholesterol, 105 mg sodium, 4 g dietary fiber
Diet Exchanges: 1 fruit, 1 bread, 1 fat
Carb Choices: 2

BLUEBERRY-GINGER CRUMB PIE

One of the sweetest things about berries is that they have large amounts of fiber. When shopping for fresh blueberries, look for plump, firm berries with an indigo-blue color and a silvery frost. Rinse fresh berries just before you're ready to use them.

Prep time: 10 minutes • Cook time: 18 minutes

CRUST

1 cup gingersnap cookies (about 7 ounces)	2 tablespoons butter, melted
1 ½ tablespoons brown sugar	

FILLING

5–6 cups fresh or frozen and thawed blueberries	¼ cup water
4 tablespoons cornstarch	½ cup granulated sugar

To make the crust: Preheat the oven to 325°F. Place the gingersnaps in a food processor and process until the crumbs are fine. Add the brown sugar and butter and pulse the processor until the mixture is just combined.

Press into a 9" pie plate and bake for 8 to 10 minutes. Let cool.

To make the filling: Place the blueberries, cornstarch, and water in a medium saucepan. Bring to a simmer over medium heat until slightly thickened. Add the granulated sugar and heat on low for 10 to 12 minutes, until the sugar is dissolved. Remove from the heat and cool slightly. Pour the filling into the prepared crust. Cool completely before cutting.

Makes 8 servings

Per serving: 220 calories, 2 g protein, 45 g carbohydrates, 5 g fat, 10 mg cholesterol, 135 mg sodium, 3 g dietary fiber
Diet Exchanges: 1 fruit, 2 ½ bread, 1 ½ fat
Carb Choices: 4

FALL FRUIT CRISP

Surely there's no sweeter way to increase your fiber intake. Studies have shown that eating 40 grams of fiber a day will block the absorption of 160 calories. This medley of vibrant fruits is a painless way to do it.

Prep time: 20 minutes • Cook time: 45 minutes

FRUIT

2 large Granny Smith apples, peeled, cored, and thinly sliced

2 large ripe pears, peeled, cored, and thinly sliced

½ cup fresh or frozen cranberries, thawed

2 tablespoons packed brown sugar

2 tablespoons ground cinnamon

TOPPING

¾ cup old-fashioned rolled oats

1½ tablespoons whole grain pastry flour

3 tablespoons packed brown sugar

1½ tablespoons butter, cut into small pieces

1½ tablespoons pure maple syrup

½ teaspoon ground cinnamon

2 tablespoons chopped walnuts

To make the fruit: Preheat the oven to 375°F. In a large bowl, combine the apples, pears, cranberries, sugar, and cinnamon. Toss to combine. Turn the fruit mixture into a shallow 2-quart baking dish and spread evenly.

To make the topping: In the same bowl, combine the oats, flour, sugar, butter, maple syrup, and cinnamon. With your fingers, mix until crumbly. Stir in the walnuts. Sprinkle the topping over the fruit mixture. Cover the dish loosely with foil. Bake for 20 minutes. Uncover and bake 25 minutes longer, or until the fruit is tender when pierced with the tip of a sharp knife. Let cool on a rack and serve warm.

Makes 6 servings

Per serving: 210 calories, 3 g protein, 42 g carbohydrates, 5 g fat, 10 mg cholesterol, 25 mg sodium, 6 g dietary fiber
Diet Exchanges: 1 ½ fruit, 2 bread, 1 ½ fat
Carb Choices: 4

PEACH AND RASPBERRY CROSTATA

Indulge your sweet tooth with a slice of this wholesome confection! With their velvet skin and succulent flesh, peaches are popular summertime fare and are good sources of fiber.

Photo on page 292.

Prep time: 40 minutes • Cook time: 45 minutes • Stand time: 30 minutes

CRUST

1 ½ cups whole grain pastry flour

¼ teaspoon salt

¼ cup vegetable shortening

2 ounces reduced-fat cream cheese

2 teaspoons lemon juice

4–5 tablespoons ice water

TOPPING

3 tablespoons shredded bran cereal

1 tablespoon whole grain pastry flour

¼ teaspoon ground cinnamon

6 tablespoons sugar

1 ¾ pounds fresh peaches, peeled and pitted (see note)

1 cup fresh raspberries

To make the crust: In a large bowl, combine the flour and salt. Cut in the shortening and cream cheese until the mixture resembles coarse crumbs. In a cup, stir the lemon juice together with 2 tablespoons of the water. Drizzle over the crumb mixture and mix until moistened. Mix in the remaining water 1 tablespoon at a time, until the texture resembles cottage cheese and it can be pressed into a firm ball.

Press the dough into a 6" disk. Wrap in plastic wrap and refrigerate at least 30 minutes before using.

Place a wide sheet of foil onto a large baking sheet and coat with cooking spray. Fold the edges of the foil up ½" to form a rim. Roll the dough out between sheets of lightly floured waxed paper to a 13" circle. Place onto the prepared baking sheet, cover with plastic wrap, and refrigerate until using.

To make the topping: Preheat the oven to 400°F.

In a food processor or blender, combine the cereal, flour, cinnamon, and 4 tablespoons of the sugar. Process until the cereal is finely ground. Sprinkle the cereal mixture over the pastry, leaving a 2" border. Arrange the peaches over the cereal mixture. Fold the pastry border over the fruit. Sprinkle the remaining 2 tablespoons of sugar over the fruit and the pastry edge.

Bake for 45 to 50 minutes, or until the crust is golden brown and juices are bubbly. Cool in the pan on a rack. Sprinkle on the raspberries.

Note: To substitute frozen peaches, use 1 ½ pounds dry-packed sliced peaches, thawing in a single layer on paper towels to absorb excess liquid.

Makes 10 servings

Per serving: 181 calories, 3 g protein, 30 g carbohydrates, 6 g fat, 5 mg cholesterol, 90 mg sodium, 4 g dietary fiber
Diet Exchanges: 1 fruit, 1 bread, 1 fat
Carb Choices: 2

STRAWBERRY-RHUBARB CRISP

Rhubarb is an excellent source of fiber. When shopping, pick the redder stalks, which are less sour. *Photo on page 293.*

Prep time: 25 minutes • Cook time: 35 minutes • Stand time: 20 minutes

2 pints strawberries, hulled and quartered lengthwise

2 cups fresh or frozen and thawed rhubarb (cut into ½" pieces)

1–2 tablespoons quick-cooking tapioca, or

½–1 tablespoon cornstarch (see note)

¼ teaspoon ground ginger

¾ cup sugar

1 teaspoon ground cinnamon

⅓ cup whole grain pastry flour

Pinch of salt

2 tablespoons butter

½ cup old-fashioned rolled oats

1½ tablespoons honey

In a 2-quart baking dish, combine the strawberries, rhubarb, tapioca or cornstarch, ginger, ½ cup of the sugar, and ¼ teaspoon of the cinnamon. Spread the fruit mixture level, and let stand for 20 minutes.

Meanwhile, preheat the oven to 400°F. In a medium bowl, stir together the flour, salt, and the remaining ¼ cup sugar, and ¾ teaspoon cinnamon. Cut in the butter until the mixture is the texture of fine meal. Stir in the oats until combined. Drizzle the honey on top and stir until the mixture is crumbly. Sprinkle over the fruit in an even layer.

Bake for 35 to 40 minutes, or until the fruit is bubbly and the topping is golden brown. Serve warm or at room temperature.

Note: If the berries are not very juicy, use the minimum amount of cornstarch suggested in the recipe.

Makes 6 servings

Per serving: 232 calories, 3 g protein, 47 g carbohydrates, 5 g fat, 10 mg cholesterol, 0 mg sodium, 5 g dietary fiber
Diet Exchanges: 1 fruit, 2 bread, 1 fat
Carb Choices: 3

ROASTED PEARS WITH ORANGE-CARAMEL SAUCE

FAST PREP

This scrumptious dessert features the mellow sweetness of pears, the zesty tang of orange, and an impressive amount of fiber, which will help keep your blood sugar balanced.

Photo on page 294.

Prep time: 20 minutes • Cook time: 50 minutes

- **2 tablespoons hazelnuts, chopped**
- **1 tablespoon butter**
- **⅓ cup sugar**
- **4 ripe pears, halved and cored**

- **¼ cup orange juice, at room temperature**
- **4 dried figs, stemmed and chopped**
- **1 tablespoon orange liqueur (optional)**

Place the hazelnuts in a dry skillet and cook over medium heat for 4 minutes, or until fragrant. Be sure to stir the nuts frequently to prevent burning. Set aside.

Preheat the oven to 400°F. Spread the butter in the bottom of a 13" × 9" × 2" baking dish. Sprinkle with 2 tablespoons of the sugar. Place the pear halves cut side down in the prepared baking dish. Bake for 35 to 40 minutes, or until the pears are tender when pierced with the tip of a knife.

Meanwhile, place the remaining sugar in a small saucepan. Cook over medium-high heat, swirling the pan frequently, for 5 minutes, until the sugar melts and turns amber in color. Remove the pan from the heat and slowly pour in the orange juice to avoid sputtering hot liquid. Return the pan to medium-low heat. Cook the sauce, stirring constantly, for 5 minutes, until the sauce thickens slightly. Stir in the figs and liqueur, if using. Set the sauce aside.

Remove the pears from the baking dish to serving plates. Add any juices remaining in the baking dish to the sauce.

Serve the pears warm or at room temperature. Spoon the sauce over the pears and sprinkle with the hazelnuts. If the sauce thickens after sitting, rewarm it over low heat.

Makes 4 servings

Per serving: 260 calories, 2 g protein, 54 g carbohydrates, 6 g fat, 10 mg cholesterol, 20 mg sodium, 6 g dietary fiber
Diet Exchanges: 2 ½ fruit, 1 ½ bread, 1 fat
Carb Choices: 4

CHOCOLATE-HAZELNUT FONDUE

Indulge your chocolate cravings by taking a dip in this rich, creamy sauce. With the saturated fats and calories cut back, you won't have those "morning after" regrets.

Prep time: 15 minutes • Cook time: 6 minutes

½ ounce unsweetened chocolate, chopped

1 can (14 ounces) fat-free sweetened condensed milk

2 tablespoons unsweetened cocoa powder

Pinch of salt

3 tablespoons chocolate-hazelnut spread

½ teaspoon vanilla extract

Assorted cubed or sliced fresh fruit and angel food cake cubes

In a small nonstick saucepan, combine the chocolate and about half of the condensed milk. Heat over medium heat for 3 minutes, stirring until the chocolate is melted. Remove from the heat and stir in the remaining milk. Sift the cocoa and salt on top. Stir until blended.

Return to the heat and cook, stirring, for 3 minutes longer, or until the fondue just begins to simmer. Remove from the heat. Stir in the chocolate-hazelnut spread and vanilla until smooth. Serve warm with the fruit and cake cubes.

Note: The fondue can be made ahead (up to 4 days in advance) and reheated in a saucepan or in the microwave on medium power, stirring occasionally. If needed, thin the fondue by adding hot water by teaspoonfuls, until the desired dipping consistency.

Makes 8 servings (1 ⅓ cups)

Per serving: 220 calories, 6 g protein, 45 g carbohydrates, 2 g fat, 5 mg cholesterol, 80 mg sodium, 1 g dietary fiber
Diet Exchanges: 3 bread
Carb Choices: 3

DARK CHOCOLATE PUDDING

Here is a healthier, more sophisticated version of the ultimate comfort food. The creamy and satisfying texture is all you need for finishing a perfect meal. *Photo on page 295.*

Prep time: 10 minutes • Cook time: 12 minutes • Chill: 2 hours

¼ **cup sugar**

¼ **cup malted milk powder**

3 **tablespoons unsweetened cocoa powder**

2 **tablespoons cornstarch**

1 **teaspoon instant coffee powder**

2 **cups 1% milk**

1 **ounce unsweetened chocolate, finely chopped**

1 **teaspoon vanilla extract**

In a medium saucepan, whisk together the sugar, malted milk powder, cocoa, cornstarch, and coffee powder until blended. Gradually whisk in the milk.

Cook over medium heat, stirring constantly, for 10 minutes until the pudding thickens and comes to a boil. Reduce the heat to low and add the chocolate. Cook, stirring constantly, for 1 minute, until the chocolate melts. Remove from the heat and stir in the vanilla. Pour the pudding into 4 custard cups. Cover with plastic wrap and refrigerate until cold, at least 2 hours.

Note: A heatproof rubber spatula works well for stirring the pudding to prevent it from scorching on the bottom.

Makes 4 servings

Per serving: 250 calories, 8 g protein, 46 g carbohydrates, 6 g fat, 5 mg cholesterol, 125 mg sodium, 4 g dietary fiber
Diet Exchanges: ½ milk, 3 bread, ½ fat
Carb Choices: 3

BROWN RICE PUDDING

You'll love this dessert's unique coupling of nutty and sweet flavors. We've used brown rice so you get even more nutritious fiber.

Prep time: 20 minutes • Cook time: 1 hour 20 minutes • Chill time: 4 hours or overnight

1 1/4 cups water

1 tablespoon grated lemon peel

1/4 teaspoon salt

1/2 cup brown rice

3 cups 2% milk

1 tablespoon vanilla extract

3 tablespoons packed brown sugar

Chopped mango or papaya (optional)

1/4 cup shredded sweetened coconut (optional)

In a large saucepan, combine the water, 1 1/2 teaspoons of the lemon peel, and the salt. Bring to a boil and add the rice. Reduce the heat and simmer, covered, for 40 minutes, or until the rice is tender and most of the water is absorbed.

Stir in the milk, vanilla, sugar, and the remaining lemon peel. Bring to a boil. Reduce the heat to low and simmer for 40 to 45 minutes, stirring frequently to prevent sticking, especially toward the end of the cooking time, until the pudding thickens and the rice is very tender. (It will thicken more on standing.) Pour the pudding into a bowl and let cool to room temperature, stirring occasionally. Cover with plastic wrap and refrigerate 4 hours (or overnight) until chilled.

To serve, spoon the pudding into 6 individual serving dishes. Top with the mango or papaya, if using, and coconut, if using.

Makes 6 servings

Per serving: 141 calories, 5 g protein, 25 g carbohydrates, 2 g fat, 5 mg cholesterol, 160 mg sodium, 1 g dietary fiber
Diet Exchanges: 1/2 milk, 1 1/2 bread
Carb Choices: 2

SPICED KAHLÚA CUSTARDS

Turn a standard cup of joe into a satisfying treat. This puddinglike dessert is as creamy and delicious as traditional custards but without the usual fat and calories.

Prep time: 20 minutes • Cook time: 45 minutes • Chill time: 4 hours to overnight

2 **cups unsweetened light soymilk**	2 **eggs**
½ **cup brewed coffee**	2 **egg whites**
¼ **cup coffee liqueur (such as Kahlúa)**	¼ **cup sugar**
1 **tablespoon instant coffee powder**	⅛ **teaspoon salt**
1 **teaspoon ground cinnamon**	**Chocolate-covered espresso beans (optional)**
½ **teaspoon ground allspice**	

Preheat the oven to 350°F. Set six 6- or 8-ounce custard cups into a 13" × 9" baking dish.

In a medium saucepan, combine the soymilk, coffee, liqueur, instant coffee powder, cinnamon, and allspice. Set over medium heat and cook for 4 minutes, or just until bubbles form around the edge of the pan. Remove from the heat. In a large bowl, whisk together the eggs, egg whites, sugar, and salt until well blended. Gradually stir in the milk mixture until blended. Ladle the mixture into the custard cups, dividing evenly. Add boiling water to the baking dish to come halfway up the sides of the custard cups.

Bake for 40 to 45 minutes, or until a knife inserted into the center of a custard comes out clean. Carefully remove the cups from the water and cool on a rack. Cover with plastic wrap and refrigerate for 4 hours (or overnight) until chilled. Garnish with espresso beans, if using.

Makes 6 servings

Per serving: 135 calories, 5 g protein, 20 g carbohydrates, 2 g fat, 70 mg cholesterol, 135 mg sodium, 0 g dietary fiber
Diet Exchanges: ½ milk, 1 bread, ½ meat
Carb Choices: 1

GINGER FROZEN YOGURT WITH SWEET PLUM SAUCE

Frozen yogurt typically has less fat and calories than its full-fat cousin, ice cream. Adorn it with high-fiber plums and a sprinkling of almonds, and you've made your frozen yogurt even healthier and more satisfying. *Photo on page 296.*

Prep time: 10 minutes • Cook time: 35 minutes

¼ **cup sliced almonds**

1 **pint fat-free vanilla frozen yogurt, slightly softened**

2–4 **tablespoons finely chopped crystallized ginger**

1 **pound ripe plums (4 large), pitted and sliced**

3 **tablespoons sugar-free grape jam**

1 **tablespoon sugar**

Preheat the oven to 300°F. Spread the almonds on a baking sheet. Bake for 10 minutes, or until lightly toasted. Let cool, then coarsely chop the almonds.

In a large bowl, combine the frozen yogurt and ginger. Quickly stir to combine. Return the yogurt to the freezer.

In a medium saucepan, combine the plums, jam, and sugar. Bring to a simmer over medium heat. Reduce the heat to low, cover, and simmer for 12 minutes, until the plums soften and break down. Uncover and simmer for 5 minutes, until the sauce thickens slightly. Pour the sauce into a bowl and let cool. Cover with plastic wrap and refrigerate until cold.

To serve, spoon the sauce into 4 individual serving dishes. Top with scoops of the frozen yogurt and sprinkle with the almonds.

Makes 4 servings

Per serving: 200 calories, 6 g protein, 39 g carbohydrates, 4 g fat, 0 mg cholesterol, 80 mg sodium, 2 g dietary fiber
Diet Exchanges: 1 fruit, 2 ½ bread, 1 fat
Carb Choices: 4

RED WINE–BERRY SORBET

High-fiber fruit never looked so elegant! Cleanse your palate with this refreshing dessert.

Prep time: 15 minutes • Cook time: 1 minute • Stand time: 1 hour • Chill time: Overnight

1 bottle (750 ml) fruity red wine, such as
Beaujolais

1 cup sugar

¾ cup water

1 cup fresh or frozen raspberries

1 cup fresh or frozen strawberries, hulled
and halved

1 cup fresh or frozen blueberries

1 tablespoon lemon juice

In a large saucepan, combine the wine, sugar, and water. Bring to a boil, then boil for 1 minute. Remove the pan from the heat and add the raspberries, strawberries, and blueberries. Cover and let stand for 1 hour.

With a slotted spoon, remove the berries to a blender. Set the wine mixture aside. Blend the berries until pureed. Pour the puree into a sieve set over a bowl and stir to remove the seeds. Discard the seeds. Stir the puree and the lemon juice into the reserved wine mixture. Pour into a shallow baking dish. Cover with plastic wrap and freeze overnight.

With a spoon, break the wine mixture into chunks. Process briefly in a food processor, in batches, until smooth but still frozen. Serve immediately, or spoon into a food storage container and freeze until ready to serve.

Makes 12 servings (1 ½ quarts)

Per serving: 126 calories, 0 g protein, 22 g carbohydrates, 0 g fat, 0 mg cholesterol, 0 mg sodium, 2 g dietary fiber
Diet Exchanges: ½ fruit, 1 bread, 1 fat
Carb Choices: 1

INDEX

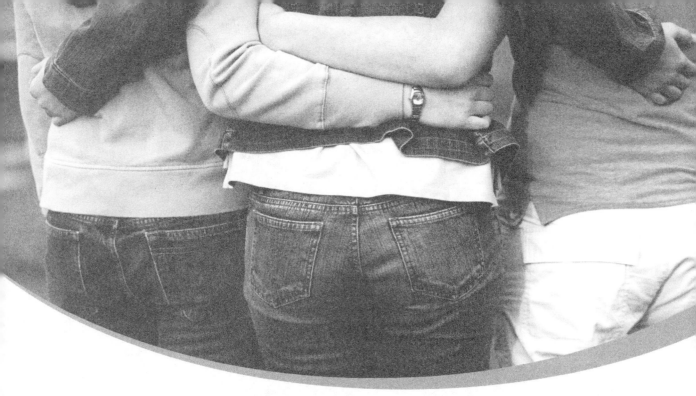

Find all the support you need to lose all the pounds you don't.

Introducing The Sugar Solution Online.

Your body. Your preferences. Your schedule. And all the features to put your goals within reach:

- Message boards that let you share tips and inspiration with other Sugar Solution Online members
- Recipes and menu plans based on your food preferences
- A customized fitness program based on your goals
- Shopping lists to save time at the grocery
- Free e-newsletter with added tips and weight loss help

Log on today for a FREE TOUR:
sugarsolutiononline.com

From the Editors of *Prevention*